Notes on
Operative Dentistry
and
Endodontics

Second Edition

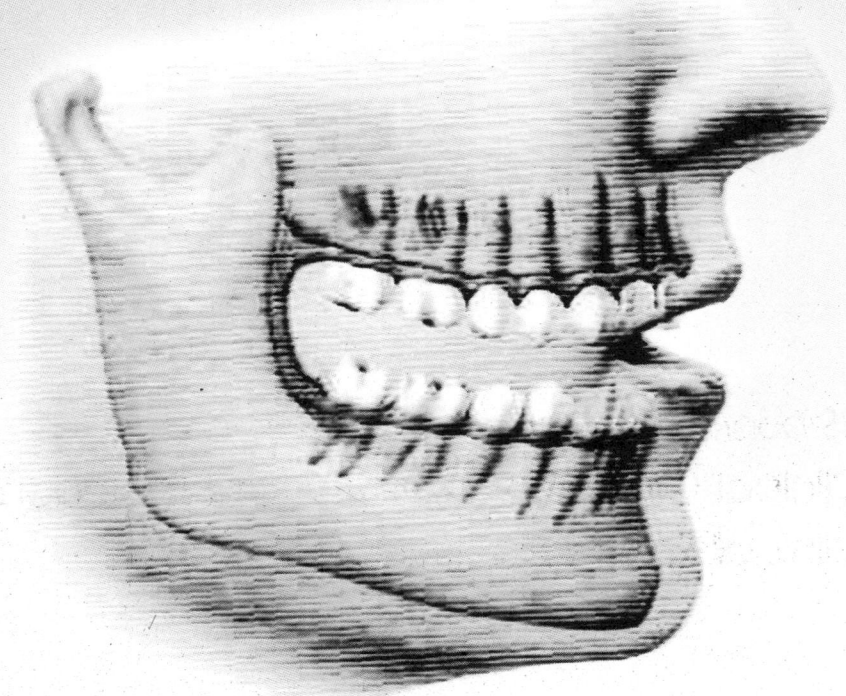

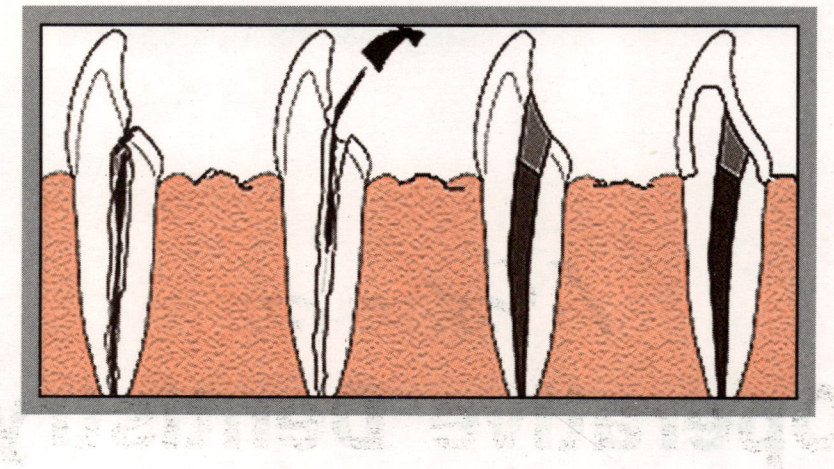

Notes on

Operative Dentistry and Endodontics

Second Edition

Narendranatha Reddy P.
Vanitha N.

Bangalore

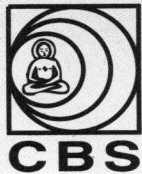

CBS

CBS Publishers & Distributors Pvt. Ltd.

New Delhi • Bangalore • Pune • Chennai • Cochin

ISBN : 81-239-1432-6

Second Edition : 2007
Reprint : 2008, 2009, 2011, 2013

Published by Satish Kumar Jain and produced by V.K. Jain for
CBS Publishers & Distributors Pvt. Ltd.,
CBS Plaza, 4819/XI Prahlad Street, 24 Ansari Road, Daryaganj,
New Delhi - 110002, India.   • Website: www.cbspd.com
e-mail: delhi@cbspd.com, cbspubs@airtelmail.in
Ph.: 23289259, 23266861, 23266867   • Fax: 011-23243014

Branches:

• ***Bengaluru:*** Seema House, 2975, 17th Cross, K.R. Road,
  Bansankari 2nd Stage, Bengaluru - 560070
    • Ph.: +91-80-26771678/79 • Fax: +91-80-26771680
    • E-mail: cbsbng@gmail.com, bangalore@cbspd.com
• ***Pune:*** Bhuruk Prestige, Sr. No. 52/12/2+1+3/2,
  Narhe, Haveli (Near Katraj-Dehu Road By-pass), Pune - 411041
    • Ph.: +91-20-64704058/59, 32342277   • E-mail: pune@cbspd.com
• ***Kochi:*** 36/14, Kalluvilakam, Lissie Hospital Road,
  Kochi - 682018, Kerala • Ph.: +91-484-4059061-65
    • Fax: +91-484-4059065   • E-mail: cochin@cbspd.com
• ***Chennai:*** 20, West Park Road, Shenoy Nagar, Chennai - 600030
  Ph.: +91-44-26260666, 26208620   • Fax: +91-44-42032115
    • E-mail: chennai@cbspd.com

Printed at :
Diamond Agencies Pvt. Ltd., Noida (UP)

to
Our
Parents

Preface to the Second Edition

Encouraged by the remarkable success of the first edition, we have embarked upon the second edition of this title. This edition is definitely a vast improvement over the first edition, and the outstanding feature of this book is the two-colour printing format which makes a more esthetic and pleasant presentation to the reader.

This second edition continues to retain the primary objective of the first edition, being a concise, reader-friendly and bridging the gap between what a student knows and what he/she ought to know to write in the theory examination.

The chapter sequence of the first edition remains unchanged, but the new text material has been incorporated wherever considered necessary. All the illustrations have been revised and redrawn with an added dimension of professionalism.

This time we have introduced separate indexes for the Operative Dentistry and Endodontics sections to make it more reader-friendly.

Constructive suggestions and comments from the readers are sincerely invited and shall be duly acknowledged.

Dr. Narendranatha Reddy P.
Dr. Vanitha N.

drpnnreddy@hotmail.com
drvanithan@hotmail.com

Preface to the First Edition

The aim of the compilers was to produce a book on the Operative Dentistry and Endodontics, which should fully meet the requirements of the undergraduate students who are preparing for the final BDS degree examination.

No doubt there are several books available on this subject, but it is a fact that none exclusively satisfies in full the needs of the final BDS students.

This book aims at bridging the gap between what a student knows and what he ought to know to write in the theory examination.

The scheme of our book is very simple. It has been divided into two main sections: *Operative Dentistry* and *Endodontics*. We have started each section with an elementary and basic concepts and then have passed on to the details in the subsequent chapters.

It is sincerely hoped that this modest effort will prove useful to the final BDS students for whom it is primarily intended.

Every effort has been made to present the matter in a simple manner. However, suggestions for the improvement of this book will be gratefully accepted.

Dr. Narendranatha Reddy P.
Dr. Vanitha N.

Acknowledgements to the Second Edition

First and foremost, we express our heart-felt appreciation towards Mr. Babu Prasad MP, our friend, well wisher, professional DTP composer and graphic illustrator, who went beyond limits to complete the book in time.

We solicit our special thanks to our friend and supporter Dr. Jenny M John who generously came forward to copy-edit the manuscripts, in spite of her busy clinical practice.

We also remember Dr. Roopa V Reddy, Dr. Ambika and Ms. Soumya MP for their efforts in proofreading the text for which we express our deepest thanks to them.

We sincerely acknowledge Mr. S K Jain of CBS Publishers and Distributors for his faith and interest in this project. Mr. Y N Arjuna, Publishing Director, CBS Publishers and Distributors, deserves special thanks for his untiring efforts for this project.

We are also indebted to Mr. Deepak Rao, General Manager, CBS Publishers and Distributors, Bangalore Branch, for his cooperation in this project.

And finally, once again we acknowledge our parents and family members for their tolerance of our absence and their unflinching support for this seemingly endless task.

Dr. Narendranatha Reddy P.
Dr. Vanitha N.

Acknowledgements to the First Edition

No book can be completed without the help of many individuals. Hence, we owe thanks and gratitude to all of them for help in various ways in the completion of this work.

First and foremost, we wish to thank our HoD, Dr. Vipool Malkan MDS, who encouraged us to go forward. His principles of emphasising clear writing and his uncompromising standards of accuracy continue to guide us. His mark on this book remains indelible.

Words are inadequate to express our gratitude to our beloved friend Dr. M. Lokeswara Reddy, who inspired us to do this work and who has been constantly encouraging us. Our sincere thanks to our beloved teacher Dr. Girish, whose grace made us conceive this project.

Our special thanks to Dr. Rufus Allwyn MDS, Assistant Professor, Department of Conservative Dentistry and Endodontics, Vydehi Dental College, Bangalore; Dr. Rayeesa Saleern MDS, Professor; Dr. Srinidhi MDS, Reader; Dr. Satish Abraham MDS, Sr. Lecturer; Dr. Arundhathi, Dr. Geetha, Lecturers, Department of Conservative Dentistry and Endodontics, Sri Rajiv Gandhi Dental College, Bangalore, for their excellent teaching and guidance.

We owe thanks to Dr. Yellappa MDS, Prof. and HoD, Department of P and SD; Dr. Arun Jacob Silas MDS, Prof. and HoD, Department of Paedodontics; Dr. Mohammed Saleem MDS; Associate Professor, Department of Prosthodontics, Sri Rajiv Gandhi Dental College, Bangalore; Dr. Thimma Reddy MDS, Prof. and HoD, Department of Paedodontics, SP Dental College, Wardha, Maharashtra, for their support and encouragement.

We are thankful to our friends Dr. Revanth, Dr. Srinivas V, Dr. Harikiran, Dr. Usha, Dr. Manju, KSR Prasad, Nidhi Sinha, Sarath, Sumathi JK, Sandhya, Jenny, Lakshmi, Chitra, Rishu Tiwari, Shashikanth, Apoorva, Rishidhar, Sridevi, Srinivas P and Vijaya Sekhar for their cooperation and encouragement.

Our deepest thanks to Mr. D. Naveen for his technical and financial assistance. We thank our college librarian Mr. Basavaraju who enriched our knowledge with a lot of literature on the dentistry. A special debt of gratitude goes to Mr. Bhaskar Reddy M., Bangalore, for his timely help in the preparation of this book, and also to Dr. Rajeswara Reddy M.S., Assistant Professor, S.J.M. Medical College, for his encouragement.

Our deepest gratitude to Mr. Babu Prasad, who undertook the desktop work and did a marvelous job and heartfelt 'thank-you' to our Advocate Mr Surya Prakash for his tireless cooperation.

We particularly thank Mrs. Nalini, on whose shoulders lay the burden of orchestrating the flow of manuscripts, galley proofs, page proofs and illustrations. Her help has been indispensable in the completion of the book on schedule. We also thank Mrs. Kalpana for her assistance in data entry. We wish to thank Mr. G.V. Murthy for his cooperation and encouragement. We are also indebted to our printer Mr. Ramesh Babu, S.L.N. Printers, and others in the press who participated in the production of the book.

Undoubtedly there are many other `unsung heroes' who should be recognized for their contributions — our thanks to all of them and ask forgiveness for their not being individually singled out.

And finally, once again we acknowledge our parents and family members for their tolerance of our absences and their unflinching support of this seemingly endless task.

CONTENTS

Preface to the Second Edition   vii

Preface to the First Edition   viii

Section I
OPERATIVE DENTISTRY

Chapter 1
INTRODUCTION TO OPERATIVE DENTISTRY   3
Definition of Operative Dentistry   3
Aims and Objectives   3

Chapter 2
FUNDAMENTAL CONCEPTS   4
Tooth Numbering Systems   4
Tooth Surface Designations   6
Nomenclature of Cavity Preparation   6
Walls of Cavity Preparation   7
Angles of Cavity Preparation   8
Principles of Cavity Preparation   10
Restorations   14
Enamel Patterns   15

Chapter 3
DENTAL BIO-MATERIALS   16
Dental Amalgam   16
Dental Cements   25
Agents for Pulp Protection   31
Dental Investments and Die Materials   33
Dental Casting Procedures   35
Dental Ceramics   40

Chapter 4
DENTAL CARIES   43
Definition of Dental Caries   43
Classification of Dental Caries   43
Theories of Dental Caries   45
Caries Activity Tests   45
Diagnosis of Dental Caries   46
Identification of Occlusal and Proximal Caries   46
Zones of Dentinal Carious Lesion   46
Direct Pulp Capping   48
Indirect Pulp Capping   48
Prevention of Caries   49
Pit and Fissure Sealants   49

Enameloplasty *50*
Prophylactic Odontotomy *50*

Chapter 5
OPERATIVE DENTISTRY ARMAMENTARIUM   51
Classification of Operative Dental Instruments *51*
Hand Cutting Instruments
    Parts of an Instrument *52*
    Nomenclature of Instrument *52*
    Instrument Formula *52*
    Instrument Design *52*
    Classification *54*
    Advantages *56*
Instrument Grasps, Rests and Guards *56*
Rotary Instrumentation
    Characteristics *57*
    Rotary Instrument Design
        Hand Piece *58*
        Tools for Removal of Tooth Structure *58*
            Dental Cutting Burs *58*
            Dental Abrasive Stones *61*
    Uses and Limitations *62*
    Low Speeds *62*
    High Speeds *62*
Ultrasonic Instruments *63*
Restoring Instruments *63*
Finishing and Polishing Instruments *64*
Maintenance of Cutting Instruments *64*

Chapter 6
THE OPERATING FIELD   68
Basic Instrument Tray Setup *68*
Positioning of the Dental Team and the Patient
    Objectives *68*
    Zones of Operating Field *68*
    Positioning of the Operator *69*
    Operator's Chair Position *69*
    Positioning of the Dental Assistant *69*
    Positioning of the Patient *69*
Isolation of the Operating Field
    Goals of Isolation *69*
    Methods of Isolation *70*
        Gingival Tissue Retraction *70*
    Rubberdam *71*
Infection Control *77*

Chapter 7
CONTACTS AND CONTOURS   79
Embrasures *79*
Height of Contour *80*
Marginal Ridges *80*
Mamelon *80*
Overhang *80*
Consequences of Faulty Reproduction of Contacts
        and Contours *80*
Separation of the Teeth *81*
Matrices *82*
Wedges *84*

Chapter 8
DENTAL AMALGAM RESTORATIONS   86
Class 1 Cavity Preparation *86*
Class 2 Cavity Preparation *88*
Modifications in Tooth Preparation for
    Class 2 Cavity *91*
Class 3 Cavity Preparation *92*
Class 5 Cavity Preparation *92*
Failures of Amalgam Restorations *93*
Finishing and Polishing of Amalgam Restorations *93*

Chapter 9
COMPLEX AMALGAM RESTORATIONS   94
Pin Retained Amalgam Restorations *94*
Slot Retained Amalgam Restorations *97*
Amalgapin *98*

Chapter 10
ESTHETIC RESTORATIONS   99
Esthetic Restorative Materials *99*
Composites
    Composition *100*
    Indications *100*
    Contraindications *100*
    Advantages *100*
    Disadvantages *100*
    Classification *100*
    Conventional *100*
    Microfilled *101*
    Hybrid *101*
    Flowable *101*
    Packable *102*

Composites for Posterior Restorations 102
Polymerization of Composites 102
Acid Etching 103
Conditioning of the Cavity 104
Dental Adhesion
Concepts of Adhesion 104
Enamel Bonding Agents 104
Smear Layer 104
Hybrid Layer 105
Classification of Dentin Bonding Agents 105
Pulpal Protection 106
Tooth Preparations
Class III Cavity Preparation 107
Class IV Cavity Preparation 108
Class V Cavity Preparation 109
Class I and II Cavity Preparations 109
Finishing and Polishing of Composites 110
GIC Restorations 110
Veneers 111
Diastema Closure 113
Miscellaneous
Abfraction 113
Golden Proportion 114
Sandwich Technique 114
Differences between the Class II Cavity Preparation for Amalgam and Composite Restorations 115

Chapter 11
DIRECT FILLING GOLD (DFG) 116
Indications 116
Contraindications 116
Advantages 116
Disadvantages 116
Forms/Types of DFG 116
Characteristics of Gold 117
Manipulation of DFG 118
Steps for Insertion of DFG 120
Tooth Preparations
Class I Cavity 121
Class II Cavity 122
Class III Cavity 124
Class V Cavity 126
Finishing and Polishing of Direct Gold Restorations 128

Chapter 12
CAST RESTORATIONS 129
Inlay 129
Class II Inlay 129
Indications for Inlays 129
Onlay 129
Class II Onlay 129
Indications for Onlays 129
Cast Restorations
Indications 129
Contraindications 130
Advantages 130
Disadvantages 130
Materials for Cast Restorations 130
Principles of Tooth Preparation for Cast Restorations 130
Bevels 131
Flares 131
Finishing Lines 132
Tooth Preparation for Class II Cast Metal Inlays 133
Proximal Margin Designs 134
Impression Procedures for Cast Metal Restorations 135
Finishing and Polishing of Cast Metal Restorations 135
Differences between the Class II Cavity Preparation for Silver Amalgam and Cast Restorations 136

Chapter 13
NON-CARIOUS LESIONS 137
Attrition 137
Abrasion 138
Erosion 139

Chapter 14
DENTIN HYPERSENSITIVITY 140
Definition 140
Theories of Dentin Hypersensitivity 140

Chapter 15
MISCELLANEOUS 143
CAD-CAM Systems 143
Copy Milling Process 143
LASERS 144
Micro and Macro Abrasion 144
Air Abrasion 145
Microleakage 145
Nanoleakage 145
Finishing and Polishing of the Restorations 146
Reaction of the Pulp to Irritating Stimuli 146

Section II
ENDODONTICS

Chapter 1
INTRODUCTION TO ENDODONTICS   *151*
Definition *151*
Aims and Objectives *151*
Scope of Endodontics *151*

Chapter 2
DENTAL PULP AND PERIRADICULAR TISSUES *152*
Zones of Pulp *152*
Anatomy of the Pulp Cavity *154*
Types of Root Canal Configurations *155*
Normal Periradicular Tissues *155*
Morphology of the Pulp *156*
Apical Closure *156*

Chapter 3
DISEASES OF THE DENTAL PULP   *158*
Causes of Pulp Disease *158*
Classification of Pulp Diseases *159*
Barodontalgia *160*
Pathways of Bacterial Invasion of the Pulp *160*
Reversible Pulpitis *160*
Irreversible Pulpitis *161*
Chronic Hyperplastic Pulpitis *161*
Internal Resorption *161*
Pulp Degeneration *162*
Necrosis of Pulp *162*
Cracked Tooth Syndrome *163*

Chapter 4
DISEASES OF THE PERIRADICULAR TISSUES *164*
Classification *164*
Acute Alveolar Abscess *164*
Acute Apical Periodontitis *165*
Acute Exacerbation of a Chronic Lesion *165*
Chronic Alveolar Abscess *165*
Granuloma *166*
Radicular Cyst *166*
Condensing Osteitis *166*
External Root Resorption *167*

Chapter 5
ENDODONTIC MICROBIOLOGY   *168*
Root Canal Flora *168*
Bacteriologic Examination *168*

Chapter 6
CLINICAL DIAGNOSTIC METHODS   *170*
History and Record *170*
   Subjective Symptoms *170*
   Objective Symptoms *171*
Pulp Vitality Tests *173*

Chapter 7
ENDODONTIC ARMAMENTARIUM   *176*
Classification of Endodontic Instruments *176*
Standardization of Endodontic Instruments *177*
Exploring Instruments *177*
Extirpating Instruments *178*
Instruments for Cleaning and Shaping of
      Root Canals *178*
Obturating Instruments *180*
Motions of Instrumentation *180*
Mechanical Instrumentation *182*
Sotokawa's Classification of Instrument Damage *183*

Chapter 8
PRINCIPLES OF ENDODONTIC TREATMENT   *184*
Principles of Endodontics *184*
Trephination *185*
Chemical Irritation *185*

Chapter 9
STERILIZATION   *186*
Sterilization of Endodontic Instruments *186*
Causes of Sterilization Failure *187*
Monitoring Sterilization *188*

Chapter 10
RATIONALE OF ENDODONTIC TREATMENT   *189*
Fish Zones *189*

Chapter 11
RCT : AN OVERVIEW   *191*

Chapter 12
SELECTION OF CASES FOR ENDODONTIC TREATMENT 193
Local Contraindication 193
General Contraindication 193
Chemoprophylaxis 194

Chapter 13
PRINCIPLES OF ENDODONTIC CAVITY PREPARATION 195
Coronal Cavity Preparation 195
Radicular Preparation 197

Chapter 14
ROOT CANAL IRRIGANTS 198
Ideal Properties 198
Irrigating Solutions 198
Sodium Hypochlorite 199
Combination Solutions 199

Chapter 15
WORKING LENGTH DETERMINATION 200
Definition 200
Objectives 200
Methods
    Radiographic Methods 200
    Non-Radiographic Methods 200
Master Apical File Determination 203

Chapter 16
CLEANING AND SHAPING (BIOMECHANICAL PREPARATION) OF THE ROOT CANAL 204
Cleaning and Shaping 204
Schilder's Mechanical Objectives 204
Motions of Cleaning and Shaping 204
Purpose of Cleaning and Shaping 205
Techniques of Radicular Cavity Preparation
    Step-Back Preparation 205
    Step-Down Technique 206
Recapitulation 207
Evaluation Criteria for Apical Preparation 207

Chapter 17
DISINFECTION OF THE ROOT CANAL 208
Disinfection 208
Intracanal Medicaments 208
Frequency of Medication 210
Electrosterilization 210

Chapter 18
TEMPORARY FILLING MATERIALS 211
Materials
    Cavity 211
    Intermediate Restorative Material 211
    Term 211

Chapter 19
ROOT CANAL SEALERS/CEMENTS 212
Ideal Properties 212
Classification 212

Chapter 20
OBTURATION OF THE ROOT CANAL 215
Objectives 215
Obturating Materials 215
Master Cone Selection 217
Obturation Techniques for Gutta-Percha 217
Metal Core Obturation 221
Removal of Root Canal Fillings 222
Miscellaneous
    Obtura II 222
    Thermafil 223
    Under Filling of Root Canal 223
    Over Filling of Root Canal 223

Chapter 21
RESTORATION OF THE ENDODONTICALLY TREATED TEETH 224
Dowel (Post) 224
Core 225
Coronal Restoration 226
Pre-fabricated Post and Core System 226
Cast Post Systems 227

Chapter 22
ENDODONTIC PROCEDURAL MISHAPS 228
Ledge Formation 228
Perforation 229
Separated Instruments and Foreign Objects 230
Hypochlorite Accident 231

Chapter 23
FAILURES OF ENDODONTIC TREATMENT 232
Pre-operative Causes 232
Operative Causes 232
Post-operative Causes 233
Instruments for Retrieving Broken Instruments
    and Posts 233

Chapter 24
SINGLE-VISIT ENDODONTICS   **234**
Oliet's Criteria for Case Selection *234*
Indications *234*
Contraindications *234*

Chapter 25
ENDODONTIC EMERGENCIES   **235**
Acute Reversible Pulpitis *235*
Acute Irreversible Pulpitis *235*
Acute Alveolar Abscess *236*
Acute Periodontal Abscess *236*
Emergencies During Treatment *236*
Crown Fracture *237*
Fractured Root *237*
Tooth Avulsion *238*

Chapter 26
PAEDIATRIC ENDODONTICS   **239**
Pulpotomy *239*
Pulpectomy *241*
Apexification *241*
Apexogenesis *242*

Chapter 27
DENTAL INJURIES AND MANAGEMENT   **243**
Classification *243*
Soft Tissue Injuries *244*
Tooth Fracture *244*
Luxation Injuries *246*

Chapter 28
ENDODONTIC REPLANTATION,
TRANSPLANTATION AND IMPLANTATION   **248**
Replantation *248*
Transplantation *250*
Endodontic Implants *250*

Chapter 29
BLEACHING OF DISCOLOURED TEETH   **252**
Classification of Tooth Discolouration *252*
Causes of Tooth Discolouration *252*
Bleaching Agents *253*
Techniques for Bleaching of Pulpless Teeth/
   Endodontically Treated Teeth/
   Non Vital Teeth *254*
Techniques for Bleaching of Vital Teeth *254*
Complications of Bleaching *256*

Chapter 30
ENDODONTIC–PERIODONTIC
INTERRELATIONSHIP   **257**
Classification *257*
Perforations *258*

Chapter 31
SURGICAL ENDODONTICS   **259**
Objective *259*
Indications *259*
Contraindications *259*
Classification of Endodontic Surgical Procedures *260*
Types of Incisions and Flaps *260*
Retrograde Filling *261*
Radisectomy/Root Resection *262*
Hemisection *263*
Bicuspidization/Bisection *263*
Apicoectomy *264*
Repair *264*
Complications of Endodontic Surgery *264*

REFERENCES/BIBLIOGRAPHY   **265**

INDEX   **267**

Section I

Operative Dentistry

CHAPTER 01

INTRODUCTION TO OPERATIVE DENTISTRY

– Historically, Operative Dentistry has been the primary nucleus of the dental practice. It includes everything from the prevention of caries and reminerlization of initial carious attacks to complex restorative treatments. More than a century of clinical experience has provided tradition for the treatment that are deep rooted in the dental profession.

DEFINITION OF OPERATIVE DENTISTRY

– *Operative Dentistry is the art and science of the diagnosis, treatment, and prognosis of defects of teeth that do not require full coverage restorations for the correction. Such treatment should result in the restoration of proper tooth form, function, and esthetics while maintaining the physiologic integrity of the teeth in a harmonius relationship with the adjacent hard and soft tissues, all of which should enhance the general health and welfare of the patient.*

AIMS AND OBJECTIVES

1. Diagnosis of the extent and location(s) of the lesions.

2. Prevention of the disease.

3. Interruption, i.e. prevention of further loss of the tooth structure.

4. Preservation of the vitality and important anatomy of the remaining sound tooth structure.

5. Restoration of health.

6. Preservation of esthetics.

"Father of Modern Operative Dentistry" and "The Grand Old Man of Dentistry" – *Dr. G.V. Black.*

CHAPTER 02

FUNDAMENTAL CONCEPTS

– There are over 12 systems are available for the recording of different teeth and teeth surfaces. Different notations are used for the permanent and deciduous dentition.

– Most systems divide the mouth into four quadrants, and the dental arch is expressed by a cross. Four sides of the cross are used to denote four quadrants as follows:

UPPER RIGHT	UPPER LEFT
LOWER RIGHT	LOWER LEFT

Sometimes it is simplified to denote *upper right* as ⌐|, *upper left* as |⌐, *lower right* as ⌐| and *lower left* as ⌐.

– Currently three numbering systems are more popular in dentistry. They are described below,

1. UNIVERSAL / NATIONAL SYSTEM

– Approved by American Dental Association (ADA).

(A) *Primary Dentition*

– Capital letters 'A' through 'T' are used to designate the Primary dentition.

– Numbering begins with the right side of the upper arch at maxillary right second molar as 'A', following the arch to the maxillary left second molar (J) and then continuous to the mandibular left second molar (K), following the arch to the right side and terminates at the second molar as 'T'.

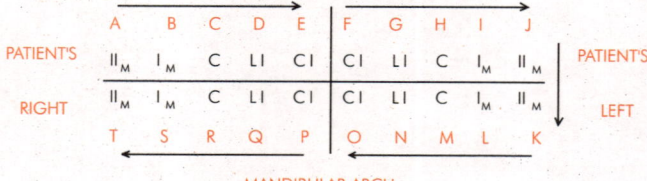

CI - Central Incisor, LI - Lateral Incisor, C - Canine, I_M - First Molar, II_M - Second Molar.

(B) *Permanent Dentition*

– Teeth are numbered from 1 to 32 starting with the third molar (1) on the right side of the upper arch, following around the arch to the third molar (16) on the left side, descending to the lower third molar (17) on the left side and following that arch to the lower right third molar (32).

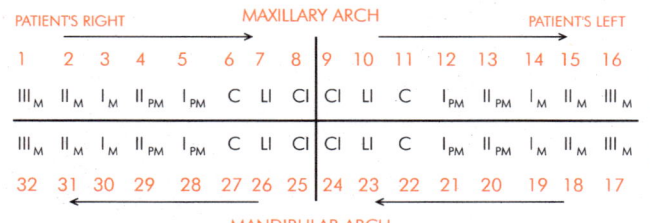

CI - Central Incisor , LI - Lateral Incisor, C - Canine,
I_{PM} *- First Premolar,* II_{PM} *- Second Premolar,* I_M *- First Molar,* II_M *- Second Molar,* III_M *- Third Molar.*

2. ZSIGMONDY/PALMER SYSTEM

- *Oldest and most widely used method.*
- This notation designates each tooth based on its location in a quadrant.
- A horizontal line separates the maxillary and the mandibular arches.
- A vertical midline separates the patient's right and left side of the mouth.

(A) *Primary Dentition*

- Deciduous teeth are designated with the capital letters beginning with the central incisor (A) to the second molar (E) in each quadrant.

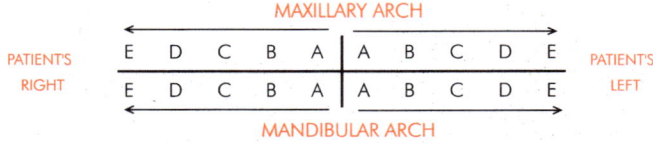

(B) *Permanent Dentition*

- Permanent teeth are numbered from 1 – 8 in each quadrant, beginning with the central incisor (1) to the third molar (8).

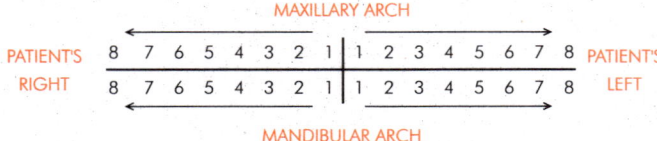

- Identifying a specific tooth by this system combines the quadrant grid with the tooth number in reference to the midline. Thus, the tooth number is written within the angle. Ex: Permanent maxillary right canine as 3⌋ and Deciduous mandibular left second molar as ⌈E .

3. FEDERATION DENTAIRE INTERNATIONAL (FDI) / INTERNATIONAL NUMBERING SYSTEM / TWO DIGIT SYSTEM / ISO SYSTEM

- In this system 2 digits are used for each tooth.
- First digit indicates the quadrant, i.e.

PERMANENT TEETH		DECIDUOUS TEETH	
Maxillary right	*- 1*	*Maxillary right*	*- 5*
Maxillary left	*- 2*	*Maxillary left*	*- 6*
Mandibular left	*- 3*	*Mandibular left*	*- 7*
Mandibular right	*- 4*	*Mandibular right*	*- 8*

- Second digit indicates the specific tooth within the quadrant (1 to 8 for permanent teeth, 1 to 5 for deciduous teeth).
- Thus, in this system combination of numbers from 11 through 48 represent permanent teeth and numbers from 51 through 85 represent deciduous teeth.
- The digits should be pronounced separately, i.e. permanent cuspids are teeth one-three, two-three, three-three and four-three.

(A) *Primary Dentition*

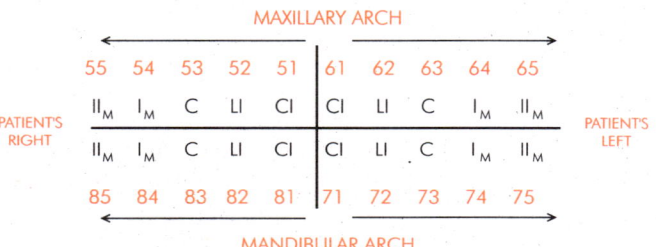

(B) *Permanent Dentition*

Advantages

1. simple to understand and to teach.
2. easy to pronounce during conversation.
3. easy to translate into computer.
4. easy to adapt to standard charts used in general practice.

THE SAFEST METHOD

- Out of the existing systems for noting the dentition, there is no system which is full-proof.
- The safest method is to write full description of the teeth. Ex: Upper left first permanent Molar.

TOOTH SURFACE DESIGNATIONS

– The coronal portion of each tooth is divided into surfaces that are named according to related anatomic landmarks, i.e.

Mesial	-	*toward the anterior midline.*
Distal	-	*away from the anterior midline.*
Buccal	-	*toward the cheek. [Facial (refers to either buccal or labial)]*
Labial	-	*toward the lip [facial (refers to either buccal or labial)]*
Lingual	-	*toward the tongue.*
Occlusal	-	*masticating surface of a bicuspid or molar.*
Incisal	-	*functional edge of anterior tooth.*
Cervical	-	*related to cervix or neck of tooth.*
Gingival	-	*close to or in proximity of gingiva.*

– The naming is further simplified by representing by the first letter of the surface or by numbering as follows (Table 1.1, Fig. 1.1):

Surface	Letter	Numerical exponent
Mesial	1	M
Distal	2	D
Labial/Buccal (Facial)	3	F
Lingual	4	L
Occulusal/Incisal	5	O/I

Table 1.1

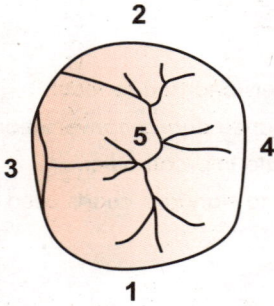

Fig. 1.1

– The occlusal surfaces of some teeth are divided by an oblique or transverse ridge of enamel extending from buccal to lingual surface. Ex: Maxillary first molar, Maxillary second molar and Mandibular first bicuspid.

The numerical exponent 5 is used to indicate the mesial occlusal surface and the exponent 6 indicates the distal occlusal surface (Fig. 1.2)

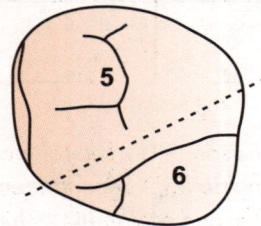

Fig. 1.2

– Combining the tooth number and the surface exponent or letter is used to designate the location of the carious lesion. Ex: A mesial proximal carious lesion of the mandibular left first molar is indicated by 19^1 or 19M. The site of the proposed cavity preparation is therefore designated as 19^{1-5} or 19 MO. When the buccal groove of this tooth involved as an extension of the occlusal it is indicated as 19^{1-5-3} or 19 MOB.

NOMENCLATURE OF THE CAVITY PREPARATION

1. **Angle:** The union of two surfaces.
2. **Line angle:** The union of two surfaces along a definite line.
3. **Point angle:** The union of two surfaces along of three surfaces at a point.
4. **Axial line angle:** A line angle running parallel with the long axis of the tooth.
5. **Pulpal line angle:** A line angle running horizontally to the long axis of the tooth.
6. **Cavo surface angle:** The angle formed by the junction of the walls of the cavity with the surface of the tooth.
7. **Margin:** The junction of the walls of a cavity with the surface of a tooth.
8. **Marginal out line:** The shape of the cavity along its margins.
9. **Cavo surface margin:** The surface periphery of the cavity preparation, which is the junction between the cavity wall (floor) and the adjacent tooth surface.
10. **Floor:** Refers to those portions of the preparation which are almost at right angles to the surrounding walls. Floors are usually composed of dentin only (pulpal floor), but they can be formed of enamel and dentin (gingival floor).

11. **Seat:** The bottom or floor in simple cavities, either the axial or pulpal wall; in proximo incisal and proximo occlusal cavities, the gingival wall.

12. **Step:** The auxillary portion of the compound mortise form, consisting of the axial and pulpal walls in complex cavities.

13. **Wall:** One of the internal boundaries of a cavity.

14. **Enamel wall:** That part of a cavity wall composed of enamel.

15. **Dentin wall:** That part of a cavity wall consisting of dentin.

16. **Sub pulpal wall:** When the pulp is removed the pulpal wall disappears and the base of the pulp chamber becomes the sub pulpal wall.

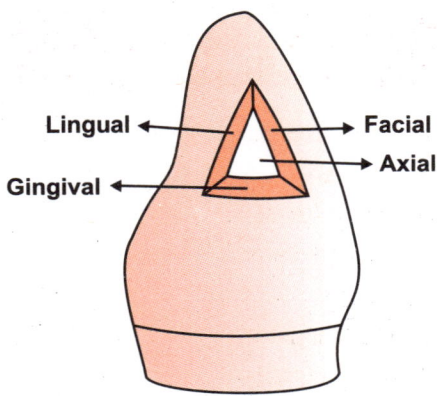

4. **For a Class-IV preparation:** It has 6 walls, i.e. Mesial, Facial, Axial, Lingual, Pulpal and Gingival.

WALLS OF THE CAVITY PREPARATION

— Extra coronal cavity walls carry the name of the surface that is reduced and the intracoronal walls of the preparation also take the name of the surface from which they are derived.

1. **For an Occlusal Class - I preparation:** It has 4 surrounding walls, i.e. Distal, Mesial, Facial and Lingual.

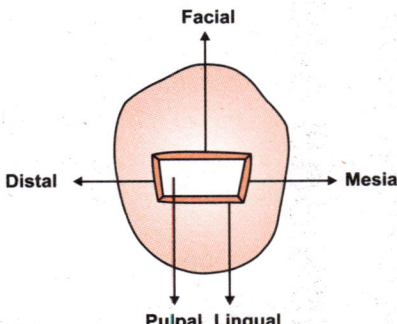

2. **For a Class - II (MO) preparation:** It has 6 walls, i.e. Distal, Lingual, Facial, Pulpal, Axial and Gingival.

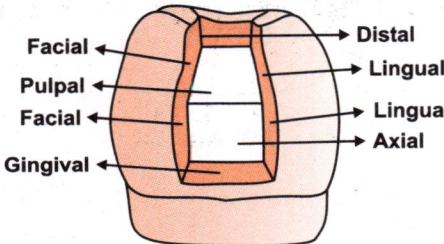

3. **For a Class - III preparation:** It has 4 walls, i.e. Facial, Lingual, Gingival and Incisal wall (only occasionally)

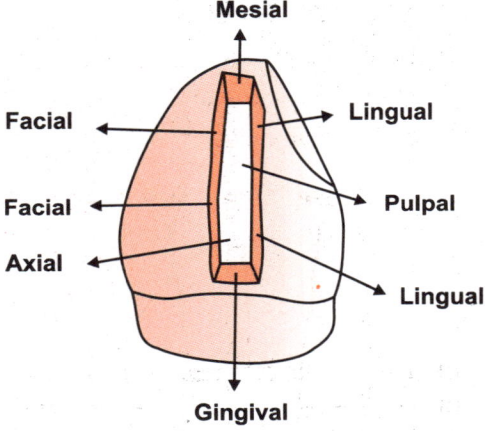

5. **For a Class-V preparation:** It has 5 walls, i.e. Incisal, Mesial, Axial, Gingival and Distal.

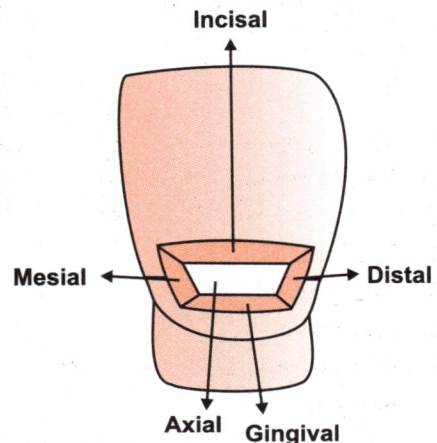

6. **For a Class-VI preparation:** Same as an occlusal class-I preparation.

ANGLES OF THE CAVITY PREPARATION

1. **For an Occlusal Cavity: (Class-I)**
   A. **Line angles : (8)**
      (1) Mesio facial
      (2) Mesio lingual
      (3) Disto facial
      (4) Disto lingual
      (5) Facio pulpal
      (6) Linguo pulpal
      (7) Mesio pulpal
      (8) Disto pulpal

   B. **Point angles: (4)**
      (1) Mesio facio pulpal
      (2) Distofacio pulpal
      (3) Mesio linguo pulpal
      (4) Disto linguo pulpal

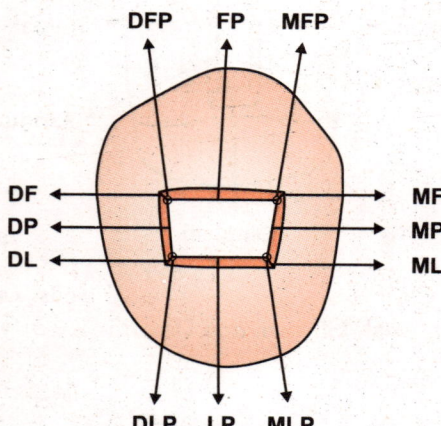

2. **For a Buccal or Lingual cavities on Posterior teeth**
   A. **Line angles: (8)**
      (1) Mesio gingival
      (2) Disto gingival
      (3) Mesio occlusal
      (4) Disto occlusal
      (5) Axio gingival
      (6) Axio mesial
      (7) Axio occlusal
      (8) Axio distal

   B. **Point angles: (4)**
      (1) Axio mesio gingival
      (2) Axio mesio occlusal
      (3) Axio disto gingival
      (4) Axio disto occlusal

3. **For a Proximo Occlusal cavity: (Class-II)**
   There are 11 line angles and 6 point angles, i.e.

   (i) **In the mesial or distal portion: (5 line and 2 point angles)**
   A. **Line angles**
      (1) Bucco gingival
      (2) Linguo gingival
      (3) Bucco axial
      (4) Linguo axial
      (5) Gingivo axial

   B. **Point angles**
      (1) Gingivo bucco axial
      (2) Gingivo linguo axial

   (ii) **In the step portion: (5 line and 2 point angles)**
   A. **Line angles**
      (1) Bucco distal (or mesial)
      (2) Linguo distal (or mesial)
      (3) Disto (or mesial) pulpal
      (4) Linguo pulpal
      (5) Bucco pulpal

   B. **Point angles**
      (1) Disto - (or mesio -) bucco pulpal
      (2) Disto - (or mesio -) linguo pulpal

   – Also an *axiopulpal line angle* and *pulpolinguo axial* and *pulpo bucco axial point angles* may be named.

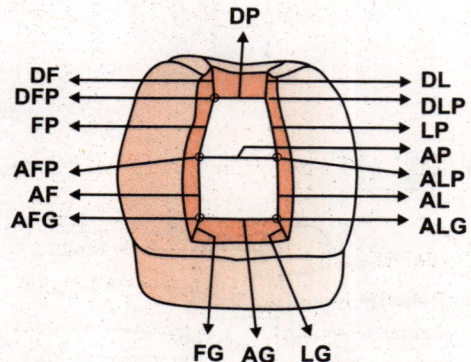

4. **For Mesial and Distal cavities on Anterior teeth (Class - III)**
   A. **Line angles: (6)**
      (1) Labio [facio] gingival
      (2) Linguo gingival

(3) Axio incisal

(4) Axio labial [facial]

(5) Axio lingual

(6) Axio gingival

B. Point angles: (3)

(1) Axio labio gingival

(2) Axio linguo gingival

(3) Axio incisal

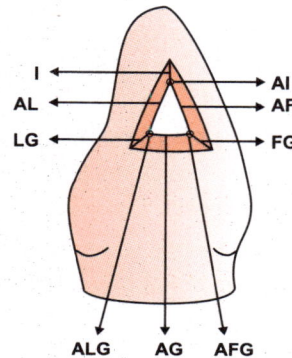

5. For Proximo Incisal cavity: (Class - IV)
A. Line angles: (11)

(1) Mesio - (or disto -) labial

(2) Mesio - (or disto -) lingual

(3) Pulpo distal (or - mesial)

(4) Pulpo lingual

(5) Pulpo labial

(6) Pulpo axial

(7) Axio gingival

(8) Facio gingival

(9) Linguo gingival

(10) Axio facial

(11) Axio pulpal

B. Point angles: (6)

(1) Mesio - (or disto -) pulpolabial

(2) Mesio - (or disto -) pulpo lingual

(3) Axio - facio - gingival

(4) Axio - linguo - gingival

(5) Axio - facio - pulpal

(6) Axio - linguo - pulpal

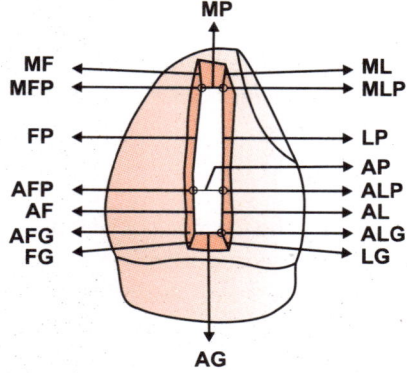

6. For a Class-V cavity
A. Line angles : (8)

(1) Axio incisal

(2) Mesio incisal

(3) Axio mesial

(4) Mesio gingival

(5) Axio gingival

(6) Disto gingival

(7) Disto incisal

(8) Axio distal

B. Point angles : (4)

(1) Axio disto incisal

(2) Axio mesio incisal

(3) Axio mesio gingival

(4) Axio disto gingival

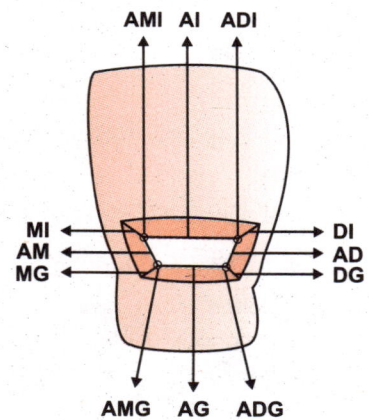

PRINCIPLES OF THE CAVITY PREPARATION

CAVITY: Refers to *a defect in enamel or in enamel and dentin, resulting from the pathologic process of dental caries.*

CAVITY PREPARATION

Defined as *"the mechanical alteration of defective, injured or diseased tooth inorder to best receive restorative materials which will reestablish the form, function and esthetics".* Or also defined as *"the orderly operating procedure required to establish in a tooth the biomechanically acceptable form necessary to receive and retain a restoration".*

OBJECTIVES OF CAVITY PREPARATION

1. To remove all the defects and to give necessary protection to the pulp.
2. To locate the margins of the restoration in a consecutive manner.
3. To form the cavity, that will not allow the fracture of the tooth or restoration and the displacement of the restoration.
4. To allow for the esthetic and functional placement of a restoration.

FACTORS AFFECTING CAVITY PREPARATION

1. **Diagnosis**
   - Caries, fractured teeth, esthetics.
   - Occlusal relationships.
   - Risk potential.
2. **Knowledge of dental anatomy**
3. **Patients factors**
   - Age, economic status.

STAGES OF CAVITY PREPARATION

1. **1st STAGE: Initial cavity preparation**

   Includes the mechanical alteration of the tooth which is extended to enamel, supported by, non - carious dentin in all directions but into a limited pulpal depth.

2. **2nd STAGE: Final cavity preparation**

   Includes the completion of the cavity, i.e. excavation of remaining infected carious dentin, removal of the old restorative material, finishing of the walls, cleaning, inspection and varnishing of the cavity.

STEPS IN CAVITY PREPARATION: (G.V. BLACK)

I. **Initial cavity preparation stage**
   1. Obtaining outline form and initial depth.
   2. Obtaining primary resistance form.
   3. Obtaining primary retention form.
   4. Obtaining convenience form.

II. **Final cavity preparation stage**
   1. Removal of carious tooth portion and old restoration if any.
   2. Secondary resistance and retention form.
   3. Finishing of external walls.
   4. Debridement of the preparation.

1. *OUTLINE FORM AND INITIAL DEPTH*

- Outline form is *the shape of the area of the tooth surface included within the cavo surface margins of the prepared cavity.*
- Outline form usually varies according to the type of restorative material and to the class of preparation.
- Initial depth varies from 0.2–0.8 mm pulpally of the DEJ.

Principles of establishing outline form are

1. All weakened enamel should be removed.
2. All faults should be included.
3. All margins should be placed in esthetically pleasing position.

Factors determining the outline form are

1. Extent of caries, defect or faulty or old restoration.
2. Occlusal condition.
3. Cavo surface marginal configuration.
4. Adjacent tooth contour.
5. Esthetic consideration.

Significance of outline form

Provides sufficient access for the proper cavity preparation and for the placement and finishing of the restoration.

2. *PRIMARY RESISTANCE FORM*

- Defined as *the shape given to the preparation that enables the restoration and remaining tooth structure to withstand masticatory stresses without fracture.*
- This property is chiefly obtained by the bulk of the cavity form in an axio - pulpal direction; the bulk in

turn produces thickness for the restoration and the optimum compressive and tensile strengths.

- Primary resistance is obtained by the following features during cavity preparation, i.e.

    1. Flat pulpal and gingival wall.
    2. Box shaped cavity.
    3. Inclusion of weakened tooth structure.
    4. Restricting the extension of external walls.
    5. Preservation of cusps and marginal ridges.
    6. Rounding internal line angles.
    7. Providing adequate thickness of restorative material.
    8. Reduction of cusps for capping when indicated.
    9. Parallelism of the walls.

3. PRIMARY RETENTION FORM

- Defined as *the shape given to the preparation that resists displacement or removal of the restoration from the tipping or lifting forces.*

- Retention means are divided into principal and auxillary types according to their efficiency in retaining the restoration.

A. Principal means of Retention

(i) Frictional Retention

It can be obtained (i) by increasing the surface area of contact between tooth structure and restorative material (ii) by creation of opposing walls or surfaces (iii) by producing parallelism between opposing walls (iv) by bringing the restorative material closer to tooth structure during insertion.

(ii) Elastic deformation of dentin

It can be done by changing the position of dentinal walls and floors microscopically by using condensation energy within the dentin's proportional limit.

It creates more gripping action by the tooth on the restorative material.

(iii) Undercuts or inverted truncated cones

Usually placed in the point angles of the cavity.

(iv) Dove - tail retention

Dove - tail is *a widened or fanned - out portion of the prepared cavity, usually established to increase the retention and resistance form.*

B. Auxillary means of Retention

(i) Grooves: cut in dentin without undermining the adjacent enamel whenever bulk allows.

(ii) Internal boxes: have definite walls and floors.

(iii) Posts: are made from wrought or cast metal and placed in the root canals.

(iv) Pins: are made from cast or wrought metal. They may be parallel or non - parallel, vertical or horizontal, threaded or cemented.

(v) Triangular areas: are placed within the dentin and are located laterally without undermining overlying enamel plates.

(vi) Acid conditioning or Etching of enamel creates mechanical locks and increases surface areas of contact between tooth structure and the restorative material. Sometimes, it is considered as a principal retention mode.

(vii) Cements or Luting agents: Least effective auxillary means of retention.

4. CONVENIENCE FORM

Defined as, *the shape given to a tooth preparation or modification added to the basic preparation, to facilitate proper instrumentation for the preparation of the cavity or insertion of the restorative material.*

(i) Modifications in tooth preparation: include flaring of some walls more than otherwise necessary for resistance or retention to decrease distortion errors during the fabrication of intermediate materials (castings); decreasing the roundness of some walls more than normally needed; extension of margins more than otherwise necessary.

(ii) Instrument modification: includes contra-angling, bayonetting or the addition of several angles to the shank of an instrument.

(iii) Separation: includes the use of wedges interproximally during proximal surface instrumentation.

5. REMOVAL OF CARIOUS TOOTH PORTION AND OLD RESTORATION IF ANY

- Removal of caries is the mechanical elimination of carious dentin and debris from the cavity preparation.

- If the decay is soft, removal should be done with the broadest discoid or spoon excavator, directing it with scooping actions from the cavity peripheries to the center.

- If the decay is hard, a large round bur is used in addition to excavator. Bur should be in slow revolving motion, used with brushing strokes from the peripheries of the cavity preparation to the center, with a lot of water coolant.

6. SECONDARY RESISTANCE AND RETENTION FORM

- After the removal of infected dentin and/or old restorative material, pulpal protection is provided.
- Now, Resistance and Retention features are necessary for the preparation.
- The secondary resistance and retention forms are of 2 types: (A) Mechanical preparation features and (B) Treatments of the preparation walls with etching, priming and adhesive materials.

A. Mechanical Features

I. Retention Locks, Grooves and Coves

1. Retention locks

Proximal retention locks in the axiofacial and axiolingual line angles significantly *strengthen the isthmus of a class-II restoration* and are superior to axiogingival grooves in *increasing the restoration's fracture strength*, and *prevents the proximal displacement of the restoration.*

Characteristics

There are 4 characteristics or determinants of proximal locks, i.e.

1. Position
2. Translation
3. Depth and
4. Occlusogingival orientation

Position refers to the axiofacial and axiolingual line angles of initial tooth preparation (0.2mm axial to DEJ). *Retention locks should be placed 0.2mm inside the DEJ, regardless of the depth of the axial walls and axial line angles.*

Translation refers to the direction of movement of the axis of the bur.

Depth refers to the extent of translation (i.e 0.5 mm at gingival floor level).

Occlusogingival orientation refers to the tilt of the No. 169 L bur which dictates the occulusal height of the lock, given a constant depth.

Preparation

- To prepare a retention lock, use a No.169 L bur with air coolant (to improve vision) and reduced speed (to improve tactile 'feel' and control).
- The bur is placed in the properly positioned axiolingual line angle and directed to bisect the angle approximately parallel to the DEJ. This positions the retention lock 0.2 mm inside the DEJ, thus maintianing the enamel support.

- The bur is titled to allow cutting to the depth of the diameter of the end of the bur at the point angle and permit the lock to diminish in depth occlusally, terminating at the axiolinguopulpal point angle.
- In a similar manner facial lock is prepared in the axio facial line angle.
- If the axial line angle is too shallow, the lock may undermine the enamel of dentinal support.
- If the line angle is too deep, preparation of the lock may result in exposure of the pulp.

2. Retention grooves

- Grooves are for cast metal restorations and also root surface tooth preparation in composites.
- Grooves are horizontally oriented.
- Are prepared in most class - III and V preparations for amalgam and in some root surface tooth preparations for composite.

1. In Class-II Amalgam

- Prepare the retention grooves with a No. ¼ bur into the occluso axial and gingivo axial line angles, 0.2 mm inside the DEJ or 0.3 to 0.5 mm inside the cemental cavosurface margin.
- The depth of these grooves is one half the diameter of the bur head (i.e 0.25 mm).
- The bur is directed to bisect the angle formed by the junction of occlusal (or gingival) and axial walls.
- Ideally, the direction of the occlusal groove is slightly more occlusal than axial, and the direction of a gingival groove would be slightly more gingival than axial.

2. In Class-III Amalgam

- Prepare the gingival retention groove by placing a No. ¼ bur in the axio faciogingival point angle.
- It is positioned in the dentin to maintain 0.2 mm of dentin between the groove and the DEJ.
- Move the bur lingually along the axiogingival line angle with the angle of cutting generally bisecting the angle between the gingival and axial walls.

3. In Class-V Amalgam

- Use a No. ¼ bur to prepare two retention grooves, one along the inciso axial line angle and the other along the gingivoaxial line angle.

- The handpiece is positioned so that the No. ¼ bur is directed generally to bisect the angle formed at the junction of the axial wall and the incisal (or occlusal) wall.

- The depth of the grooves should be approximately 0.25mm which is half the diameter of the bur.

4. In Class-III Composite

- Groove retention may be necessary in root surface preparations.

- The retention groove created helps in (1). Minimizing the negative effects of polymerization shrinkage (2) enhance the marginal seal by resisting flexural forces placed on the cervical portion of the restoration.

- A continuous retention groove can be prepared in the internal portion of the external walls using a No. ¼ round bur.

- The groove is located 0.25 mm from the root surface and is prepared to a depth of 0.25 mm.

- This groove is directed as the bisector of the angle formed by the junction of the axial wall and the external wall. For its entire length, the groove should be parallel to the root surface.

5. In Class-IV Composite

- A gingival retention groove can be prepared using a No. ¼ round bur.

- It is prepared 0.2 mm inside the DEJ at a depth of 0.25 mm and at an angle bisecting the junction of the axial wall and gingival wall.

- The groove should extend the length of the gingival floor and slightly up the facioaxial and linguoaxial line angles.

6. In Class-V Composite

- Retention grooves are prepared with a No. ¼ bur along the full length of the gingivo axial and inciso axial (occluso axial) line angles.

- These grooves are prepared 0.25 mm in depth into the external walls and next to the axial wall at an angle that bisects the junction between the axial wall and the gingival or occlusal (or incisal) wall.

3. Retention coves

Retention coves are appropriately placed undercuts for the incisal retention of class III amalgams, occlusal portion of some amalgam restorations, some class V amalgams and occasionally for facilitating the start of insertion of certain gold foil restorations.

1. In Class - III Amalgam

- If less retention form is needed, two gingival coves may be used, as opposed to a continuous groove.

- One each may be placed in the axiogingivo facial and axiogingivo lingual point angles.

- The diameter of the bur is 0.5 mm and the depth of the groove should be half this diameter or 0.25 mm.

- Prepare an incisal retention cove at the axiofacio incisal point angle with a No. ¼ bur in dentin, being careful not to undermine the enamel.

- It is directed similarly into the incisal point angle and prepared to one half the diameter of the bur.

- Undermining the incisal enamel (or incisal canopy) should be avoided.

2. In Class-I Amalgam

- No. 33 ½ bur may be used to prepare a retention cove in the faciopulpal line angle.

- The tip of the No. 245 bur held parallel to the long axis of the tooth crown also might be used to prepare this cove.

- This retention cove is recommended only if occlusal convergence of the mesial and distal walls of the occlusal portion is absent or inadequate.

3. In Class - V Amalgam

- Four retention coves may be prepared, one in each of the four axial point angles of the preparation.

- Using four coves instead of two full length grooves conserves dentin near the pulp.

II. Groove Extensions

- These are obtained by extending the preparation for molars onto the facial or lingual surface to include the facial or lingual groove.

- These extensions are given for cast metal restorations.

- This feature enchances resistance for the remaining tooth.

III. Skirts

- Skirts are preparation features that extend the preparation around the line angles of the tooth.

- Skirts increase the resistance form by enveloping the tooth.

- Used in cast gold restorations.

IV. Beveled Enamel Margins

- These are primarily used to provide a better junctional relationship between the metal and the tooth.

- Bevel provides increased surface area for etchable enamel in composite restorations.
- Used in cast gold/metal restorations.

V. Pins, Slots, Steps and Amalgapins

- These are indicated when there is unusually great need for increased retention form.
- Mostly for amalgam restorations.

B. Placement of Etchant, Primer or Adhesive on Prepared Walls

Along with mechanical alterations, certain etchants and primers are used for increased retention and resistance.

1. Enamel wall etching

- Etching results in microscopically roughened surface to which the bonding material is mechanically bound.
- Enamel walls are etched for porcelain, composite and amalgam materials.

2. Dentin treatment

- Dentin surface require etching and priming for bonded porcelain, composite or amalgam restorations.

7. FINISHING OF EXTERNAL WALLS

Objectives

1. To create best marginal seal between restorative material and tooth structure.
2. To afford a smooth marginal structure.
3. To provide maximum strength to the tooth and the restorative material near the margin.

For an ideal enamel wall, *Noy* formulated certain structural requirements. They are,

1. The enamel wall must rest upon sound dentin.
2. The enamel rods which form the cavosurface angle must have their inner ends resting on sound dentin.
3. The enamel rods which form the cavosurface angle must be supported, or be resting on sound dentin and their outer ends must be covered by the restorative material.
4. The cavosurface angle must be trimmed or beveled so that the margins will not be exposed to injury in condensing the restorative material against it.

8. DEBRIDEMENT (TOILET) OF THE PREPARATION

- Defined as *the act of freeing the preparation walls and margins from objects that may interfere with the proper adaptability and behaviour of the restorative material.*

- It includes the freeing of all preparation walls, floors and margins from enamel and dentin chips resulting from excavation and grinding; drying the preparation walls, floors and margins from any introduced moisture; sterilization of preparation of walls and floors.

Methods

1. Water, air or combinations of air–water jets, using the water–air syringe is very efficient in removing.
2. Dry cotton pellets is a safer way to dry the cavity.
3. Cavity cleaners which are solutions of very low concentration of citric, ascorbic and acetic acids are sometimes used to remove the debris. They should be used in shallow cavities and should be followed by long period of water jet rinsing.
4. A dilute solution of hydrogen peroxide is a very efficient debris removing agent.
5. Scrapping preparation walls, floors and margins with sharp hand instruments especially chisels is most effective way of freeing the lodged debris.
6. Smear layer of the preparation can be removed by a solution of 10% EDTA.

RESTORATIONS

- Restoration is defined as *filling material or prosthesis used to restore or replace a tooth, a portion of a tooth, multiple teeth or other oral tissues.*

Classification

I. Based on fabrication
1. Direct Restoration
2. Indirect Restoration

II. Based on Longevity
1. Intermediate / Temporary
2. Permanent

1. Direct Restoration

Defined as a *cement, metal or resin - based composite that is placed and formed intra orally to restore teeth or enhance esthetics.*

Ex: Amalgam, GIC, Composite, DFG, etc.

2. Indirect Restoration

Defined as a *ceramic, metal, metal-ceramic, or resin-based composite used extra orally to produce prosthesis, which replace missing teeth, enhance esthetics and/or restore damaged teeth.*

3. Intermediate / Temporary Restoration

Defined as *a tooth filling or prosthesis that is placed for a limited period, from several days to months, and is designed to seal teeth and maintain their position until a long-term restoration is placed.*

4. Permanent Restoration

Defined as *a long-lasting replacement or restoration for missing damaged or discolored teeth.*

Indications for Restorations

1. Caries
2. Replacement or repair of old restorations
3. Fractured teeth
4. To restore form and function
5. Esthetic desire
6. To fulfil other restorative needs

Factors affecting the placement of the restoration

1. Extent of caries.
2. Strength of remaining tooth structure.
3. Patient's oral hygiene and dental caries history.
4. Economic status.
5. Ability of the dentist to perform the procedure.
6. Preferences of the dentist and the prevailing standard of care.
7. Patient's acceptance.

ENAMEL PATTERNS

1. DIRECTION OF THE ENAMEL RODS (PRISMS)

– For better understanding purpose, *the long axis of the crown* is taken as the reference point.

– Directions of the enamel rods relative to the long axis of the crown are described as follows,

1. Rods at the center of the occlusal surface: always lean to pits or fissures towards the long axis of the crown. The stronger the inclination of the cusps, the greater the degree of such slants.

2. On the periphery of the occlusal surfaces (near the tips of the cusps and crests of the marginal ridges): The rods are inclined toward cusp tips and crests, away from the long axis of the crown.

3. In between the center and periphery of the occlusal surfaces: The rods are parallel to the long axis of the crown.

4. Rods at the incisal or occlusal third of the axial surface: incline incisally or occlusally making an average of plus (plus means toward incisal or occlusal) with the perpendicular to the long axis of the crown at this area.

5. Rods at the gingival third of the axial surface: incline by an average of minus (toward the gingival) from the perpendicular to the long axis of the crown at this area.

6. Rods at the middle third of the axial surface: Perpendicular to the long axis of the crown.

2. THICKNESS PATTERN OF ENAMEL

– *Enamel has its maximum thickness at the tips of the cusps and at the crests of triangular, marginal and crossing ridges.*

– Its thickness decreases from occlusal surface to the depth of the pits, fissures and grooves.

– Enamel thickness decreases towards gingivally on the axial surface, with its least thickness at the CEJ.

– *For anterior teeth, the maximum thickness of enamel is at the incisal edge (slopes in the canine).*

– Lingual enamel plates are generally thinner than the facial and which is more apparent in anterior teeth than the posterior teeth.

– As age increases, the thickness of the enamel decreases at the occluding areas with the result of attrition and also as the mineralization and dehydration of the enamel increases by the age, the brittleness and erasing tendency of enamel is also increases.

CHAPTER 03

DENTAL BIOMATERIALS

DENTAL AMALGAM

- Dentists have more than a century of experience using amalgam as a direct filling material.

- Dental amalgam has a much longer service record, than most drugs and bio materials in use today and except for gold, all other dental restorative materials.

- There is more information about dental amalgam than about any other dental restorative material presently used, yet concerns are raised periodically about the safety of dental amalgam relative to one of its ingredients - elemental mercury.

DEFINITION

- *Amalgam* is an alloy of mercury with another metal or metals.

- *Dental amalgam* is produced by mixing liquid mercury with solid particles of an alloy of silver, tin, copper and some times zinc, palladium, indium and selenium. This combination of solid metals is called *Amalgam alloy*.

- The reaction between mercury and alloy follows mixing is termed an *amalgamation* reaction. It results in the formation of a hard restorative material of silver-grey appearance.

APPLICATIONS

- *It is the strongest and most widely used filling material*.

- It is used in /as,

  1. Class - I and Class - II cavities on the posterior teeth.

  2. Class - V cavities where esthetics are not considered.

  3. Core build up for crown preparation in a grossly destructed tooth.

  4. Retrograde root canal filling.

  5. Preparation of dies.

  6. Combination with retentive pins to restore a crown in which one or two walls of cavity are missing.

  7. Restoration of disto-facial cusps of canine.

  8. The patients where moisture control is difficult.

ADVANTAGES

  1. Easy to manipulate

  2. Least technique sensitive

  3. Self sealing property

  4. Good strength

5. Long lasting

6. Economic

7. Good wear resistance

8. Applicable in a broad range of clinical situations

9. Less chair side time required

10. Direct restorative material

11. Easy to repair

12. Durable

DISADVANTAGES

1. Cannot be used in esthetic zones.

2. More brittle and less tough.

3. Do not bond to the tooth structure.

4. Mercury toxicity.

5. Galvanic action.

6. Prone to tarnish and corrosion.

7. Marginal breakdown.

8. Microleakage.

9. Delayed expansion and resultant pulpitis.

10. Some destruction of sound tooth structure.

CLASSIFICATION

I. Based on size of alloy particle

1. Microcut

2. Macrocut

II. Based on shape of alloy particle

1. Lathecut

2. Spherical

3. Spheroidal / Admixed (Spherical with irregular surface)

III. Based on number of alloying metals

1. Binary: two metals - silver, tin.

2. Ternary: three metals - silver, tin, copper.

3. Quaternary: Four metals - silver, tin, copper, indium.

IV. Based on noble - metal content

1. Non noble metal alloys.

2. Noble metal alloys.

V. Based on Copper content

1. **Low copper / conventional / Traditional alloys:** Contain less than 6% of copper.

2. **High copper alloys:** Contain more than 6% of copper.

These are classified into,

 i. *Admixed / Dispersed / Blended alloys*

It is a mixture of spherical eutectic high copper alloy and lathecut low copper alloy.

 ii. *Single / Uni composition alloys*

6. Based on Zinc content

 1. *Zinc containing alloys*

Contain more than 0.01% of zinc.

 2. *Zinc free alloys*

Contain less than 0.01% of zinc.

COMPOSITION

– According to *ADA specification No.1,*

Silver - 69.4%

Tin - 26.2%

Copper - 3.6%

Zinc - 0.8%

ROLE OF MAJOR COMPONENTS IN AMALGAM

1. Silver

   – Major element

   – Whitens the alloys

   – Decreases the creep

   – Increases the strength

   – Increases the setting expansion

   – Reduces tarnish and corrosion

2. Tin

   – Controls the reaction between silver and mercury.

   – Reduces strength and hardness of the amalgam.

   – Reduces tarnish resistance of the amalgam.

3. Copper

   – Increases strength and hardness.

   – Increases setting expansion.

   – Decreases the brittleness of the alloy.

4. Zinc

   – Acts as a **scavenger or deoxidizer**: prevents the oxidation of silver, copper and tin during manufacture of alloy powder.

   – Adds plasticity to the mix.

- Zinc less alloys are more brittle.
- Zinc causes delayed expansion if its content is > 0.01%.

5. Platinum and Palladium
- Increases the hardness and whitens the alloy.

6. Mercury
- Necessary for the reaction to form plastic mass.

MANUFACTURING OF ALLOY

1. Lathe - cut powder
- The metal ingredients are heated and protected from oxidation until melted, then poured into a mold to form an ingot.
- Lathe-cut alloys are normally subjected to two heat treating procedures.
- The first is a **homogenization** heat treatment, normally carried out on the alloy ingot before lathecutting and designed to produce homogenous grains in which the $Ag_3Sn(\gamma)$ intermetallic compound predominates. Homogenization ensures that each filing has similar composition and properties. The heat treatment involves heating to about 420°C for several hours. The resulting alloy contains relatively larger grains of γ – phase material.
- The second is **heat treatment** which is carried out after lathe-cutting.
- This is a lower temperature treatment typically involving heating the alloy powder to approximately 100°C for about 1 hour. This treatment is called as 'alloy ageing' ; it is to remove residual stresses introduced during cutting and ensures that the alloy remains stable during future storage.

2. Spherical Powder
- Manufactured by **atomization** process.
- All the desired elements are melted together. The liquid alloy is then sprayed, under high pressure of an inert gas, through a fine crack in a crucible into a large chamber. The droplets of alloy solidify as they falldown. The produced particles are either spherical or spheriodal in nature.

3. Particle size
- The average particle size of amalgam is 15-35 microns.
- Average small particle size alloys have high strength and produce rapid hardening.

4. Comparison of Alloy - Powder particles
- Lathecut and Admixed alloys require more condensation pressure and tend to resist condensation better than spherical alloys.
- Spherical alloy amalgams are more plastic.
- Spherical alloy requires less mercury than lathe cut alloys.

5. Admixed alloys
- These alloy powder particles contain both lathe cut and spherical alloy particles.
- Contain 30 to 55 wt% spherical high-copper powder.

DIFFERENCES BETWEEN *LOW COPPER* AND *HIGH COPPER* ALLOYS

Low Copper Alloys	High Copper Alloys
1. Less compressive strength (presence of γ_2 phase).	1. High compressive strength.
2. Less corrosion resistance.	2. High corrosion resistance.
3. Less marginal integrity.	3. High marginal integrity.
4. High creep: 0.8 – 8%.	4. Low creep: 0 – 1%.

DIFFERENCES BETWEEN *LATHE-CUT* ALLOYS AND *SPHERICAL* ALLOYS

Lathe – Cut Alloys	Spherical Alloys
1. Particles are irregular in shape.	1. Particles are in spherical shape.
2. Manufactured by milling an annealed ingot of alloy.	2. Manufactured by atomization of molten alloy.
3. Less plastic and resists condensation pressure.	3. More plastic.
4. More mercury required hence has inferior properties.	4. Requires less mercury hence has better properties.

ADVANTAGES AND DISADVANTAGES OF *ADMIXED* AND *SPHERICAL* HIGH COPPER AMALGAMS

Admixed High Copper Amalgam	Spherical High Copper Amalgam
Advantages:	Advantages:
1. Longer working time.	1. Sets faster.
2. Less dimensional change.	2. Lower residual mercury.
3. Displacement of matrix.	3. Lower creep.
	4. Faster finishing.
	5. Higher early strength.
	6. Low condensation pressure.
Disadvantages:	Disadvantages:
1. Slower set.	1. Less working time.
2. High residual mercury.	2. Greater dimensional change.
3. Higher creep.	
4. Less early strength.	
5. Harder to finish.	

SETTING REACTIONS AND STRUCTURE (AMALGAMATION PROCESS)

Phases in amalgam alloys and set dental amalgam	Stoichiometric formula
γ (gamma)	Ag_3Sn
γ_1	Ag_2Hg_3
γ_2	$Sn_{7-8}Hg$
ε (epsilon)	Cu_3Sn
η (eta)	Cu_6Sn_5
Silver – copper eutectic	$AgCu$

γ_1 - *noble phase*, γ_2 - *weakest phase*.

A. Low copper alloys

– Silver and Tin can form an intermetallic compound of formula $Ag_3Sn(\gamma)$ which contains 73.15% silver and 26.85% Tin.

– The reaction is,

$$Ag_3Sn + Hg \rightarrow Ag_2Hg_3 + Sn_{7-8}Hg + \underset{(unreacted)}{Ag_3Sn}$$

$$\quad\gamma \qquad\qquad\qquad \gamma_1 \qquad \gamma_2 \qquad \gamma$$

– **Structure of set material:** a core of unreacted γ and a matrix of the γ_1 and γ_2 compounds.

– The percentages are γ_1 - 54% to 56%; γ_2 - 11% to 13%; γ - 27% to 35% by volume.

– Mercury has limited solubility for silver (0.035 wt%) and tin (0.6 wt%).

– Because the solubility of silver in mercury is much lower than that of tin, the γ_1 phase precipitates first and the γ_2 phase precipitates later.

– γ_1 has Body-centred cubic structure and γ_2 has Hexagonal structure.

– The more unconsumed $Ag - Sn$ particles that are retained in the final structure, the stronger the amalgam.

– γ_2 phase is least stable to corrosion environment and suffer corrosion attack especially at 'crevices' of the restorations.

B. High - Copper Admixed Alloys

– It has Silver - Copper eutectic alloy (71.9wt% Silver and 28.1 wt% Copper).

– **Main feature:** The set structure is essentially free of γ_2 phase.

– The reactions are,

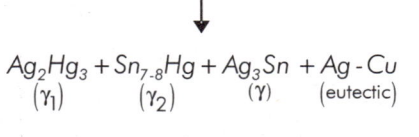

$$(1) \quad \underset{(\gamma)}{Ag_3Sn} + \underset{(eutectic)}{Ag - Cu} + Hg$$

$$\downarrow$$

$$\underset{(\gamma_1)}{Ag_2Hg_3} + \underset{(\gamma_2)}{Sn_{7-8}Hg} + \underset{(\gamma)}{Ag_3Sn} + \underset{(eutectic)}{Ag - Cu}$$

$$(2) \quad \underset{(\gamma_2)}{Sn_{7-8}Hg} + \underset{(eutectic)}{Ag - Cu} \longrightarrow \underset{(\eta)}{Cu_6Sn_5} + \underset{(\gamma_1)}{Ag_2Hg_3}$$

– **Set material:** consists of a core of Ag_3Sn and $Ag - Cu$ surrounded by a halo of Cu_6Sn_5 and a matrix of γ_1.

C. High - Copper Unicomposition Alloys

– **Main feature:** The set structure is free of γ_2 phase.

– The reaction is,

$$Ag_3Sn + Cu_3Sn + Hg \rightarrow Ag_2Hg_3 + Cu_6Sn_5$$
$$(\gamma) \qquad (\varepsilon) \qquad\qquad (\gamma_1) \qquad (\eta)$$

- **Set material:** consists of a core of Ag_3Sn and and Cu_6Sn_5 is present in the γ_1 matrix rather than as a halo.

PROPERTIES OF AMALGAM

- **ADA Specification No: 1 for Amalgam Alloys** lists three physical properties as a measure of amalgam quality: *Creep, Compressive strength and Dimensional change.*

- According to ADA, when a cylindrical specimen is 7 days old, a 36 Mpa stress is applied in a environment. The maximum allowable creep is 3%. The minimum allowable compressive strength 1 hour after setting, when a cylindrical specimen is compressed at a rate of 0.25 mm/min is 80 Mpa. The dimensional change between 5 min and 24 hrs. must fall within the range of 20 μm/cm.

1. Creep

- *Creep is the time-dependent strain or deformation that is produced by a stress.*

- Creep can cause an amalgam restoration to extend out of the cavity preparation, there by increasing its susceptibility to marginal breakdown.

- Creep values of low-copper amalgams: 0.8% - 8% and of high - copper amalgams: < 0.1%.

- Creep rates increase with higher γ_1 and γ_2 volume fractions.

- Creep also increases with high mercury / alloy ratio and low condensation pressure.

2. Compressive Strength

- Set amalgam has a very weak tensile and a very high compressive strength.

- The following factors affect the strength of the amalgam,

  #### 1. Temperature

  It loses 50% of its room temperature strength when its temperature is elevated to 600°C (as when hot coffee flows over it).

  #### 2. Trituration

  Under - trituration and over - triturartion decreases the strength.

  #### 3. Mercury

  Higher the residual mercury, lower the strength.

4. Condensation

Greater the condensation pressure, higher the strength.

5. Porosity

It results from under - trituration, under - condensation, irregularly shaped particles of the alloy powder, insertion of too large increments into the cavity, delayed insertion.

6. Gamma 2 Phase

Its reduction or the prevention of its formation can definitely increase the strength.

3. Dimensional change

- During setting, amalgam undergoes three distinct dimensional changes, i.e.

- **Stage -1: Initial contraction:** Results from the absorption of the mercury into the interparticular spaces of the alloy powder.

- **Stage - 2: Expansion:** due to the formation and growth of the matrix crystals.

- **Stage - 3: Limited, delayed contraction of the mass:** results from the absorption of unreacted mercury.

- The following are the factors affect the Dimensional change,

1. Constituents

The more the basic gamma - phase, the more the expansion.

Greater traces of Tin produce lesser expansion.

2. Mercury

More mercury produces a more prolonged second stage of amalgamation (expansion).

3. Particle Size

Smaller the particle size, the less the expansion.

4. Trituration

Good trituration causes no apparent expansion.

5. Condensation

Higher condensation pressure induces more contraction.

6. Contamination with moisture

If it contaminate, causes delayed expansion.

4. Corrosion

- The order of corrosion resistance of the different stages of amalgamation are,

$$Ag_2Hg_3 > Ag_3Sn > Ag-Cu > Cu_3Sn >$$
$$\underset{(\gamma_1)}{} \qquad \underset{(\gamma)}{} \qquad \qquad \underset{(\varepsilon)}{}$$
(Most resistant)

$$Cu_6Sn_5 > Sn_{7-8}Hg \,(Least\ resistant)$$
$$\underset{(\eta)}{} \qquad \underset{(\gamma_2)}{}$$

1. Low-Cu system

- In the Low - Copper amalgam system, the most corrodable phase is the γ_2 phase.
- Corrosion results in the formation of tin oxychloride from the tin in the γ_2 phase and also liberates mercury.

$$Sn_{7-8}Hg + \frac{1}{2}O_2 + H_2O + Cl^- \rightarrow Sn_4(OH)_6 Cl_2 + Hg$$

2. High - Cu System

- $Cu_6Sn_5\,(\eta)$ is the least resistant phase.
- The corrosion product is $CuCl_2 . 3Cu(OH)_2$.

$$Cu_6Sn_5 + \frac{1}{2}O_2 + H_2O + Cl^- \rightarrow CuCl_2 . 3Cu(OH)_2 + SnO$$

5. Delayed Expansion / Secondary Expansion

- Defined as *the gradual expansion of a zinc containing amalgam over weeks to months which is associated with hydrogen gas development caused by contamination of the plastic mass with moisture during its manipulation in a cavity preparation.*
- The expansion usually starts after 3 to 5 days and may continue for months, reaching values greater than 400 μm (4%).

Complications

- Protrusion of the restoration out of the cavity.
- Increased microleakage space around the restoration.
- Restoration perforation.
- Blister formation on the restoration surface.
- Increased flow and creep.
- Pulpal pressure pain.

TECHNICAL CONSIDERATIONS

- The following steps are involved in the building up of an amalgam restoration.

1. Choice of the Alloy and Mercury

- Select an alloy certified by the ADA.
- High-Copper amalgam is recommended because of its superior clinical performance.

- There is no decision in the choice of mercury except that it should follow the USP specifications.
- Alloys are available in powder, tablet and pre proportioned forms.
- Most operators prefer diposable capsules.

2. Proportioning of the alloy and mercury

- Two techniques are available for the purpose of proportioning.

1. High - mercury technique

- Also called as *increasing dryness technique.*
- The initial amalgam mix contains a little or more mercury than needed for the powder (52-53% Hg) producing a very plastic mix.
- It is necessary to continue squeezing the mercury out of the mix increments being introduced during build - up of the restoration so that each increment will be dryer than the previous one.

2. Minimum mercury technique

- Also called as *1:1 technique* or *'Eame's technique'* or *'No - Squeeze cloth technique'.*
- It is more popular technique.
- The initial amalgam mix contains equal amounts of mercury and powder alloy.
- With this techniques one can assume that 50% or less mercury will be in the final restoration.
- Proportioning of the alloy and mercury should be done by weight.

3. Trituration

- Defined as *the process of mixing the amalgam alloy particles with mercury in an amalgamator.*

Objectives

1. To achieve a workable mass of amalgam in a minimum time.
2. To remove oxides from the surface of powder particles.
3. To pulverize the pellets into particles that can be easily wetted by the mercury.
4. To reduce particle size so as to increase the surface area of the alloy particles per unit volume.
5. To dissolve the particles or part of the particles of the powder in mercury, which initiate the formations of the matrix crystals.
6. To keep the amount of γ_1 or $\gamma_1 - \gamma_2$ matrix crystals as minimal as possible.

Methods of Trituration

- The two methods of trituration are,

1. Hand Trituration

– Alloy and mercury are triturated by hand with a mortar and pestle: its use is diminishing nowadays.

2. Mechanical Trituration

– Used universally.

– Has a metal or plastic capsule to contain the powder and mercury which serves as a mortar.

– A cylindrical metal or plastic piston of smaller diameter than the capsule is inserted into the capsule and this serves as the pestle.

– The *three* basic movements of mechanical triturators are,

   i. The mixing arm carrying a capsule moves back and forth in a straight line at varying speeds.

   ii. The mixing arm travels back and forth in a figure of 8 at varying speeds.

   iii. The mixing arm travels in a centrifugal fashion.

Normal Mix

– Appears shiny and separates in a single mass from the capsule.

– Has maximum strength.

– Carved surface retains its lustre after polishing.

– Mix may be warm (not hot) when it is removed from the capsule.

Under - triturated mix

– Appears dull and crumbly.

– Mix is rough and grainy.

– Susceptable to tarnish after carving.

– Less strength.

Over - triturated mix

– Appears soapy and tends to stick to the inside of the capsule.

– Decreased working time.

– Results in higher contraction of amalgam.

– Increased creep.

4. Mulling

– It is a continuation of trituration.

– *It is done to improve the homogenity of the mass and to assure a consistent mix.*

– There are two ways to accomplish the mulling, i.e.

   i. The mix is enveloped in a dry piece of rubber dam and vigorously rubbed between the index finger and thumb or the thumb of one hand and palm of another hand. This process should not exceed 2 to 5 sec.

   ii. After trituration pestle is removed from the capsule and the mix in triturated in the pestle free capsule for 2 to 3 seconds. In addition to fulfilling the objectives of mulling, this process delivers the mix in one single coherent and consistent mass.

5. Condensation

– Defined as *the process of compaction of the alloy into the prepared cavity to attain greatest possible density with adequate mercury present to ensure maximum continuity of the noble phase* (Ag_2Hg_3) *between the remaining alloy particles.*

1. Objectives

1. To adapt amalgam intimately to the prepared walls and margins.

2. To produce a uniform and viod-free restoration as possible.

3. To minimize the residual mercury content.

4. It brings the strongest phase of amalgam close together, there by increasing the strength of the restoration.

– Condensation should be done immediately after trituration.

– Condensation can be done by the hand or mechanical condensers.

– It is shown that mechanical condensation is superior to hand condensation.

– Condensers are available in different shapes and sizes, i.e. round, parallelogram, diamond etc., and as well as in various angulations to facilitate access.

– The face or nib of the condenser is inversely proportional to the square of its surface area.

– *Condensation pressure : 66.7 N.*

2. Condensation of non-spherical alloy

– Amalgam should be inserted in small increments and condensed with small condensers, to eliminate voids, to bind the increments together and to facilitate the filling of minor details of the prepared cavity.

– Once the surface of the preparation is reached, larger condensers should be used to avoid undue pressure on the enamel at the cavo surface.

– Condensation forces should be applied at 45° to walls and floors, i.e. bisecting line angles and trisecting point angles.

– Further increments are condensed at 90° to the previous portion to avoid shear force that may displace the already condensed amalgam.

- *Amalgam should be condensed from its center to periphery to avoid overlapping or bridging of voids at critical areas.*

- Excess mercury or splashy amalgam which appears on the surface should be excavated and discarded before inserting another increment.

3. Condensation of spherical alloy

- Here, increments are taken in such a way so as to fill the entire cavity or a large part of the cavity.

- Largest condenser is used to prevent the lateral escape of the spherical particles during condensation pressure toward the cavity floor.

4. Blotting mix

- After completely filling the prepared cavity and covering the cavosurface anatomy, an over dried amalgam mix (made by squeezing off mercury in squeezing cloth) is condensed heavily over the restoration using the largest condensers possible for the involved tooth. This mix is called the blotting mix.

- It serves to blot excess mercury from the critical marginal and surface area of the restoration and to adapt amalgam more intimately to the cavosurface anatomy.

- The mix is excavated and discarded after its use.

5. Delayed condensation

- It results in a mix with increased residual mercury, less strength, higher creep, decreased plasticity and the mix does not adapt well to the cavity walls.

- Higher concentrations of mercury is located around the margins of the restorartions.

6. Burnishing or Surfacing

- *It is the process of rubbing usually performed to make a surface shiny or lustrous.*

- Immediately, after discarding the blotting mix, a large rounded burnisher is used for burnishing.

- Burnishing proceeds from the amalgam surface to the tooth surface on the occlusal and other conspicuous portions of the restoration.

- Inaccessible areas, such as the proximal portion of the restoration are burnished with a beaver tail burnisher and / or Sprately burnisher or T-burnisher.

Objectives

1. As a continuation of condensation to reduce the voids.

2. To bring out excess mercury to the surface.

3. To adapt the amalgam further to cavosurface anatomy.

4. Condition the surface amalgam to the carving step.

Pre Carve burnishing

- It is a form of condensation done to improve the benefits of condensation.

- It produces a denser amalgam at the margins of occlusal preparations restored with high-copper amalgam and initiates carving.

Post Carve burnishing

- Done to improve smoothness and to produce a Satin (not shiny) appearance.

- To improve marginal integrity of high copper amalgams.

- Produces denser amalgam at the margins of occlusal preparation restored with low-copper amalgam.

7. Carving

- Defined as *the anatomical sculpturing of the amalgam material.*

Objectives

1. To produce a restoration with no underhangs.

2. To produce a restoration with the proper physiological contours.

3. To produce a restoration with minimal flash.

4. To produce a restoration with functional, non-intefering occlusal anatomy.

5. To produce a restoration with adequate, compatible marginal ridges.

6. To produce a restoration with physiologically compatible embrasures.

- Carving can be achieved by Hollenbeck carvers, Ward's carvers, Diamond carvers, Cleiod, Discoid carvers, etc.

- Under carving leaves thin portions of amalgam (subjected to fracture) on the unprepared tooth surface. Such margins give the appearance that the amalgam has expanded beyond the preparation. *The thin portion of amalgam extending beyond the margin is referred to as `flash'.*

MERCURY TOXICITY

- OSHA has set a Threshold Limit Value (TLV) of 0.05 mg/m^3 as the maximum amount of mercury vapour allowed in the work place.

- The lowest dose of mercury that elicits a toxic reaction is 3 to 7 μg/kg body weight.

- The dosage of mercury to cause death is 4000 μg/kg body weight.

- The maximum allowable level of mercury in the blood is 3 μg/l.
- Free mercury should not be sprayed or exposed to the atmosphere.
- Mercury hazard can arise during trituration, condensation, finishing and polishing of the restoration and also during the removal of old restoration at high speed.
- Skin contact with mercury should be avoided as it can be absorbed by the skin.
- Dentists and dental assistants are having the high risk of mercury intoxication.
- Mercury vapour can be inhaled.

Effects of Mercury Toxicity

1. CNS disturbances: Tremors, Headache, Depression, Insomnia.
2. Excessive salivation.
3. Glossitis, Stomatitis
4. Dark opaque line on the free gingival margin

Precautions

- Air contamination is managed by proper ventilation.
- Mercury from the carpets is removed by sprinkling the sulphur (Sulphur reacts with mercury to form cinnabar which can be easily disposed).
- Excess mercury removed during condensation, mulling, trituration is stored in well sealed jars.
- Adequate use of water or coolant during polishing will minimize the inhalation of mercury vapour.
- Skin contacted with mercury should be thoroughly washed with soap and water.
- Excess mercury should not be thrown into sinks.
- The alloy mercury capsules should have a tightly fitting cap to avoid leakage.
- The excess amalgam spilled on the floor is picked and stored in well sealed containers.

BONDED AMALGAM

- It is a newly introduced concept.
- Amalgam bonding systems are used to seal underlying tooth structure and bond amalgam to enamel and dentin.
- Amalgam is strongly hydrophobic whereas enamel and dentin are hydrophilic. Therefore the bonding system is modified with a wetting agent which has the capacity to wet both hydrophobic and hydrophilic surfaces.

- The frequently used bonding system is 4-META (4 Methyloxy Ethyl Trimellitic Anhydride).
- The bonding system is applied in thicker layers (10 to 50 μm) to improve micro mechanical bonding.

Indication

- Indicated when weakened tooth structure remains and bonding may improve the overall resistance form of the restored tooth.

Advantages

1. Dentin sealing
2. Improved resistance form

Disadvantages

- Poor micromechanical bonding at the interface of amalgam with the bonding system.

GALLIUM ALLOYS

- These are developed to overcome the toxic effects of the mercury.
- In this, Gallium is used as the liquid instead of mercury and then it is triturated with a silver - tin - copper alloy powder in the same fashion as dental amalgam.

Gallium Amalgam

- It is a product formed by the reaction of an alloy powder (silver - tin - copper) with a gallium - based liquid alloy (gallium - indium - tin).

Composition
Powder

Silver	- 50%
Tin	- 25.7%
Copper	- 15%
Palladium	- 9%
Trace elements	- 0.3%

Liquid

Gallium	- 65%
Indium	- 18.95%
Tin	- 16%
Trace elements	- 0.5%

- Indium and Tin are added to the Gallium liquid to decrease its melting temperature.

Structure

- The structure of set alloy consists of a reaction zone of $CuGa_2$ and $PdGa_5$, surrounded by the unreacted zone, which consists of a matrix of Ag_9In_4 and islands of Ag_9Ga_3 and beta - tin particles.

Properties

– Measured at 24 hours.

1. Compressive strength   -   383 Mpa.
2. Tensile strength   -   57 Mpa.
3. Creep   -   0.17%.
4. Dimensional change   -   16 μm/cm.

DENTAL CEMENTS

– Cements are widely used in dentistry for a variety of applications, i.e. for lining, luting, restorative purposes, etc.

Classification

I. Cements based on Phosphoric acid

1. Zinc phosphate cements.
2. Silicophosphate cements.
3. Copper phosphate cements.

II. Cements based on Organometallic chelate compounds

1. Zincoxide eugenol cements.
2. Ortho-ethoxybenzoic acid (EBA) Cements.
3. Calcium hydroxide cements.

III. Cements based on Polyalkenoic Acids

1. Polycarboxylate cements.
2. Glass ionomer / polyalkenoate cements.

ZINC PHOSPHATE CEMENT

– *Oldest of the luting cements.*
– It is the traditional crown and bridge cement used for alloy restorations.

COMPOSITION AND SETTING

Powder

ZnO	:	90.2%
MgO	:	8.2%
SiO_2	:	1.4%
Bi_2O_3	:	0.1%
Miscellaneous	:	0.1%

(BaO, Ba_2SO_4, CaO)

Liquid

– Phosphoric acid (free acid) - 38.2%.
– Phosphoric acid (combined with Al and Zn)-16.2%.

Al	-	2.5%
Zn	-	7.1%
H_2O	-	36.0%

– Water controls the ionization of the acid, which in turn influences the rate of the liquid-powder (acid - base) reaction.
– The set cement is a cored structure consisting primarily of unreacted zinc oxide particles embedded in a cohesive amorphous matrix of zinc aluminophosphate.

MANIPULATION

1. *Powder / Liquid Ratio:* 1.4 g powder to 0.5 ml liquid.
2. *Mixing:* The cement is mixed over a large area of the cooled slab to dissipate the heat of the reaction (exothermic reaction).
3. *Mixing Time :* 60–90 Sec.
4. *Setting Time:* According to ADA Specification No: 96, it is 2.5–8 min.

PROPERTIES

1. *Consistency and film thickness*
   Luting 25 μm (max).
2. *Strength*
   i.   Compressive strength: 96 - 133 Mpa
   ii. Tensile Strength: 3.1 - 4.5 Mpa
3. *Retention*
   Bonding occurs by mechanical inter locking at interfaces, not by chemical interactions.
4. *Biological*
   Pulp response is **moderate** as compared with *silicate cement*.
   The pH of the cement two minutes after the start of the mixing is 2.14. The pH then increases rapidly to 5.5 at 24 hour.

APPLICATIONS

1. For luting permanent metal restorations.
2. As a base.
3. For the cementation of orthodontic brackets.

ADVANTAGES

1. Easy manipulation.

2. Sharp setting.
3. Adequate strength after setting.

DISADVANTAGES

1. Pulp irritation.
2. No antibacterial action.
3. Brittleness
4. No adhesion property.
5. Solubility in oral fluids.

SILICO PHOSPHATE CEMENT

– This is a hybrid of zinc phosphate and silicate materials.
– They are supplied as powder and liquid.
– Powder is a mixture of zinc oxide and aluminosilicate glass.
– Liquid is an aqueous solution of phosphoric acid containing buffers.
– The set cement contains a matrix of zinc and aluminium phosphates enclosing unreacted cores of zinc oxide and glass particles.
– It has anticariogenic property.
– Used primarily as luting cements for porcelain crowns because of their extra translucency at the margins.
– Used as temporary filling materials also.

COPPER CEMENT

– Not widely used nowadays.
– They are closely related to the zinc phosphate cements.
– Supplied as powder and liquid.
– Powder is a mixture of zinc oxide and black copper oxide.
– Liquid is an aqueous solution of phosphoric acid.
– It possess bactericidal effect due to the copper.
– They can be used in primary teeth where complete excavation of caries is not possible.
– Used for cementation of splints and orthodontic appliances.

ZINC OXIDE EUGENOL CEMENT

– It is the least irritant among all dental materials (pH is 7 at the time of placement).

COMPOSITION AND SETTING

Powder

ZnO	-	69.0%
White Rosin	-	29.3%
Zinc Stearate	-	1.0%
Zinc Acetate	-	0.7%

Liquid

Eugenol	-	85.0%
Olive Oil	-	15.0%

– The setting of ZOE cements is a chelation reaction in which an *amorphous zinc eugenolate* is formed.
– The set material consists of a matrix of amorphous zinc eugenolate that binds the unreacted zinc oxide particles together.

TYPES OF ZOE

– According to ADA Specification No. 30,

Type - I	:	Temporary cementation.
Type - II	:	Long term cementation of fixed prosthesis.
Type - III	:	Temporary fillings, Thermal insulating bases.
Type - IV	:	Intermediate restorations.

ADVANTAGES OF ZOE

1. Bland and Obtundent effect on pulp.
2. Good sealing ability.
3. Resistance to marginal penetration.

DISADVANTAGES OF ZOE

1. Low strength and abrasion resistance.
2. Solubility in oral fluids.
3. Little anticariogenic action.

MODIFICATIONS OF ZOE

– Two compositional changes have been used to increase the strength of the cement for luting purposes.

1. Polymer reinforced ZOE

– Contains 80% zinc oxide and 20% poly methyl methacrylate in the powder and eugenol in the liquid.
– Can be used for final cementation of fixed prosthesis, cement bases, cavity liners and provisional restorations. Ex : IRM (Type III).

Advantages

1. Minimal biologic effects.
2. Good sealing property.
3. Adequate strength for final cementation.

Disadvantages

1. Higher solubility.
2. Hydrolytic instability.
3. Possible discoloration.

2. *EBA - Alumina - reinforced ZOE*

   – Contains 70% zinc oxide and 30% alumina by weight in the powder.
   – The liquid contains 62.5% ortho EBA by weight and 37.5% eugenol by weight.
   – It is stronger than reinforced ZOE.
   – Has lower solubility.
   – Forms a suitable cavity lining for amalgam due to their adequate strength and resistance.
   – Primarily used as luting agent.

   Advantages

   1. Easy manipulation.
   2. Long working time.
   3. Good flow.
   4. Low irritation to pulp.

   Disadvantages

   1. Critical proportioning.
   2. Hydrolytic instability.
   3. Poor retention.

MANIPULATION

– Supplied as a powder and liquid or as two pastes.

   Mixing time :   30 to 60 sec

   Setting Time :   4 to 10 min

   (ADA Specification No. 30)

PROPERTIES

1. *Film thickness*

   For permanent cementation: 25 μm (max).

   For temporary cementation : 40 μm (max).

2. *Strength*

   Compressive strength: 35 Mpa.

3. *Retention*

   By mechanical retention.

4. *Biological*

   Pulp response is *mild* when compared to *silicate cement.*

APPLICATIONS

1. Cement bases
2. Lining of deep cavities
3. As obtundent
4. Temporary cementation
5. Permanent cementation
6. Provisional restorations
7. Endodontic sealers

CALCIUM HYDROXIDE

COMPOSITION AND SETTING: (BASE)

– It is supplied as two pastes system,

1. *Paste - I*

Calcium Hydroxide	-	50%
Zinc Oxide	-	10%
Zinc Stearate	-	0.5%
Ethyltoluene sulphonamide	-	39.5%

2. *Paste - II*

Glycol salicylate	-	40%
Titanium dioxide		
Calcium sulphate		
Calcium tungstate		

– The setting reaction occurs between calcium hydroxide and salicylate and yields calcium disalicylate.

pH

– Above 12
– The high pH of calcium hydroxide leads to extreme cytotoxicity of bacteria and there by it is bactiricidal.

COMPOSITION AND SETTING (LINER)

– Calcium hydroxide, used as a cavity liner is suspended in a solvent carrier with a thickening agent.
– When it is placed on the pulpal floor, the solvent evaporates and leaves a thin film of calcium hydroxide.
– It can neutralize acids that migrate toward the pulp and in the process, induce the formation of reparative dentin.

APPLICATIONS

1. Pulp capping procedures
2. Reparative dentin formation
3. Liners
4. Root canal sealer

5. Low strength base
6. Perforation repairs

ADVANTAGES

1. Easy manipulation
2. Rapid setting in thin layers
3. Good sealing property
4. Beneficial effects on carious dentin and exposed pulp

DISADVANTAGES

1. Low strength
2. Plastic deformation
3. Moisture senstitivity
4. Soluble in acidic conditions

ZINC POLYCARBOXYLATE CEMENT

- It is also called as *Zinc Poly Acrylate Cement.*
- *It is the first cement system that developed an adhesive bond to tooth structure.*

COMPOSITION AND SETTING

Powder

Zinc Oxide (Mainly)

Magnesium oxide

Stannous fluoride (Small quantities)

Liquid

- An aqueous solution of polyacrylic acid or a copolymer of acrylic acid with other carboxylic acids, such as itaconic acid.
- The acid concentration varies from 32% to 42% by weight.
- The set cement is a zinc polyacrylate ionic gel matrix that unites unreacted zinc oxide particles.

MANIPULATION

1. Powder / Liquid Ratio

1.5 parts of powder to 3 parts of liquid by weight.

2. Mixing

The powder is rapidly incorporated into the liquid in large quantities.

- If good bonding to tooth structure is to be achieved, the cement must be adapted against the tooth surface before it looses its glossy appearance.

- The glossy appearance indicates a sufficient amount of free carboxylic acid groups on the surface of the mixture that are vital for bonding to tooth structure.

3. Mixing Time: 30 - 60 sec

4. Setting Time: 6 - 9 min

(ADA Specification No. 96)

PROPERTIES

1. Consistency and Film thickness : 25 - 48 µm.

2. Strength

Compressive strength : 57 - 99 MPa

Tensile Strength : 3.6 - 6.3 MPa

3. Bonding to Tooth Structure

- It bonds chemically to the tooth structure.
- The polyacrylic acid is believed to react with calcium ions via carboxyl groups on the surface of enamel or dentin. *Thus the bond strength to enamel is greater than that to dentin.*

4. Biological

- Pulp response is **mild** when compared with *silicate cement*.
- The pH of Zinc polycarboxylate cement is higher than that of a zinc phosphate cement.
- Its mild irritation is due to that, the larger size of the poly acrylic acid molecule compared with phosphoric acid molecule may limit its diffusion through the dentinal tubules.

APPLICATIONS

1. Primarily for luting permanent alloy restorations and as bases.
2. Also used for cementation of orthodontic bands.

ADVANTAGES

1. Adhesion to tooth structure
2. Less irritation
3. Easy manipulation
4. Strength
5. Film thickness properties

DISADVANTAGES

1. Critical proportioning
2. Lower compressive strength
3. Requires clean surface

GLASS IONOMER CEMENT

– It is *"an aqueous based material that hardens following an acid- base reaction between fluoroalumino silicate glass powder and a polyacrylic acid solution"* - also referred to as conventional GIC.

SYNONYMS

1. Poly alkenoate cement
2. ASPA (Alumino Silicate Polyacrylic Acid)

TYPES

Type - I	:	*for luting*
Type - II	:	*for restorations*
Type - III	:	*liners and bases*

COMPOSITION AND SETTING

Powder

– It is an acid soluble calcium fluoroaluminosilicate glass.

Silica	-	41.9%
Alumina	-	28.6%
Aluminium fluoride	-	1.6%
Calcium fluoride	-	15.7%
Sodium fluoride	-	9.3%
Aluminium phosphate	-	3.8%

– *Lanthanum, Strontium, Barium* or zinc oxide are added to provide radiopacity.

Liquid

– Earlier, the liquids for GIC were aqueous solutions of polyacrylic acid in a concentration of about 40% to 50%. The liquid was quite viscous and tends to gel over time.

– In most of the current cements liquid contains,
  – Polyacrylic acid in the form of copolymer with itaconic, maleic or tricarboxylic acids.
  – Tartaric acid
  – Water

– On mixing the powder and liquid, the acid slowly degrades the outer layers of the glass particles releasing Ca^{2+} and Al^{3+} ions.

– During the early stages of setting, Ca^{2+} is released more rapidly and is primarily responsible for reacting with the poly acid to form a reaction product. Al^{3+} is released more slowly and becomes involved in setting at a later stage, often referred to as a secondary reaction stage.

– The set cement consists of an agglomeration of unreacted powder particles surrounded by a silica gel in an amorphous matrix of hydrated calcium and aluminium polysalts.

– Water serves as the reaction medium initially and then slowly hydrates the cross linked matrix, thereby yielding a stable gel structure that is stronger and less susceptible to moisture.

– If freshly mixed cements are exposed to ambient air with out any protective covering, the surface will craze and crack as a result of desiccation.

– Any contamination by water that occurs at this stage can cause dissolution of the matrix forming cations and anions in the surrounding areas.

– Therefore conventional GIC must be protected against desiccation and water changes in the structure during placements.

MANIPULATION

1. *P/L Ratio :* Manufacturer's recommendation to be followed.

2. *Mixing :* is done on the paper pad with an agate or lastic spatula. Metal spatula is not used because it corrodes the formed matrix.

3. *Mixing time :* 45 to 60 sec.

4. *Setting time :* According to ADA specification No. 96, it is 2.5 to 6.0 min.

PROPERTIES

1. *Film thickness*

   Luting : 15 μm

   Restorative : 50 μm

2. *Strength*

   Compressive strength : 93 - 226 Mpa

   Tensile strength : 4.2 - 5.3 Mpa

3. *Mechanism of Adhesion*

   – The mechanism has not been clearly identified.

   – It primarily involves chelation of carboxyl groups of the poly acids with the calcium in the apatite of the enamel and dentin.

   – The bond strength to enamel is always higher than that to dentin because of the greater inorganic content of enamel and its greater homogenicity.

4. *Biological*

   – Pulp response is *mild* to *moderate*.

   – They elicit a greater pulp reaction than ZOE but generally less than that from zinc phosphate cement.

5. Anticariogenic

- They release fluoride in amounts comparable to those released initially from silicate cement and continue to do so over an extended period.

- In addition, due to its adhesive effect they have the potential for reducing infiltration of oral fluids at the cement tooth interface, there by preventing secondary caries.

APPLICATIONS

1. Anterior esthetic restorative material for Class - III cavities

2. For eroded areas and Class - V restorations

3. Luting agents

4. Liners and bases

5. Orthodontic bracket adhesives

6. Pit and fissure sealants

7. Intermediate resorations

ADVANTAGES

1. Esthetics

2. Low thermal conductivity

3. No galvanic reaction

4. Direct restoration

5. Minimal removal of sound tooth structure

DISADVANTAGES

1. Technique sensitive

2. Moisture sensitive

MODIFICATIONS OF GIC

1. Metal reinforced GIC

2. Resin modified GIC (Hybrid Ionomer)

3. Compomer

1. METAL REINFORCED GIC

They were introduced to improve the strength, fracture toughness and resistance to wear.

Types

1. Silver alloy admixed / miracle mix

Spherical amalgam alloy powder is mixed with type - II GIC Powder.

2. Cermet

Prepared by fusing glass powder to silver particles through sintering.

Properties

- Nearly same as conventional GIC.

- Metallic fillers have little or no influence on the mechanical properties of restorative glass ionomers.

- They release appreciable amount of fluoride initially, but the magnitude decreases substantially over time.

Applications

1. Restoration of small Class - I cavities as an alternative to amalgam or composites.

2. For core build up of grossly destructed teeth (not be used wherever the cement will constitute greater than 40% of the total core building).

2. RESIN MODIFIED GIC (RMGIC)

Also called as *'Hybrid Ionomer'*.

Developed to overcome the moisture sensitivity and low early strength of GIC'S.

Composition and Setting Reactions

Powder

- Ion leachable fluoro aluminosilicate glass particles.

- Initiatos for light curing and / or chemical curing.

Liquid

- Water and polyacrylic acid or polyacrylic acid modified with methacrylate and hydroxyethyl methacrylate (HEMA) monomers.

- The initial setting reaction of the material occurs by the polymerization of methacrylate groups. The slow acid base reaction will ultimately be responsible for the unique maturing process and the final strength.

Advantages

1. Improved Translucency.

2. Fluoride release at the same level as conventional GIC .

3. Higher tensile strength.

4. Higher bond strength to tooth structure.

Disadvantages

1. Polymerization shrinkage

2. Microleakages

Applications

1. Liners and bases

2. Fissure sealants

3. Core buildups

4. Restoratives

5. Adhesives for orthodontic brackets

6. Repair materials for damaged amalgam cores or cusps

7. Retrograde root filling materials

8. Cervical lesions

9. Sandwich technique

10. Root caries

11. High caries risk patients

3. COMPOMER

Also known as *Poly acid modified composites*.

Developed to get the properties of fluoride releasing capability of conventional GIC and the durability of composites.

Composition and Setting Reaction

1. Single Component System

- Provides as a one paste, light curable material for restorative applications.

- It consists of silicate glass particles, sodium fluoride and polyacid - modified monomer with out any water.

- Setting is initiated by photopolymerization of the acidic monomer that yields a rigid material.

- During the service life of the restoration, the set material begins to absorb water in the saliva that contributes the acid base reaction between the acidic functional groups with in the matrix and silicate glass particles. This reaction eventually sustains fluoride release.

- Because of the absence of water in the formulation the cement mixture is *not self adhesive like conventional GIC and hybrid GIC.*

2. Two Component System

- Consists of powder and liquid or of two pastes.

- Used for luting applications.

- The powder is composed of strontium aluminium fluorosilicate, metallic oxides and chemically activated and / or light activated initiators.

- The liquid contains polymerizable methacrylate / carboxylic acid monomers, multifunctional acrylate monomers and water.

- The pastes have same ingredients as powder and liquid.

- Because of the presence of water in the liquid, these materials are self adhesive and an acid base reaction starts at the time of mixing.

Advantages

1. High bond strength

2. High compressive strength

3. High flexural strength

4. Low solubility

5. Sustained fluoride release

Disadvantages

1. Less fluoride release

2. Physical properties inferior to composites.

Applications

1. Class I and II restorations in children.

2. Cervical lesions.

3. Cementation of cast alloy crowns and bridges, porcelain fused to metal crowns and bridges, gold cast inlays and onlays.

4. Orthodontic bonding.

AGENTS FOR PULP PROTECTION

CAVITY VARNISHES

- Cavity varnishes are natural gums, such as copals, resins, or synthetic resins dissolved in an organic solvent, such as acetone, chloroform or ether.

- They form a coating on the tooth by evaporation of the solvent.

- *Varnishes are applied on all the surfaces of the cavity preparation including the margins.*

- Minimum of two layers of varnish is applied to attain a uniform and continuous coating. When the first layer dries, small pinholes develop. A second or third application fills in most of these voids and there by producing a more continuous coating.

- *Varnish is not indicated for adhesive materials, such as GIC and resin based composite.*

Uses

1. Reduces microleakage around the margins of newly placed amalgam restorations there by reducing post operative sensitivity.

2. Prevent penetration of corrosion products of amalgams into the dentinal tubules there by reducing the tooth discoloration.

3. Reduces the passage of irritants into the dentinal tubules from the overlying restoration or base.

4. Used as a surface coating over certain restorations to protect them from dehydration or contact with oral fluids.

5. Applied on the metallic restorations as a temporary protection in cases of galvanic shock.

Properties

– Varnishes neither possess mechanical strength nor provide thermal insulation because of inadequate film thickness.

– Contact angles of varnishes on dentin range from 53 to 106 degrees.

CAVITY LINERS

– *Liners are applied only onto the pulpal floor.*

Composition

– Liners are suspensions of calcium hydroxide in an organic liquid such as methyl ethyl ketone or ethyl alcohol or in an aqueous solution of methyl cellulose. On evaporation of the volatile solvent, the liner forms a thin film on the prepared tooth surface.

Properties

– Liners neither possess mechanical strength nor provide any significant thermal insulation.

– Calcium hydroxide liners are soluble and should not be applied at the margins of restorations.

Uses

1. To provide a barrier against the passage of irritants from cements or other restorative materials.

2. To reduce the sensitivity of freshly cut dentin.

3. To accelerate the formation of reparative dentin (due to the presence of calcium hydroxide).

Other Liners

1. Type III glass ionomer
2. Type IV ZOE

CEMENT BASES

Cement base

– It is a *material used in the cavity preparation to restore internal outline form and to provide chemical and thermal insulation.*

Intermediary Base

– It is a *material used in the cavity preparation to act as a protective barrier between dentin and the restorative material or to provide some therapeutic benefit to the tooth.*

Classification of Cement Bases

I. Low Strength Bases

– Have minimum strength and low rigidity.

– Main function is to act as a barrier to irritating chemicals and to provide therapeutic benefit to the pulp.

Ex: Calcium Hydroxide , ZOE.

II. High Strength Bases

– Used to provide thermal protection for the pulp and mechanical support for a restoration.

Ex: Zinc phosphate, Zinc polycarboxylate, Glass ionomer, Hybrid ionomer, Compomer, Polymer reinforced ZOE.

Functions

1. To prevent thermal shock
2. To prevent galvanic shock
3. To prevent chemical irritation
4. To support forces of condensation
5. To support the restoration under masticatory load
6. To provide therapeutic action

Thickness of the Base: *0.5 to 0.75 mm*

Clinical Considerations

– The selection of a base depends to an extent by the design of the cavity, the type of restorative material used and the proximity of the pulp relative to the cavity wall.

1. For Amalgam restorations

Calcium hydroxide or ZOE.

2. For Direct filling gold

Zinc phosphate , Zinc polycarboxylate or GIC.

3. For Resin based composites

Calcium hydroxide, GIC.

Principles of Intermediary Basing

1. Do not apply the intermediary base material on margins or surrounding walls but confine it to pulpal and axial walls only.

2. Confine the intermediary base material to the deepest part of the pulpal floor and or the axial walls.

3. Apply in minimal thickness to fulfill the objectives.

4. Therapeutic bases are always very weak so they should be covered with a stronger and more durable base.

Effective Depth

– It is the "*area of minimum thickness of sound dentin separating the pulpal tissues from the carious lesion or the thickness of the dentin bridge between the floor of the cavity and the roof of the pulp chamber*".

– The lesser the effective depth, the nearer the irritating ingredients to the pulp, so the more destructive the pulpal reaction will be.

Effective depth	Reaction on Pulp –Dentin organ
1. ≥ 2 mm	Healthy reparative reaction.
2. 0.8 to 2 mm	Unhealthy reparative reaction.
3. < 0.3 to 0.8 mm	Pulpal destruction.

Determination of effective depth

– Radiographic method is the most reliable method.

Procedure

On the radiograph, measure the dentin bridge at its deepest portion and the thickness of any clinically measurable anatomical landmark of the tooth. Ex. enamel thickness at the periphery of the preparation on the tooth measure the same anatomical mark. Then follow the following equation.

$$\frac{\text{Effective depth in the radiograph}}{\text{Enamel thickness in the radiograph}} = \frac{\text{Actual effective depth}}{\text{Actual enamel thickness}}$$

$$\text{Actual effective depth} = \frac{\text{Effective in radiograph} \times \text{Actual enamel thickness}}{\text{Enamel thickness in the radiograph}}$$

Disadvantage

– Radiograph is a two dimensional measure rather than three dimensional.

DENTAL INVESTMENTS AND DIE MATERIALS

DENTAL INVESTMENTS

– Investment is defined as a *ceramic material that is suitable for forming a mold into which a metal or alloy is cast. The operation of forming the mold is described as investing*.

IDEAL PROPERTIES

– It should,

1. Be easily manipulated.
2. Have sufficient strength at room temperature.
3. Have stability at higher temperatures.
4. Have sufficient expansion.
5. Have beneficial casting temperatures.
6. Be adequately porous.
7. Have smooth surface.
8. Be inexpensive.

COMPOSITION

– In general an investment is a mixture of three distinct types of materials, i.e.

1. **Refractory material**
   – Usually a form of silicon oxide such as quartz, tridymite or cristoballite or a mixture of these.
   – The purposes are to act as a material that can withstand high temperatures and to regulate the thermal expansion.

2. **Binder material**
   – It sets and bind together the particles of refractory substance.
   – The common binder used for dental casting gold alloy is α – calcium sulfate hemihydrate.

3. **Other chemicals**
   – Other chemicals such as sodium chloride, boric acid, potassium sulfate, graphite, copper powder or magnesium oxide are often added in small quantities to modify various physical properties.

Types

– There are three types of investment materials, i.e.

1. *Gypsum bonded investments.*
2. *Phosphate bonded investments.*
3. *Ethyl silica bonded investments.*

— They all contain silica as the refractory material, but the type of binder used is different.

1. GYPSUM BONDED INVESTMENTS

Classification

— According to ADA specification No: 2,

Type I	:	*Inlay thermal, for casting inlays and crowns.*
Type II	:	*Inlay hygroscopic, for casting inlays and crowns.*
Type III	:	*Partial denture, thermal*

Uses:

— Limited to gold castings and other low fusing alloys.

2. PHOSPHATE BONDED INVESTMENTS

— Supplied as a powder containing silica, primary Ammonium phosphate ($NH_4 H_2 PO_4$) and Magnesium oxide (MgO).

— The setting reaction in aqueous solution is,

$$NH_4H_2PO_4 + MgO \longrightarrow NH_4MgPO_4 + H_2O$$

Classification

— According to ADA specification No: 42,

Type I	:	*For inlays, crowns and other fixed restorations.*
Type II	:	*For partial dentures and other cast removable restorations.*

Uses

— Used for high fusing alloys (i.e. palladium and base metal alloys) with porcelain.

3. ETHYL SILICA BONDED INVESTMENTS

— Used for high fusing alloys.

Disadvantages

— Gives off flammable components during processing.

— Expensive.

DIE, CAST AND MODEL MATERIALS

DIE: Defined as *a reproduction of a prepared tooth made from a gypsum product, epoxy resin, a metal or a refractory material.*

CAST: Deifned as *a reproduction of the shape and features of a surface made from an impression of the surface.*

MODEL: Defined as *a positive full-scale replica of teeth, soft tissues and restored structures used as a diagnostic aid for construction of orthodontic and prosthetic appliances.*

— Dental stones plaster, electroformed silver and copper, epoxy resin and casting investment are some of the materials used to make casts or dies from dental impressions.

— Impressions in agar or alginate hydrocolloid can be used only with a gypsum material such as plaster, stone or casting investment.

— Compound impressions can be used to produce dies of plaster stone or electroformed copper.

— Various rubber impression materials can be used to prepare gypsum, electroformed or epoxy dies.

1. DENTAL STONES

— The most commonly used die materials are type IV (dental stone, high strength) and type V (dental stone, high strength, high expansion) improved stones.

— Type IV stones have a setting expansion of 0.1% or less and type V has 0.3% in accordance with ADA specification No.25.

— The greater expansion is useful for compensation of the relatively large solidification shrinkage of base metal alloys.

Advantages

1. Relatively inexpensive.
2. Easy to use.
3. Compatible with all impression materials.
4. Good strength.

Disadvantages

1. Brittle
2. Susceptibility to abrasion of edges and occlusal surface.

2. ELECTROFORMING

— Also known as *electroplating or electrodeposition*.

— Electroforming is a process by which a thin coating of metal is deposited on the impression.

— Metals used for electroforming are copper and silver; plating can be done for individual tooth impression, full arch impression; plating is done on compound impression; (usually copper plated) polysulphide impression (usually silver plated) and silicone impression.

– Hydrocolloid impressions are extremely difficult to electroplate and the process is not feasable for dental use.

Components

1. *Cathode:* The impression to be coated.

2. *Anode:* The metal to be deposited, i.e. copper or silver.

3. *Anode holder* and *cathode holder*

4. *Electrolyte:* The solution through which the electric current is passed.

5. *Ammeter:* Registers the current in milliamperes.

6. *Plating tank:* Made of glass or rubber with well fitting cover to prevent evaporation.

Procedure

1. Wash and dry the impression.

2. Attach the impression to the cathode holder with an insulated wire.

3. *Metallizing* the impression to make it to conduct electricity. In this process a thin layer of metal such as silver powder is deposited on the surface of the impression material. The metallizing agents are bronzing powder, aqueous suspensions of silver powder and powdered graphite.

4. The surface of the copper ring or impression tray is covered by wax, 2mm beyond the impression margin to avoid the plating of ring or the tray.

5. With a dropper, the impression is filled with the electrolyte without air bubbles.

6. The electrode is attached to the cathode and the impression is immersed in the electrolyte bath.

7. The direct current is applied for approximately 10 hr.

8. The current is disconnected. The impression is washed, then the die is completed by pouring dental stone. When the stone hardens, the impression is removed and the die is trimmed.

Advantages

1. Excellent abrasion resistance.

2. Moderately high strength.

3. Dimensional accuracy.

Disadvantages

1. Difficult to trim.

2. Health hazard from silver bath.

3. Not compatible with all impression materials.

3. EPOXY RESINS

– They are most effective with rubber impression materials.

Advantages

Tougher and more abrasion resistant than die materials.

Disadvantages

1. Slight shrinkage

2. Viscous

3. More setting time (may take upto 24 hrs)

4. DIVESTMENT

– It is a *Die stone Investment combination*.

– This is a combination of die material and investing medium.

– A gypsum bonded material called divestment is mixed with a colloidal silica liquid. A die is prepared from the mix and a wax pattern is constructed on it. Then the wax pattern together with die is invested in divestment

Advantages

1. Possibility of distortion of wax pattern during removal from the die or during setting of the investment is minimized.

2. Highly accurate technique for conventional gold alloys especially for extra coronal preparations.

Disadvantages

Not recommended for high fusing alloys.

Ex: Metal ceramic alloys (as it is a gypsum bonded material).

5. DIVESTMENT PHOSPHATE OR DVP

– This is a phosphate bonded investment that is used in the same manner as divestment.

– Suitable for high fusing alloys.

DENTAL CASTING PROCEDURES

– *Casting* can be defined as *"The act of forming an object in a mould"*.

– The casting procedure is used to make dental restorations such as inlays, onlays, crowns, bridges and removable partial dentures.

– The steps involved in the casting procedure are,

1. *Tooth /teeth preparation*
2. *Die preparation*
3. *Waxing*
4. *Spruing*
5. *Casting ringlining*
6. *Investing*
7. *Burnout*
8. *Casting process*
9. *Cleaning and finishing of the casting*

1. TOOTH/TEETH PREPARATION

- The tooth/teeth are prepared by the dentist to receive a cast restoration.

2. DIE PREPARATION

- A die is prepared from die stone or the impression is electroformed. A die spacer is coated or painted over the die which provides space for the luting cement.

3. WAXING/FORMATION OF THE WAX PATTERN

- There are two fundamental ways to prepare a wax pattern for a dental restoration.
- They are,
  I. *Direct wax pattern*
  II. *Indirect wax pattern*

I. Direct wax pattern

- In this direct method, the pattern is prepared on the tooth in the mouth.
- This method can only be used for small inlay restorations.

Technique

- Type-I Inlay wax is used.
- It is heated sufficiently to have adequate flow and plasticity under compression to reproduce all the details of the prepared cavity.
- Over heating of the wax should be avoided to prevent tissue damage, discomfort to the patient and difficulty in compression of the over heated wax.
- The heating and annealing of the wax is accomplished in a dry-heat oven.
- Wax may be annealed in water that is at a proper temperature and the storage for longer periods should be avoided under these conditions.
- Prolonged heating of the wax in water, especially at high temperatures, may result in a crymply mass.

- Ample time for cooling (from the working temperature to mouth temperature) should be allowed.
- Adequate compression of the wax is required for forming direct wax patterns.
- Carving instruments should be sufficiently warmed as desirable to soften, but not melt, the wax as the marginal adaptation and contour are developed and to minimize the formation of stresses in the wax.

II. Indirect wax pattern

- In this method, a model (die) of the tooth is first made, and then the pattern is made on the die.
- This method is used for all types of restorations.

Technique

- A metal or stone die is used in indirect method, which is the positive replica of a portion of the surrounding tooth structure and the cavity preparation.
- Type II Inlay wax is used.
- The advantage of the indirect method is, it makes the property of flow less critical, because pattern may be removed at a lower temperature and with greater ease from the die.
- A lubricant is applied to the die to release the wax pattern from the die (In the mouth saliva or dentinal fluid acts as lubricant). Excess seperator should be avoided as it results in the inaccuracies in the wax pattern and poor surface of the cast alloy.
- The wax may be adapted to the die either by the flowing of small melted increments from a spatula to build up the desired contour or by the compression method as in direct method.
- The metal die is warmed throughout to near body temperature, so that the wax solidifies more evenly throughout its mass, resulting in better adaptation.
- The die can be warmed by placing it under an electric lamp or on an electric heating pad that is at a suitable temperature.
- The wax pattern is carved with a warm instrument, to minimize the formation of stresses in the wax.

4. SPRUING

I. **Definition:** Sprue is defined as *"The mold channel through which molten metal or ceramic flows into the mold cavity"*.

II. *Purpose of Spuruing*

1. To form a mount for the wax pattern.
2. To create a channel for the elimination of wax during burn out.

3. To form a channel for the flowing - in of molten alloy during casting.

4. To compensate for alloy shrinkage during solidification procedure.

III. Sprue size and design

– Large inlays require sprues that are 14 - gauge (4 to 5 mm long) and small inlays require 16 - gauge (3 to 4 mm long) sprues.

– Large crowns require 10 - gauge sprues and small crowns require 12 - gauge sprues with an average sprue length of 4 to 5 mm.

IV. Types / Selection of Sprue materials

– Several types of materials are used for sprues, depending on the type of restoration being cast.

– For small inlays, a hollow - metal sprue may be used.

– Round wax is a commonly used sprue material for many restorations of all sizes.

– Plastic sprues have also been used for casting.

V. Sprue diameter

– The sprue former should have a diameter that is approximately the same size as the thickest area of the wax pattern.

– Attaching a large sprue former to a thin delicate pattern could cause distortion.

– If the sprue former diameter is too small then the molten metal in this area will solidify before the casting itself and localized shrinkage porosity develops.

– The Y - sprue design is often used on MOD inlay restorations.

VI. Sprue location

– The ideal area for the spure former is the point of greatest bulk in the pattern to avoid distorting thin areas of wax during attachment to the pattern and to permit complete flow of the alloy into the mold cavity.

VII. Sprue Direction

– The sprue should be directed toward the margins such that it minimizes the turbulence of the flow of the molten metal and favours the fine margins of the wax pattern.

– To get a satisfactory casting it is attached at a 45 degree angle to the proximal area.

VIII. Sprue Length

– The wax pattern should be positioned approximately 6mm from the end of the casting ring.

– If it is less than 6 mm of space, there is not enough thickness of investment to keep the molten alloy from breaking through.

– If it is more than 6 mm of space, the alloy will solidify before the escape of entrapped air, resulting in rounded margins, incomplete casting, mold fracture, etc.

IX. Sprue attachment

– Once the sprue is attached to the restoration the other end of the sprue is attached to a sprue base usually made of hard rubber.

– As with the attachment of the sprue to the restoration, the base - sprue attachment should avoid sharp corners to ensure smooth non turbulent flow of the metal into the pattern during casting.

– A reservoir should be added to a sprue network to prevent localized shrinkage porosity. When the molten alloy fills the heated casting ring the pattern area should solidify first and the reservoir last. Because of its large mass of alloy and position in the heat center of the ring, the resevoir remains molten to furnish liquid alloy into the mold as it solidifies

5. CASTING RING LINING

Purposes

1. Allows for mould expansion.

2. Reduces the heat loss (as it is a thermal insulator) when the ring is transferred from the furnace to the casting.

3. Permits the easy removal of the investment after casting.

Types of Ring liners

I. Asbestos Ring liners

Use has been discontinued due to its health hazards.

II. Non - Asbestos Ring liners

1. Alumino silicate ceramic liner
2. Cellulose (paper) liner

Placement

– The ceramic paper liner is cut to fit the inside of the metal ring and is held in place with the finger.

- The ring with the liner is then dipped into water until the liner is completely wet and water is dripping from it.

- After the liner has been soaked, it should not be touched because this reduces the cushioning effect, which is needed for the lateral expansion of the investment.

- The liner is 3 mm short of the top and bottom of the ring to lock in the investment during burn out and casting.

6. INVESTING

- Investing is the process by which the sprued wax pattern is embedded in a material called an investment.

- Gypsum and phoshate bonded investment materials are the two types of materials used for this purpose.

- A casting ring is added to contain the investment while the investment material is poured carefully around the pattern.

Procedure

- A wetting agent is applied on the wax pattern to reduce air bubbles.

- Place the casting ring into the crucible former so that the wax pattern is located near the centre of the ring.

- Mix the investment in a vaccum mixer and vibrate.

- Some investment is applied on the wax pattern with a brush to reduce the trapping of air bubbles.

- The ring is reseated on the crucible former and placed on the vibrator and gradually filled with the remaining investment mix. Allow it to set for 1 hour.

7. BURNOUT

- *Burnout is the process of heating an invested mold to eliminate the embedded wax or plastic pattern.*

Purpose

1. To eliminate the wax (pattern) from the mould.
2. To expand the mould (thermal expansion).

Procedure

- Separate the crucible former from the ring; if a metallic sprue former is used it should be removed before burnout.

- Burnout is started when the mould is wet.

- The heating should be gradual. Rapid heating produces steam which causes the walls of the mould

cavity to flake and also causes cracks in the investment due to uneven expansion.

- The ring is placed in a burnout furnace and heated gradually to 400°C in 20 min. Maintain it for 30min. In the next 30 min raise the temperature to 700°C and again maintain it for 30 min.

- The casting should be completed as soon as the ring is ready. If casting is delayed the ring cools and the investment contracts and the crown becomes smaller.

8. CASTING PROCESS

- It involves the process of melting the casting alloy and forcing the molten alloy into the mold by using casting machines.

I. Melting of the Alloy

- There are two methods of alloy melting, i.e.
  i. Torch melting
  ii. Electrical melting

i. Torch Melting

- Most common method of melting.

- Used for melting of gold alloys.

- The natural gas / air is used by using a torch.

ii. Electrical melting

- It includes electric resistane melting which uses a furnace with a carbon or ceramic crucible.

- Can be used for all types of alloys.

II. Casting Machines

1. Casting Crucible

- It is a refractory device which is that part of the casting machine, upon which the alloy is seated.

- There are four types of casting crucibles are available, i.e. clay, carbon, quartz and zirconia - alumina.

- Clay crucibles are used for crown and bridge alloys.

- Carbon crucibles are used for both crown and bridge alloys and also for higher fusing gold based metal ceramic alloys.

- Crucibles made from alumna, quartz or silica are recommended for high fusing alloys of any type.

2. Types of Casting Machines

i. Centrifugal force type

- Available as spring driven or motor driven.

- It rapidly spins the mold, crucible and molten alloy in a circle. Casting occurs when the spinning starts suddenly.
- The advantages are simplicity of design and operation with the opportunity to cast both large and small castings on the same machine.

ii. *Vacuum / Air pressure type*

- Either compressed air or gases like carbon dioxide or nitrogen can be used to force the molten metal into the mould.
- The crucible and casting ring are stationary and only the molten metal moves.
- Used to make small casting.

III. Casting Procedure

- When the alloy is molten, it has a mirror like appearance like a ball of mercury.
- The hot casting ring is then shifted from the burnout furnace to the casting machine.
- Place the ring in the casting cradle so that the sprue hole adjoins the crucible.
- Sprinkle flux powder over the molten metal to reduce the oxides and increase its fluidity for casting.
- Release the arm and allow it to rotate till it comes to rest. This create centrifugal force which forces the metal into the mold cavity.

9. CLEANING AND FINISHING OF THE CASTING

1. Quenching

- It is done for Gold alloys.
- After the casting has solidified, the ring is removed and quenched in water.

Advantages

1. The alloy is left in an annealed (softened) condition for burnishing, polishing and similar procedures.
2. The investment becomes soft and granular, and is easily removed.

2. Recovery of casting

- The investment is removed and the casting is recovered.

3. Pickling

- *It is a process of removal of surface films which consists of heating the discolored casting in an acid.*
- The acids used are 50% Hydrochloric acid and Sulphuric acid.

- The disadvantages of HCl are corrosion health hazard fumes.

4. Polishing

- Minimum polishing is required if all the procedures from the wax pattern to casting are followed meticulously.

CASTING DEFECTS

- The casting defects are classified into,
  1. Distortion
  2. Surface roughness and irregularities
  3. Porosity
  4. Incomplete or missing detail

1. Distortion

- Distortion of the casting is due to the distortion of the wax pattern.
- It is minimized by the proper manipulation of wax and handling of the pattern.

2. Surface Roughness

- It is usually be traced to,
1. Air bubbles on wax pattern which can be avoided by proper mixing of investment and application of wetting agent.
2. Too rapid heating cracks the investment resulting in fins which can be avoided by heating the ring gradually to 700°C.
3. Higher w/p ratio gives rougher casting which can be avoided by using correct w/p ratio.
4. Composition of investment: proportion of quartz and binder influences the surface texture of casting.

3. Porosity

- Porosity may internal or external.
- Porosities are classified as,

1. *Solidification defects*
  i. Localized shrinkage porosity
  ii. Microporosity

2. *Trapped gases*
  i. Pin hole porosity
  ii. Gas inclusions
  iii. Subsurface porosity

3. *Residual air*
  ### i. *Localized shrinkage porosity*
  - Caused by premature termination of the flow of molten metal during solidification.

- Generally occurs near the sprue casting junction.
- Can be avoided by using sprue of correct thickness, attaching sprue to thickest portion of wax pattern and placing a reservoir close to the wax pattern.

Suck - back porosity

- Often occurs at an occluso axial line angle or inciso axial line angle that is not well rounded.
- The entering metal impinges on to the mold surface at this point and creates a higher localized mold temperature in this region known as a hot spot.
- Suck back porosity can be eliminated by flaring the point of sprue attachment and reducing the mold - melt temperature differential, i.e. lowering the casting temperature by about 300°C.

ii. Microporosity

- It results in small irregular voids.
- It occurs from rapid solidification if the mold or casting temperature is too low.
- It can be reduced by increasing the melting temperature of the metal and mould temperature.

iii. Pin hole porosity

- Results from the entrapment of gas during solidification.
- Many metals dissolve or occlude gases while they are molten. On solidification, the absorbed gases are expelled and thus pinhole porosity results.
- It can be minimized by premelting the gold alloy on a graphite crucible or a graphite block if the alloy has been used before.

iv. Gas inclusion porosity

- It is also results from the entrapment of gas during solidification and are usually much larger than pin hole porosities.
- These porosities are caused by gas occluded from a poorly adjusted torch flame or by use of the mixing or oxidizing zones of the flame rather than the reducing zone.
- It can be avoided by correctly adjusting and positioning the torch flame during melting.

v. Sub surface porosity

- They may be caused by the simultaneous nucleation of solid grains and gas bubbles at the first moment that the alloy freezes at the mold walls.
- Can be diminished by controlling the rate at which the molten metal enters the mold.

vi. Entrapped-air porosity / Back pressure porosity

- It produces large concave depressions which are caused by the inability of the air in the mold to escape through the pores in the investment or by the pressure gradient that displaces the air pocket toward the end of the investment via the molten sprue and button.
- It is frequently found in a 'pocket' at the cavity surface of a crown on mesio occlusal distal casting.
- It can be eliminated by proper burnout, an adequate mold and casting temperature, a sufficiently high casting pressure and proper P/L ratio.

4. **Incomplete Casting**

- It is due to the molten alloy that has been prevented from completely filling the mold.
- The causes are,
  - Use of insufficient alloy
  - High viscosity of the alloy
  - Premature solidification of alloy
  - Insufficient venting of the mold
  - Low casting pressure

DENTAL CERAMICS

CERAMIC

- Defined as *an inorganic compound with nonmetallic properties typically composed of metallic (or semimetallic) and non metallic elements. (Ex: Al_2O_3, CaO and Si_3N_4).*

DENTAL CERAMIC

- Defined as *an inorganic compound with nonmetallic properties typically consisting of oxygen and one or more metallic or semimetallic elements (Ex. Aluminium, calcium, lithium, magnesium, potassium, silicon, sodium, tin, titanium and zirconium) that is formulated to produce the whole or part of a ceramic based dental prosthesis.*

CLASSIFICATION

I. *According to their use or indications*

1. Anterior
2. Posterior
3. Crowns
4. Veneers
5. Post and Cores
6. FPD's
7. Stain ceramic
8. Glaze ceramic

II. *According to composition*

1. Pure alumina
2. Pure zirconia
3. Silica glass
4. Leucite-based glass-ceramic
5. Lithi-based glass ceramic

III. *According to processing method*

1. Sintering
2. Partial sintering
3. Glass infiltration
4. CAD-CAM
5. Copy milling

IV. *According to firing temperature*

1. Ultra-low fusing: < 850°C
2. Low-fusing: 850-1100°C
3. Medium-fusing: 1101°C - 1300°C
4. High-fusing: > 1300°C

V. *According to microstructure*

1. Glass
2. Crystalline
3. Crystal-containing glass

VI. *According to translucency*

1. Opaque
2. Translucent
3. Transparent

APPLICATIONS

1. Ceramics for metal crowns and FPD's.
2. All-ceramic crowns, inlays, onlays and veneers.
3. Ceramic denture teeth.

COMPOSITION

– SiO_2, Al_2O_3, CaO, Na_2O, K_2O, B_2O_3, ZnO, ZrO_2 others like barium oxide, tin oxide, lithium oxide, etc.

PROCESSING

1. Sintering / Firing

– The process of heating closely packed particles to a specified temperature (below the melting point of the main component) to densify and strengthen a structure as a result of bonding, diffusion and flow phenomena.

– It can be done either by *temperature control alone* (the furnace temperature is raised at constant rate until a specified temperature is reached) or *by controlled temperature and a specified time* (the temperature is raised at a given rate until certain levels are reached, after which the temperature is maintained for a measured period until the desired reactions are completed).

2. Glazing

Natural glaze/Auto glazed/Self-glazed

A vitrified layer that forms on the surface of a dental ceramic containing glass phase when the ceramic is heated to a glazing temperature for a specified time.

Over glaze

The surface coating of glass formed by fusing a thin layer of glass powder that matures at a lower temperature than that associated with the ceramic substrate.

Over glazing should be avoided.

Disadvantages

1. Gives unnatural shiny appearance.
2. Causes loss of contour.
3. Causes shade modification.

Advantages of Glazing

1. Reduces crack propagation.
2. Increases strength.

CERAMIC MATERIALS

1. DICOR

– It is commercially available (castable ceramic).

– It was developed by Corning Glass Works.

– Dicor is a castable glass that is formed into an inlay, facial veneer, or full-crown restoration by a lost-wax casting process similar to that employed for metals.

– Dicor glass-ceramic contains about 55 vol % of Tetra silicic fluoromica crystals.

Advantages

1. Ease of fabrication
2. Improved esthetics

3. Minimal processing shrinkage
4. Good marginal fit
5. Moderately high flexural strength
6. Low thermal expansion
7. Minimal abrasiveness

Disadvantages

1. Limited use in low-stress areas.
2. Inability to color internally.
3. Decreased translucency.

Dicor MGC

- It is Dicor-Machinable glass ceramic.
- Dicor MGC is a higher quality product provided as CAD-CAM blanks or ingots.
- It contains 70 vol% tetra silicic fluormica platelets.
- Mechanical properties are similar to Dicor but has less translucency.

2. IN-CERAM

- It is supplied in three forms, i.e.
  1. In-ceram spinell,
  2. In ceram Alumina and
  3. In-ceram Zirconia

1. In-Ceram Spinell (ICS)

- It consists of glass-infiltrated magnesium spinel ($Mg\,Al_2\,O_4$).
- It is indicated for use as anterior single-unit inlays, onlays, crowns and veneers.
- Has greater translucency but lower strength and toughness than other types.

2. In-Ceram Alumina (ICA)

- It consists of 70 wt% alumina infiltrated with 30 wt% sodium lanthanum glass.
- It is indicated for anterior and posterior crowns and anterior three-unit FPD's.
- Its advantages are moderately high flexural strength and fracture toughness, metal free structure, ability to be used successfully with conventional luting agents.
- The disadvantages are poor marginal fit, high degree of opacity, inability to be elicited, technique sensitivity.

3. In-Ceram zirconia (ICZ)

- It contains approx. 30wt% zirconia, and 70wt% alumina.
- It is indicated for posterior crowns and FPD's.
- It is the strongest and toughest of the three types.
- Its disadvantages are same as ICA.

4. ALUMINOUS PORCELAIN

- Earlier, conventional ceramics are of low strength.
- To compensate the strength, aluminous porcelain is developed which is similar to that of conventional porcelain but with increased alumina content (40–50%).
- Alumina is used to build core over which conventional body and enamel porcelain are condensed and fired.

Advantages

1. Decreased crack formation.
2. Increased strength than that of conventional porcelains
3. Less expensive than metal ceramic.
4. Increased esthetics.

CHAPTER 04

DENTAL CARIES

DEFINITION OF DENTAL CARIES

– *Dental Caries is defined as a progressive irreversible, microbial disease affecting the hard parts of the tooth exposed to the oral environment, resulting in demineralization of the inorganic constituents and dissolution of the organic constituents, there by leading to a cavity formation.*

CLASSIFICATION OF DENTAL CARIES

I. *Based on the severity and progression of the lesion*

1. *Incipient or Initial or primary carious lesion*

   – Describes the first attack on the tooth surface and is initial or original carious lesion of the tooth.

   – Are white spot lesions.

   – Reversible lesions.

   – Enamel is intact but demineralised.

   – They can be remineralised.

   – Shape and progression of the lesion depends upon the location, i.e. pit and fissures, enamel smooth suface and root surfaces.

2. *Recurrent or secondary lesion*

   – Is the one which is observed under or around the margins or surrounding walls of an existing restoration.

   – Common sites of recurrent decay are inter proximal margins of a proximal restoration not involving all of the contact area incompletely involved pits and fissures and the areas near fractured sites.

   Causes

   1. Improper cavity preparation (unable to remove all of the decay).

   2. Inadequate cavity restoration (open margins).

   3. Old restorations (microleakage).

3. *Acute or Rampant Caries*

   – Are rapidly progressing caries that usually involves several teeth.

   – Lesions are multiple, light coloured.

   – Frequently accompanied by severe pulp reactions.

   – Demineralisation exceeds remineralisation.

4. *Chronic Caries*

   – Are of variable depth, long standing and are fewer in number.

– More localized.

– Lesions are hard in consistency and dark in colour.

– Remineralisation exceeds demineralisation.

5. *Arrested caries*

– Arrested caries is the stage where the progress of the decay has stopped and is inactive.

– The softened dentin has been lost or worn away so that the discoloured (either yellow, brown or black), sound, hard dentin remains. The remaining dentin has a polished look.

– Arrested carious lesions are found most commonly on lingual and labial aspects of teeth and less common in interproximal areas.

Formation of Arrested caries

– There are a number of stages are involved in the formation of arrested caries, i.e.

1. First stage: The acids produced by advancing bacteria dissolve the mineral in the surrounding intertubular dentin. The tubule fluid becomes saturated with calcium, magnesium and phosphate ions. The lesion progresses unless the level of metabolic activity of the bacteria is reduced. If less acid is produced then the second stage can occur.

2. Second stage: If bacterial acid production is reduced and the pH increases, the salts precipitate into large crystals of tricalcium phosphate which temporarily block the tubule.

3. Third stage: If further bacterial activity is suppressed, the odontoblast secretes collagen and calcium salts. Small plate like crystals of hydroxyapatite then form and block the tubule more effectively.

6. *Active caries*

– It is the progressive carious lesion of the tooth where the demineralisation exceeds the remineralisation.

7. *Residual caries*

– It is the type of caries which is not removed during the tooth preparation either by accident, intention or neglect.

– When these caries are near the pulp, it may be covered with a pulp capping material to promote reparative dentin deposition.

– This carious dentin can be excavated at later stage.

II. Based on the pathway of caries

1. *Forward Caries (Pit Decay)*

– In this, decay starts in enamel and then it involves the dentin.

– Extent of caries is greater in enamel than in dentin.

2. *Backward Caries (Smooth surface lesion)*

– In this, decay attack the enamel from its dentinal side.

– Extent of caries is greater at DEJ than in enamel.

III. Based on the number of surfaces involved

1. *Simple*

– That involves only one surface of a tooth.

2. *Compound*

– That involves two surfaces of a tooth.

3. *Complex*

– That involves three or more surfaces of a tooth.

IV. Based on the location on the tooth surface

1. *Pit and fissure caries*

– The caries originating in the pits and fissures found on the lingual surfaces of maxillary anterior teeth, and on the buccal, lingual and occlusal surfaces of posterior teeth.

– Early lesion difficult to detect clinically.

– Appears as two cones with bases approximating each other.

– Little lateral spread occurs until DEJ is reached.

– *Occurence:* may be due to defective formation or incomplete coalescence of enamel by developmental enamel lobes or complete coalescence enamel where shallow grooves and fossa become carious due to neglect.

2. *Smooth surface caries*

– The caries originating in all surfaces without pits, fissures or grooves.

Locations

1. *Proximal surfaces cervical to the contact area.*

2. *Facial or Lingual surfaces cervical to the height of contour.*

– Caries occurs due to lack of adequate plaque removal.

– Shape is two triangles / cones.

– Base of enamel triangle is at the enamel surface.

– Apex of enamel cone contacts the base of dentin cone caries due to lateral spread at DEJ.

3. **Senile (root) caries**

   – Located exclusively on the cementum and dentin of the root surfaces of the teeth.

   – Progresses more rapidly than enamel caries.

   – Sometimes associated with partial denture clasps.

   – Associated with aging process.

V. G.V. Blacks Classification

– It is a therapeutic classification.

– It is based on the treatment and restoration design.

Class - I: Pit and fissure cavities that occur in the occlusal surfaces of bicuspids and molars; the occlusal two thirds of the buccal and lingual surfaces of the molars and the lingual surfaces of incisors. Cavities beginning in structural defects that occasionally occur on the occlusal or incisal two-thirds of all teeth.

Class - II: Cavities in the single proximal surfaces of bicuspids and molars.

Class - III: Cavities in the proximal surfaces of incisors and cuspids not involving the incisal angle.

Class - IV: Cavities in the proximal surfaces of incisors and cuspids involving the incisal angle.

Class - V: Cavities in the gingival third, not pit and fissure cavities, of the labial, buccal and lingual surfaces of all teeth.

Class - VI: Cavities on both mesial and distal proximal surfaces of bicuspids and molars that when restored will share a common occlusal isthmus or cavities on the incisal edges of anterior or cusp tips of posterior teeth.

THEORIES OF DENTAL CARIES

Endogenous Theories

1. Humoral theory
2. Vital theory

Exogenous theories

1. Chemical (acid) theory
2. Parasitic (septic) theory
3. Miller's Chemicoparasitic (Acidogenic) theory (most accepted theory)
4. Proteolysis theory
5. Proteolysis Chelation theory
6. Sucrose Chelation theory

Other Theories

1. The legend of worm
2. Autoimmune theory
3. Sulfatase theory

CARIES ACTIVITY TESTS

– They are the tests performed to detect the caries in an oral cavity.

– Caries acitivity is *the occurrence and rate at which teeth are destroyed by the acid produced by the plaque bacteria caries susceptibility*.

Different Tests

1. Lactobacillus colony count test
2. Snyder test
3. Streptococcus mutans level in saliva
4. Buffer capacity test
5. Fordick calcium dissolution test
6. Dewar test
7. Salivary reductase test
8. Cariostat test
9. Caries risk test
10. Alban's test

CRITERIA FOR THE DIAGNOSIS OF DENTAL CARIES

1. The area is carious when the explorer 'catches' or resist removal after the insertion into a pit or fissure with moderate to firm pressure and when this is accompanied by one or more of the following signs of caries:

   i. A softness at the base of the area.

   ii. Opacity adjacent to the pit or fissure as evidence of undermining or demineralisation.

   iii. Softened enamel adjacent to the pit or fissure which may be scraped away with the explorer.

2. The area is carious of there is loss of the normal translucency of the enamel, adjacent to a pit, which is in contrast to the surrounding tooth structure. This condition is considered to be reliable evidence of undermining. In some of these cases, the explorer may not catch or penetrate the pit.

3. The area is carious if surface is etched or if there is a white spot as evidence of subsurface demineralisation and if the area is found to be soft by,

   i. Penetration with explorer.

   ii. Scraping away enamel with explorer.

4. The area is sound when there is apparent evidence of demineralisation (etching or white spots) but no evidence of softness.

DIAGNOSIS OF DENTAL CARIES

1. Visual examination

– The tooth must be clean, dry and well illuminated when carrying out a visual examination.

– Discoloration gives the suspicion of decay.

– Observing a grey hue in a marginal ridge can be a suspicion of a proximal cavity under that ridge.

2. Enhanced visual examination

1. *Transillumination*

– It uses an intense beam of visible light, usually directed on the lateral surface of the tooth to transilluminate it.

– This technique is most useful in the diagnosis of anterior approximal caries and cracked teeth.

2. *Fibre - optic transillumination*

– It uses a fibre - optic light source which is placed palatal / lingual to anterior teeth and are viewed from the facial surface to diagnose the anterior approximal caries.

3. *Magnification*

– It is used most commonly in the form of magnification loupes in adjacent to clinical examination and radiographic evaluation.

3. Tactile examination

1. *Explorer*

– Any discontinuity of the enamel in which an explorer will enter is carious if it also shows other evidence of decay such as softness, shadow by transillumination or loss of translucency.

2. *Dental floss or tape*

– When a floss is inserted though a contact area and then dragged occlusally in a sawing motion against the proximal surface, if the floss fray or shread, one can suspect a cavity on this proximal surface, provided that there is no calculus or overhanging of restoration.

4. Patient complaint

– When the patient consumes hot or cold items that change osmotic pressure in the dentin, cause subjective compliants, which can be suspicion of dentinal involvement of caries.

5. Radiographic examination

– Radiographs are used to confirm a clinical suspicion of caries, to detect early lesions and for monitoring the disease activity.

– Bitewing radiographs are used for the diagnosis of occlusal and proximal caries in posterior teeth.

– Periapical radiographs are used for the anterior teeth.

6. Tooth separation method

– It is a type of visual examination.

– To see the proximal decay directly, one can use the tooth separation method.

7. Dyes

– A variety of different dyes that stain caries are currently available, which make the visualisation of caries earlier.

8. Laser fluorescence

– Lasers are used for the detection of caries especially for the early enamel lesions.

– Caries illuminated by a laser will fluoresce, the degree to which this occurs is an indicator of the disease process.

9. Electrical conduction method

– It is based on electrical conductance and the fact that sound enamel is a good electrical insulator; however, carious teeth allows the passage of an electrical current more readily, which results in a drop in the electrical resistance.

– The degree to which the resistance drops is an indicator of the extent of caries.

IDENTIFICATION OF OCCLUSAL CARIES

1. Chalkiness of enamel on the walls and the base of the pit or fissure.
2. Softened base at the pit or fissure.
3. Brownish grey discoloration under the enamel adjacent to the pit or fissure.
4. Presence of radiolucency below the occlusal enamel.

IDENTIFICATION OF PROXIMAL CARIES

1. Broken surface, which can be detectable visual or tactile methods.
2. Discoloured marginal ridge.
3. Opaque area in dentin on transillumination of the tooth.
4. Presence of radiolucency, i.e. bitewing radiographs.

ZONES OF DENTINAL CARIOUS LESION

– Any dentinal carious lesion in a vital tooth will exhibit five zones or layers, when decalcified tooth sections are examined under an optical microscope.

– The zones do not show definite demarcations; some may overlap and some may be missing.

– They differ in their dimensions, nature, contents and activities in the two types of carious processes.

- The five zones are,
  1. Decayed zone
  2. Septic zone
  3. Demineralized zone
  4. Transparent zone
  5. Opaque zone

1. Decayed Zone

- Completely devoid of minerals.
- Completely decomposed organic matrix.
- Collagen fibres if found have lost their cross striations and links.
- High concentration of micro organisms.
- The only activity in this zone is microbial.
- More pronounced in acute type.
- The colour ranges from a light yellow to a dark reddish brown, depending upon the presence and duration of chromogenic bacterial activity.
- Consistency is softer in the acute type.

2. Septic Zone

- Highest concentration of micro-organisms is found.
- Dentinal tubules are extremely widened and cavitated.
- Colour resembles that of the first zone.
- More pronounced in chronic type.
- Consistency is softer in acute type.
- Collagen fibre have fewer cross striations and links are lost.

3. Demineralized Zone

- Clinically most significant (both diagnostically and therapeutically).
- Only dentin is demineralized with the intact dentinal matrix.
- Collagen fibres show cross striations and links.
- Dentinal tubules show normal dimensions.
- Show remineralization activity.
- More pronounced in acute type.
- Microorganisms are confined to superficially in acute type but found throughout the chronic type.
- Colour of the acute type is straw yellow and for the chronic type is yellow, brown or dark brown.
- Consistency and hardness of the dentin is less in acute type.

4. Transparent Zone

- Appears transparent in ground sections and radiopaque in a radiograph.
- It is the area of undisturbed mineralization repair.
- It is the zone of dentinal sclerosis and the calcific barrier.
- More pronounced in chronic type.
- Slightly discoloured when compared to surrounding normal dentin.
- The dentin in this zone is extremely hard when compared to normal dentin.
- Harder in chronic type.

5. Opaque Zone

- Found pulpally to transparent zone.
- Characterised by intratubular fatty degeneration with lipid deposits being precipitated from fatty degeneration of the peripheral odontoblastic processes.
- More pronounced in acute type.
- Appear radiolucent on a radiograph.

INFECTED DENTIN

- It is highly demineralised
- It is unremineralisable
- It is superficial layer
- It lacks sensation
- It can be stained by,
  - 0.5% basic fuschisin
  - 10% acid red solution
  - 0.2% propylene glycol
- Intertubular dentin is greatly demineralised with irregularly scattered crystals.
- The collagen fibres are broken down and only indistinct cross bands and no inter bands are observed.
- This infected dentin should be excavated.

AFFECTED DENTIN

- Intermedially demineralised
- It is remineralisable
- It is deeper layer
- It is sensitive
- It does not stain with any solution
- Intertubular dentin is partly demineralised with distinct cross bands and inter bands.
- It should be left to remineralise.

DIRECT PULP EXPOSURE

Causes

1. Iatrogenic
2. Trauma

Type of exposure	Indication	Rx
A pin – point exposure with sound dentin at the periphery of the exposure with hemorrhage.	No inflammation or mild inflammation restricted to the exposure site.	Can be successfully repaired.
Pin point exposure with sound dentin at the periphery with a drop of blood that coagulates immediately on the cavity floor in the form of a button.	Mild pulpul inflammation restricted to exposure site	Can be successfully repaired.
Exposure with infected carious dentin at the periphery.	Inflammation beyond the exposure site	Doubtful repair.
Exposure with profuse hemorrhage.	Inflammation involving pulpal and root canals	Usually beyond repair.
Exposure with pus or inflammatory fluids.	Extensive inflammation and destruction of the pulpal and root canal.	Definitely beyond repair.

DIRECT PULP CAPPING

Definition

– *Involves the placement of a bio-compatible agent on healthy pulp tissue that has been inadvertently exposed from caries excavation or traumatic injury.*

Objective

– To seal the pulp against bacterial leakage, to encourage the formation of reparative dentin and to maintain the vitality of the underlying pulp tissue.

Indications

– Following traumatic injuries.
– Mechanical exposure less than $1mm^2$ in a asymptomatic vital young permanent tooth.

Contraindications

1. Spontaneous and nocturnal toothache.
2. Excessive tooth mobility.
3. Thickened periodontal ligament.
4. Radiographic evidence of furcal or periradicular degeneration.
5. Uncontrollable bleeding at the time of hemorrhage.
6. Purulent exudate from the site of exposure.

Materials Used

1. Calcium hydroxide
2. Unmodified Zinc oxide Eugenol

Procedure

– All undesirable and / or undermined enamel and unsound dentin should be removed.
– The cavity floor and exposure site should be gently washed and irrigated with sterile water.
– Dry with cotton pellets.
– Either calcium hydroxide or unmodified zinc oxide eugenol can be used as a capping material.
– When ZOE is used, sound dentin shavings are cut from surrounding walls and deposited at the exposure site and then covered with a creamy mix of unmodified ZOE.
– When using calcium hydroxide, a creamy mix is prepared and placed directly on the exposure site.
– The permanent restoration should be placed.
– The patient should be informed of the signs and symptoms of pulpal degeneration.
– Patient is recalled after 6-8 weeks if calcium hydroxide is placed or 8-9 weeks if the unmodified ZOE is placed.
– Radiograph is taken to evaluate the status of the tooth.

INDIRECT PULP CAPPING

Definition

– *The application of a medicament over a thin layer of remaining carious dentin, after deep excavation with no exposure of the pulp.*

Indications

1. *History*
   i. Mild discomfort from chemical and thermal stimuli.
   ii. Absence of spontaneous pain.

2. *Clinical examination*

i. Large carious lesion
ii. Absence of lymphoadenopathy
iii. Normal appearance of adjacent gingiva
iv. Normal colour of tooth

3. *Radiographic examination*

i. Deep carious lesion in close proximity to the pulp.
ii. Normal lamina dura.
iii. Normal periodontal ligament space.
iv. No inter radicular or periapical radiolucency.

Contra Indications

1. *History*

i. Sharp, penetrating pain that persists after withdrawal of symptoms.
ii. Prolonged spontaneous and nocturnal toothache.

2. *Clinical examination*

i. Excessive tooth mobility
ii. Tooth discoloration
iii. Non responsiveness to pulp tests

3. *Radiographic examination*

i. Large carious lesion with apparent pulp exposure.
ii. Interrupted or broken lamina dura.
iii. Widened periodontal ligament space.
iv. Periapical radiolucency.

Materials used

1. Calcium hydroxide
2. Zinc oxide Eugenol

Procedure

– 3 techniques are commonly used.

Technique 1 : A thin layer of calcium hydroxide paste is placed over the site of near exposure. A thick layer of zinc oxide eugenol is then applied. Patient is recalled after 6-9 weeks; the tooth is reopened and the remaining carious material removed. A sound layer of dentin should be present. Calcium hydroxide is placed as dressing and the tooth is restored by routine procedures.

Technique 2 : A thin layer of zinc oxide eugenol paste is placed over the area of near exposure. A thick layer of zinc oxide eugenol is then applied. The tooth is reopened after 6-8 weeks and the remaining carious material is removed. A sound layer of dentin should be present. Calcium hydroxide is placed as dressing and the tooth is restored by routine procedures.

Technique 3 : Routine cavity preparation is completed. Remove the gross caries. A dressing of calcium hydroxide paste with or without zinc oxide eugenol is placed over the residual caries. An amalgam restoration is placed over the dressing. Complete removal of caries is delayed for 6-8 weeks. Do not re-enter the tooth if it appears clinically and radiographically healthy.

PREVENTION OF CARIES

1. Proper general health
2. Fluoride exposure
3. Immunization
4. Proper salivary functioning
5. Antimicrobial agents
6. Balanced diet
7. Proper oral hygiene
8. Xylitol gums
9. Pit and fissure sealants
10. Restorations

PIT AND FISSURE SEALANTS

– Dental caries are highly prevalent in cases of deep pit and fissures.
– Buonocore introduced the filling of filler resin with bonded resin.
– Bodecker introduced fissure eradication technique in order to transform the retentive fissures into cleansable areas.

Classification

I. *Based on Polymerization Methods*

1. Self activation
2. Light activation

   i. First generation sealant. UV light (365 nm) Ex : Nuvaseal.
   ii. Second generation sealant. Self cure (chemical cure) Ex : Delton.
   iii. Third generation sealant. Visible light cure (430-460 nm) Ex: Fissurit.
   iv. Fourth generation sealant contain fluoride releasing agents incorporated in resins.

II. *Based on Resin Systems*

1. BISGMA
2. Urethaneacrylate

III. *Filled and unfilled resins*

IV. *Clear and tinted resins*

Recommended age groups for sealant application

– 3-4 years for primary molars.
– 6-7 years for first permanent molars.
– 11-13 years for second permanent molars.

Indications

- Newly erupted both primary molars and permanent bicuspids and molars with open or sticky grooves.
- Tooth should have erupted less than 4 years ago.

Procedure

1. Isolation of tooth.
2. Polishing is not recommended as the polish slurry would interfere with normal acid etching procedure.
3. Tooth is dried.
4. 30-50% ortho phosphoric acid is applied over recommended area using an applicator tip.
5. After a period of 60 sec tooth is washed and dried. Following studies, it has been established that waiting period of 15 sec is enough following acid etching during which time retentive property of etched surface is enhanced.
6. Then etched surface is washed and dried.
7. A characteristic chalky white and or froasty appearance is observed.
8. The sealant is applied over the etched area following which it is cured.

Test for retention

- An explorer is run along margin of treated tooth and any catch would indicate the presence of an air void in which case procedure should be repeated.

ENAMELOPLASTY

- Also called as *Dimpling*.
- It was proposed by Dr. Miles Markley.
- It is the removal of a shallow enamel developmental fissure or pit to create a smooth, saucer shaped surface that is self-cleansing or easily cleaned.
- Maximum removal of 1/3 of enamel thickness is allowed.
- Restoration cavosurface angle should not be less than 80 degrees.

PROPHYLACTIC ODONTOTOMY

- Proposed by Hyatt in 1923.
- It is characterized by minimally preparing and filling with amalgam on developmental, structural imperfections of the enamel, such as pits and fissures, to prevent caries originating in these sites.
- It is an outdated concept and hence no longer advocated as a preventive measure.

Technique

- When the tooth is erupted into oral cavity the occlusal surface was restored with amalgam or oxy phosphate cement. Later when the tooth achieves occlusion the tooth is restored with amalgam after a shallow cavity preparation.

CHAPTER 05

OPERATIVE DENTISTRY ARMAMENTARIUM

CLASSIFICATION OF OPERATIVE DENTAL INSTRUMENTS

- Operative dental instruments are classified into the following types based on their functions,

1. Cutting Instruments
   i. *Hand*
       Hatchets
       Chisels
       Hoes
       Excavators
       Others
   ii. *Rotary*
       Burs
       Stones
       Discs
       Others

2. Condensing Instruments
   Pluggers
       Hand
       Mechanical

3. Plastic Instruments
       Spatulas
       Carvers
       Burnishers
       Packing instruments

4. Finishing and Polishing Instruments
   i. *Hand*
       Orange wood sticks
       Polishing points
       Finishing strips
   ii. *Rotary*
       Finishing burs
       Mounted brushes
       Mounted stones
       Rubber cups
       Impregnated disks and wheels

5. Isolation Instruments
       Rubberdam
       Saliva ejector
       Cotton roll holder
       Evacuation tips and equipment

6. **Miscellaneous Instruments**

Mouthmirrors

Explorers

Probes

Scissors

Pliers

Others

HAND CUTTING INSTRUMENTS

PARTS OF AN INSTRUMENT

1. **Handle/Shaft**

   – It may be small, medium or large diameter; smooth, knarled or serrated.

2. **Shank**

   – Connects the shaft and the blade.

   – It may be straight or single, double or triple angled.

   – It is here where any angulation in the instrument can be placed.

3. **Blade / Nib**

   – *It is that part of the instrument that bears the cutting edge, condenser face or the like.*

   – *It is the functional end of the instrument.*

   – It begins at the angle that terminates the shank (last angle if there is more than one).

   – The blade ends in the cutting edge.

4. **Cutting edge**

   – It is the working part of the instrument.

   – It is usually in the form of a bevel with different shapes.

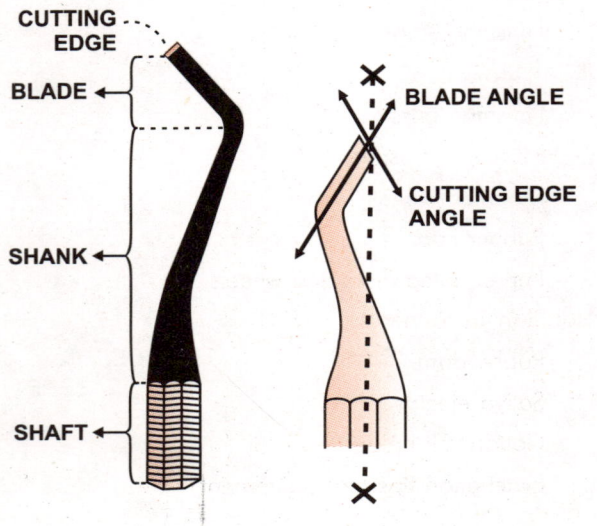

5. **Blade angle**

   – It is the angle between the long axis of the blade and the long axis of the shaft.

6. **Cutting edge angle**

   – It is an angle between the margin of the cutting edge and the long axis of the shaft.

NOMENCLATURE OF INSTRUMENT

– According to G.V. Black,

1. *Order* denotes the purpose of the instrument. Ex : Excavator.

2. *Suborder* denotes the position or manner of use of the instrument. Ex: Push or pull.

3. *Class* denotes the form of the working end. Ex : Hatchet or chisel.

4. *Subclass* denotes the angle or shape of the shank. Ex : Staight - no angle, Monangle - one angle.

INSTRUMENT FORMULA

– According to G.V. Black,

1. *The first unit* of the formula describes *the width of the blade in tenths of a millimeter.*

2. *The second unit* describes *the length of the blade in millimeters.*

3. *The third unit* describes *the angle the blade forms with the axis of the handle.* This angle is expressed in "hundredths"of a circle or in centigrades.

   Ex : *Binangle hatchet : (15-8-12)*

   – 15 = blade width 1.5 millimetres.

   – 8 = blade length 8 millimetres.

   – 12 = blade angled 12 centigrade from axis of handle or shaft.

4. A *fourth unit* is added to the basic instrument formula and is expressed in centigrades which represents the *angle formed between cutting edge and central axis of the shaft.* It is placed in the second position of the formula.

   Ex : *Gingival margin trimmer (distal):*

   12 - 92 - 10 - 8

   – 92 = the cutting edge of the blade is at an angle of 92 centigrade with the axis of the shaft.

INSTRUMENT DESIGN

– Hand instruments can be made of stainless steel, carbon steel or blades of tungsten carbide soldered to a steel handle.

— Carbide burs are the most efficient in cutting although they are brittle.

— The main principle of cutting with hand instruments is to concentrate forces on a very thin cross section of the instrument at the cutting edge. So the thinner the cross-section the more the pressure that is concentrated and the more efficient the instrument will be.

1. Direct cutting and Lateral cutting Instruments

— *Direct cutting instrument is the one in which the force is applied in the same plane as to the blade and handle. It is called as a 'Single - planed' instrument. It can be used in direct and lateral cutting.*

— *Lateral cutting instrument is the one in which the force is applied at a right angle to the plane of the blade and handle. Usually it has a curved blade and is called as 'Double Bladed' Instrument. It has angle or curve in a plane at a right angle to that of the handle. It can only be used in lateral cutting.*

2. Contrangling

— In order to gain access to use many instruments, bend the shank at one or more points to angle of the blade relative to the handle.

— The extent of this depends on the length of the blade and the degree of angulation in the shank.

— Accordingly the working point is moved out of line with the axis of the handle. If this occurs to more than 3 mm from the handle axis (its imaginary continuation), the instrument will be out of balance in lateral cutting motions, and force will be required to keep the instrument from rotating in the hand.

— To overcome this modern operative instruments are designed to possess one or more angles in the shank, placing the working point with in 3 mm from the axis of the handle. *This principle of design is called 'Contrangling'.*

— A short blade and small blade angle requires only binangle contrangling, while longer blades and greater blade angles require triple angle contrangling.

3. Right and Left Instruments

— Direct cutting instruments can be made into right or left by placing a bevel on one side of the blade. *Identification of right and left of the instrument: If the instrument is held with the cutting edge down and pointing away from the operator and the bevel is on the right side, it will be a right instrument. If the bevel is on the left it will be a left instrument. For cutting, the non beveled side of the blade should be in contact with the wall being cut.*

— Lateral cutting instruments can be made into right or left by placing the curve or angle either on the right or on the left side. *Identification of right and left of the instrument: Holding the instrument with its blade down and cutting pointing away, the instrument having that curve of the blade directed to the right is a right instrument and vice versa for the left.*

4. Single bevelled instruments

— These are single planed instruments with the cutting edge is at a right angle to the long axis of the shaft. *Identification of mesial and distal of the Instrument:* If they are beveled on the side away from the shaft, they are called *'distally beveled'*. If they are beveled on the side of the blade towards the shaft, they are called *'mesially beveled'*.

— If these instruments have no angle in the shank, or an angle of 12° or less, they can be used in push (direct cutting) and scraping motions (bevelled to non bevelled side).

— If the angle in the shank exceeds 12° the instrument could be used in pull (distally bevelled) and push (mesially bevelled) motions.

5. Bibevelled instruments

— Only hatchets and straight chisels are bibevelled.

— The blade is equally bevelled on the both sides.

— They cut by pushing them in the direction of the long axis of the blade.

6. Triple bevelled instruments

— They are made by bevelling the blade laterally, along with the end, which results in three distinct cutting edges.

— Most modern single planed instruments (especially the small ones) are of triple bevelled which can increase cutting efficiency.

7. Circumferentially bevelled instruments

— A circumferential bevel is produced by bevelling the blade at all its peripheries.

— It is usually found in double placed instruments.

8. Single - ended and Double - ended instruments

— Single ended instruments are confined to those types of instruments having only one specific function.

— Most modern instruments are double ended which incorporates the right and left or the mesial and distal form of the instrument in the same handle.

CLASSIFICATION

– Hand cutting instruments are classified into,

    I.   Excavators

    II.   Chisels

    III. Special forms of Chisels

I. EXCAVATORS

– Designed for the excavation of the carious dentin and for the shaping of the internal portions of the cavities.

– They are of five types

1. Hatchet Excavators

– Have the edge of the blade in parallel with the handle.

– Usually single - planed, bibevelled instruments.

– They cut by pushing and pull motion in the direction of the blade.

– *Use:* For cleaving the enamel in incisors.

– *Instrument Formula:* 6 - 2 - 12; 6 - 2 - 23.

2. Hoe Excavators

– Bevel is at a right angle to the shaft.

– They are available in distally bevelled and mesially bevelled types.

– Are single planed instruments with the possibility of four types of movements i.e., vertical, pull (push), right and left.

– *Use:* for cutting mesial and distal walls of premolars and molars.

– *Instrument Formula:* 6 - 2 - 10; 12 - 6 - 10.

3. Spoon Excavators

– Available in pairs, i.e. left and right.

– Cutting edge is a semi circular circumferential bevel and is sharpened to a thin edge.

– It is a double planed instrument with the possibility of right or left cutting movements only.

– *Use:* for the excavation of caries.

– *Instrument Formula:*   8 - 6 - 12 (L)

                          8 - 6 - 12 (R)

                        13 - 8 - 12 (L)

                        13 - 8 - 12 (R)

4. Discoid (Disc like) Excavators

– Have a circular blade, with a cutting edge extending around the periphery except where it joins to the shank.

– It is a double planed instrument with the possibility of right or left cutting movements only.

– *Use:* For the excavation of caries.

            for carving metallic restorations.

– *Instrument Formula:* 20 - 2 - 12.

5. Cleoid (Claw like) Excavators

– It resembles a 'claw', so the name **'Cleoid'**.

– *Use:* In amalgam carving, burnishing and finishing of cohesive and cast gold restoration and in excavation of caries from the areas of difficult access.

– It is a double planed instrument with the possibility of lateral cutting movements only.

– *Instrument Formula:* 10 - 2 - 12.

II. CHISELS

– Are used for the cutting of enamel.

– Are usually bevelled on one side only.

– They are of four types.

1. Straight Chisels

– Have a straight blade in line with the handle and shank.

– Bevel of the blade is at right angle to the shaft.

– Are single planed instruments with the possibility of five types of cutting movements, i.e. vertical, right, left, push and pull.

2. Monangle Chisels

– As a single angle between the shaft and the blade.

– Are similar to straight chisels but the blade is at an angle to the shaft.

– It may be mesially or distally bevelled.

3. Binangle Chisels

– As the name implies, there are two angles between the shaft and the blade.

– Blade is at a right angle to the shaft as in the Hoe.

– It may be mesially or distally bevelled.

– *Use:* The above mentioned three types of chisels are used for the cutting of undermined enamel.

4. Triple angle Chisel

– Has three angles in its shank.

– It may be mesially or distally bevelled.

– *Use:* Usually used to flatten pulpal floors.

– Monangle, Binangle and Triple angle chisels are single planed instruments with the

- possibility of three cutting movements, i.e. vertical, right and left.
- Mesially bevelled chisels cut in push movements and distally bevelled ones cut in pull movements.

III. SPECIAL FORMS OF CHISELS
- Are designed to perform specific functions.

1. *Enamel Hatchets*
- The shank has one or more angles or curves.
- The blade is in the same plane as with angle or angles.
- The cutting edge is parallel to the shaft.
- They may be paired, i.e. right or left or may be bibevelled.
- *Uses:* for cleaving undermined enamel in proximal cavities and on buccal and lingual walls where it is not possible to use a chisel.
- The smaller sizes are primarily used in anterior teeth, although are useful in bicuspids and molars.
- Larger sizes are mainly used in posterior teeth.
- Are single planed instruments with the possibility of four types of movements, i.e. vertical, push, pull and either right or left lateral cutting.
- *Instrument Formula:* 15 - 8 - 12 (L)
  15 - 8 - 12 (R)
  20 - 9 - 12 (L)
  20 - 9 - 12 (R)

2. *Gingival Margin Trimmers*
- Are similar to spoon excavators in both of their angles and the dimensions of their blades.
- Available in two pairs constituting a set of four.
- In a given size each pair has a right and a left bevelled instrument.
- If the cutting edge of one pair makes an acute angle with that edge of the blade away from the handle, those are *Distal GMTs*.
- If the cutting edge of the other pair makes an acute angle with that edge of the blade nearer to the handle, those are *Mesial GMTs*.
- *Uses*
  i. For trimming the margins of the various walls of the cavity preparation.
  ii. For bevelling gingival floor.

iii. For forming sharp angles in the cavity preparation.
- They are primarily lateral cutting instruments.
- *Instrument Formula*
  i. *Amalgam:* 12 - 95 - 10 - 12 (L) ⎤ D
    12 - 95 - 10 - 12 (R) ⎦
    12 - 80 - 10 - 12 (L) ⎤ M
    12 - 80 - 10 - 12 (R) ⎦
  ii. *Inlay:* 12 - 100 - 10 - 12 (L) ⎤ D
    12 - 100 - 10 - 12 (R) ⎦
    12 - 75 - 10 - 12 (L) ⎤ M
    12 - 75 - 10 - 12 (R) ⎦

L - Left; R - Right; D - Distal; M - Mesial

3. *Angle Formers*
- Bevel is at angle of 80° with the shaft (forming an acute angle with the long axis of the blade) with a pointed and linear cutting edge.
- It is considered as a combination of GMT and Chisel.
- Are single planed instruments with right or left bevelling.
- They has three cutting movements, i.e. vertical, push and pull.
- *Uses*
  - to cut line and point angles in the preparation for gold restoration.
  - to place bevel on enamel margins.
- *Instrument Formula:* 8 - 80 - 3 - 9 (L)
  8 - 80 - 3 - 9 (R)
  10 - 80 - 4 - 6 (L)
  10 - 80 - 4 - 6 (R)

4. *Wedelstaedt Chisels (Curved Chisel)*
- Resembles a straight chisel, but with a slight vertical curvature in its shank.
- Bevelled on one side of the blade only.
- If the bevel is on the side toward the curvature of the shank, it is *mesially bevelled*; If it is on the side of the blade away from the curvature, it is *distally bevelled*.
- They are single planed instruments, with three cutting motions, i.e. vertical, right and left.
- The mesially bevelled one can be used in push movements and the distally bevelled one can used in pull movements.
- *Use:* for cleaving undermined enamel and for shaping walls.
- *Instrument Formula :* 15 - 15 - 3.

5. *Off-Set Hatchets*
   – It resembles the regular hatchet, except that the whole blade is rotated a quarter of a turn forward or backward around its long axis.
   – These are single planned instruments with the same cutting efficiency as regular hatchets.
   – They available as right or left instruments.
   – However, there are two for both the right and left—One with the whole blade rotated forward and the other with the whole blade rotated backward.
   – *Use:* for creating and shaping specific angulations for cavity walls, especially in areas of difficult access.
   – *Instrument formula* : 15 - 8 - 14 - 7.

6. *Triangular Chisel*
   – Has a triangular blade with the base of the triangle away from the shaft.
   – It has a terminal cutting edge like the straight chisel.

7. *Hoe Chisel*
   – Resembles the hoe-excavator, but with the sturdier blade.

ADVANTAGES OF HAND CUTTING INSTRUMENTS

1. *They are self-limited in cutting enamel*, i.e. they will not cut sound enamel, but will cut only undermined enamel.
2. Can remove large pieces of undermined enamel quickly thus saves time and effort.
3. No vibration or heat is produced during cutting.
4. Are the most efficient way for precise intricate cutting.
5. Can create the smoothest surface of all cutting instruments.
6. Have the longest life span provided if they are resharpened.

INSTRUMENT GRASPS, RESTS AND GUARDS

I. PEN GRASP

– Instrument will be held like a pen between the thumb and first two fingers and the second finger should apply the pressure on to the instrument but not the index finger.
– This method provides very accurate control.
– Used for lower arch instrumentation.

– The action of the instruments with the pen grasp is down and away from the operator.
– Pengrasp involves the action in the wrist of the hand.

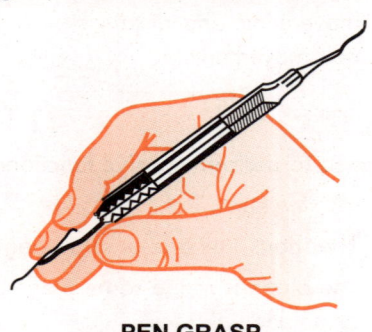

PEN GRASP

1. *Inverted pen grasp*
   – Similar to pen grasp but the hand is rotated to that the palm faces upwards.
   – Used for upper arch instrumentation.
   – Action of the instrument is up and toward the operator.

2. *Modified pen grasp*
   – Here, the fingers and the thumb engage the instrument like a grappling hook. The base of the index finger and the tip of the middle finger reciprocates each other and the thumb is placed in the middle of these two.
   – It involves the action in the fore arm of the hand.

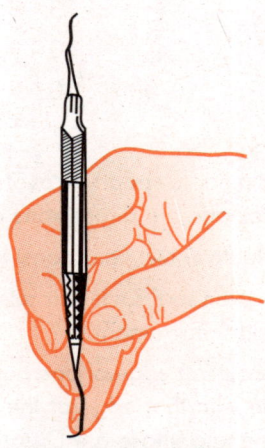

MODIFIED PEN GRASP

II. PALM AND THUMB GRASP

– The instrument is held in such a way to that is used to hold a knife to whittle a piece of wood.
– The handle of the instrument is held in the palm of the hand and is grasped by the four fingers with the thumb resting on an adjoining surface.

- Useful on maxillary teeth especially on the right side when working from the right rear chair position.

- Useful for the rotary instrumentation on anterior platalal surface.

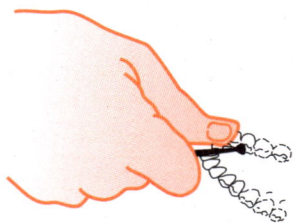

PALM AND THUMB GRASP

3. MODIFIED PALM AND THUMB GRASP

- The handle of the instrument is in contact with the tips of the four fingers on one side, opposed to which are contacts with the mesial end of the first phalanx of the thumb. The hand is only about half closed, instead of fully closed as in usual palm thumb grasp. The end of the thumb is used as rest.

- This method permits greater freedom and ease of movements and also gives a delicacy of control compared to pen grasp while preventing instrument slipping during a thrusting stroke.

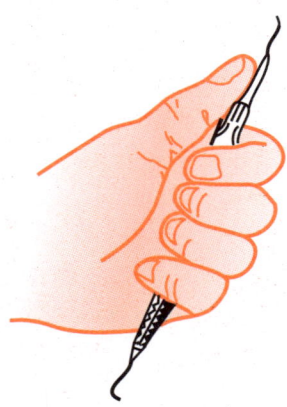

MODIFIED PALM AND THUMB GRASP

RESTS

- Rests are used to stabilize the hand, confine the instrument to the working area and prevent injury.

- Rests are made with the fingers that do not engage the instrument.

- Rests should be placed on tooth or bony support and never on soft tissues.

GUARDS

- These are hand instruments other items such as interproximal wedges that are used to protect soft tissues from contact with the sharp instruments.

ROTARY INSTRUMENTATION

- Rotary instruments are most widely used instruments for gross removal of tooth structure.

CHARACTERISTICS

1. Speed

- Refers to the surface feet per unit time of contact that the tool has with the work to be cut or revolutions per minute.

- Speeds in dentistry are classified into,

i. According to Marzouk,

1. Ultra low speed : 300–3000 RPM
2. Low speed : 3000–6000 RPM
3. Medium High Speed : 20,000–45,000 RPM
4. High Speed : 45,000–1,00,000 RPM
5. Ultra High Speed : > 1,00,000 RPM

ii. According to Charbenau,

1. Conventional or low speed: below 10,000 RPM
2. Increased or high speed: 10,000–1,50,000 RPM
3. Ultraspeed: above 1,50,000 RPM

iii. According to Sturdevant,

1. Low or slow speeds (below 12,000 RPM).
2. Medium / Intermediate speeds (12,000 to 2,00,000 RPM).
3. High / Ultrahigh speeds
   (above 2,00,000 RPM).

2. Pressure (P)

- Pressure is defined as the force per unit area.

$$P = \frac{F\,(Force)}{A\,(Area)}$$

- Using the same force F, smaller tools (burs or stones) will apply more pressure to the point of contact than larger tools.

- Clinical osbservation shows, low speed requires 2-5 pounds of force, high speed requires 1 pound of force and ultra high speed requires 1-4 ounces of force for efficient cutting.

3. Heat Production

   – Heat is directly proposed to the Pressure, RPM (Revolutions per minute) and area of tooth in contact with the tool, hence if any of the above factors is increased, heat production also increases.

   – Heat production of 113° F temperature can cause pulpitis and pulp necrosis. Temperature of 130°F results in the permanent damage of pulps.

   – To reduce the heat production coolants (such as flowing water, water-air spray or air) must be used during rotary instrumentation.

4. Vibration

   – It is the product of the equipment (hand pieces and cutting tools) used and the speed of the rotation.

   – Excess vibration causes annoyance to the patient, operator fatigue and excessive wear of instruments.

5. Patient Reaction

   – The use of coolants, intermittent application of a tool to the tooth, sharp instruments, etc. aid in minimal patient discomfort.

6. Operator fatigue

   – High speed rotary instrumentation minimises fatigue by decreasing vibrations and the time of operation.

7. Source of Power

   – Air turbine is the main power source in dental practice.

ROTARY INSTRUMENT DESIGN

– It is evaluated under two headings,

I. Hand Piece

II. Tools for the removal of tooth structure (bur, stone, etc.).

I. HAND PIECE

   – It is a device to hold rotating instruments, transmitting power to them and for intraoral positioning.

   – They are available as *straight, contra angled* and *right angled*.

   – They will retain the cutting tool by a screw in latch or friction grip type of attachment.

Evaluation Criteria

– The following criteria are used in the evaluation of hand pieces.

1. *Friction*

   – It occur in the moving parts of the hand piece especially the turbine.

   – Hand piece is unsuitable to use if the frictional heat is not prevented or counteracted.

   – Friction is reduced by equipping the hand piece with ball bearings, needle bearings, glass and resin bearings, etc.

2. *Torque*

   – Refers to the ability of the hand piece to withstand lateral pressure on the revolving tool without decreasing its speed or reducing its cutting efficiency.

   – It is depend upon the bearing type used and the amount of energy supplied to the hand piece.

3. *Vibration*

   – Excessive wear of the turbine bearings will cause centric running which creates substantial vibration.

   – So it is advised to follow the manufacturer's recommendations for the use and maintenance of handpieces to minimise turbine wear.

II. TOOLS FOR THE REMOVAL OF TOOTH STRUCTURE

– These are the units responsible for the removal of tooth structure.

They are of two types, i.e.

A. *Burs:* cutting tools.

B. *Stones:* abrading tools.

A. DENTAL CUTTING BURS

   – The Dental bur is a small milling (cutting) instrument.

Characteristics

1. *Composition and Manufacture*

– Dental burs are of two types according to their composition, i.e. *Steel burs* and *Tungsten carbide burs*.

– Steel burs are made from a blank steel stock by a rotary cutter that cuts parallel to the long axis of the bur. The bur is then hardened and tempered until its Vicker's hardness number is 800 (appox) is reached.

– Tungsten carbide burs are made from powder metallurgy technique which is a process of alloying in which only the partial fusion of the constituents will occur. The tungsten carbide powder is mixed with powdered cobalt under pressure and heated in a vacuum, so that a partial sintering of the metals takes place. A blank is then formed and the bur is cut from it with a diamond tool.

- Sometimes, only the cutting head is tungsten carbide which is welded or soldered to a steel shank.
- Vicker's hardness of number of Tungsten carbide type of bur is in the range of 1650 to 1700.
- Steel burs are used for regular speed instruments which are effective only for cutting dentin. Tungsten carbide burs are used for ultra speeds.

2. *Classification*

    i. According to Composition,

      1. Steel burs

      2. Tungsten Carbide burs

    ii. According to mode of attachment to hand piece,

      1. Latch type

      2. Friction grip type

    iii. According to the handpiece they are designed for,

      1. Contrangle bur

      2. Straight handpiece bur

    iv. According to the direction of rotation,

      1. Clockwise (right) - most common.

      2. Anticlockwise (left)

    v. According to length of the head,

      1. Long

      2. Short

      3. Regular

    vi. According to shape and size,

      1. Round burs

      2. Wheel burs

      3. Inverted cone burs

      4. Cylindrical fissure burs

      5. Tapered fissure burs

      6. Pear shaped burs

      7. End cutting burs

    vii. According to purpose,

      1. Cutting burs

      2. Finishing and Polishing burs

3. *Parts of a Bur*

- Every bur will have three parts,

    i. Head: The portion which carries the cutting blades.

    ii. Shank: The portion connecting the head to the attachment part of hand piece.

    iii. Shaft / Attachment Part: The portion which is engaged with in the hand piece, which connects the shank to the head of the bur.

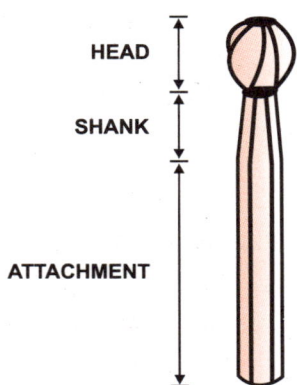

4. *General Design of Dental Bur*

  i. Bur tooth

- This terminates in the cutting edge or blade.
- It has two surfaces *(i) Tooth face*, which is the side of the tooth on the leading edge *(ii) Back or flank of the tooth*, which is the side of the tooth on the trailing edge.
- The number of teeth in dental cutting burs is usually 6-8.

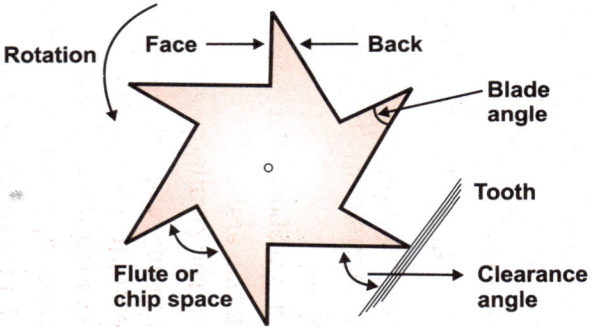

  ii. Rake angle

- Refers to *the angle that the face of the bur tooth makes with the radial line (refers to direction of rotation) from the center of the bur to the blade.*
- It is divided into three types, i.e.

  1. *Negative rake angle:* forms when the face is beyond or leading the radial line, in other words forms when the face is infront of the radial line.

  2. *Positive rake angle:* forms when the radial line leads the face, so that the rake angle is on the inside of the radial line, in other words forms when the face is behind the radial line.

3. *Radial / zero rake angle:* forms when the radial line and the tooth face coincide with each other.

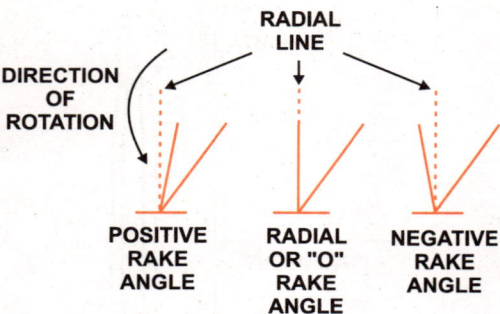

iii. *Land*
   – Refers to the plane surface immediately following the cutting edge.

iv. *Flute / Chip space*
   – Refers to the space between successive bur teeth or the blades of the bur.
   – It provides an exit for removal of the fractured matter and creates a clearance angle.

v. *Clearance angle*
   – Refers to the angle between the back of the bur tooth and the work, in other words angle between the back of the blade and the tooth surface.
   – If a land is present on the bur, it can be divided into three types, i.e.
   1. *Primary clearance angle* is the angle the land will make with work.
   2. *Secondary clearance angle* is the angle between the back of the bur tooth and work.
   3. *Radial clearance angle* is forms when the back surface of the bur tooth is curved.

5. *Common Burs*
   i. *Round burs*
   – They are numbered from ¼, ½, 1, 2 to 10.
   – They are round in shape.
   – Used for initial tooth penetration, for the placement of retentive grooves, smaller caries excavation, marginating restorations.

   ii. *Inverted cone burs*
   – They are numbered from 33 ¼, 33 ½, 34, 35 to 39.
   – They are inverted cone in shape.
   – Used for cavity extension, occasionally for establishing wall angulations and retention forms.

iii. *Cylindrical fissure / straight fissure burs*
   – Used for gross cutting, cavity extension and creation of walls.

iv. *Tapered fissure burs*
   – Are the most universally used burs in operative dentistry.
   – Used to establish and refine the tapered walls for cast gold restorations, to produce marginal bevels, to produce retention and flaring for the amalgam.

v. *Pear shaped burs*
   – They are numbered from 229 to 333.
   – They are shaped like pears.
   – Mainly used in pedodontics.

vi. *End Cutting burs*
   – They are numbered from 900 to 904.
   – They are cylindrical in shape, with just the end carrying blades.
   – Very efficient in extending preparations apically without axial reduction.

viii. *Elliptical burs*
   – Are characterised by round corners and sides with a reverse taper.

6. *Factors influencing the cutting of the Burs*
   i. *Rake angle*
   – Order of cutting efficiency: Positive rake angle > Radial rake angle > Negative rake angle.
   – Burs with a radial rake angle cut more efficiently than the burs with the negative rake angle.
   – With the burs of a negative rake angle, the cut chip moves directly away from the blade edge and often fractures into small bits or dust.
   – With the burs of a positive rake angle, the chips are larger and tend to clog the chip space.

   ii. *Clearance angle*
   – It provides clearance between the work and the cutting edge to prevent the tooth back from rubbing on the work.
   – Large clearance angle may result in less rapid dulling of the bur.

   iii. *Run-out*
   – Refers to the eccentricity or maximum displacement of the bur head from its axis of rotation while the bur takes.
   – The average value of clinically acceptable run-out is about 0.023 mm.

iv. Number of teeth or blades and their distribution

- As the number of blades decreases, the magnitude of forces at each blade increases and the thickness of the chip removed by each flute correspondingly increases.

- Fewer number of bur teeth has increased space between bur teeth and thus decreases the clogging tendency.

- Fissure bur with straight flutes produces less temperature rise than one with spiral flutes.

- The fewer the number of bur teeth, the greater the tendency for vibration.

v. Heat Treatment

- It is used to harden a bur that is made of soft steel.

- It preserves the edge placed on the bur flute by the cutter, and hardens the bur to increase its cutting life.

- This procedure is not needed for tungsten carbide burs.

vi. Design of flute ends

- Dental burs are formed with two different styles of end flutes.

- The *Revelation* cut, in which the flutes come together at two junctions near a diametrical cutting edge. It shows some superior cutting efficiency in direct cutting.

- The *Star cut*, in which the end flutes come together in a common junction at the axis of the bur.

- Both types have equal cutting efficiency in lateral cutting.

vii. Influence of the Load

- Load is the force exerted by the dentist on the tool head and not the pressure or stress induced in the tooth during cutting.

- The minimum and maximum loads for low speed are 1000 - 1500 gm and for high speed are 60 - 120 gm.

B. DENTAL ABRASIVE STONES

- Abrasive cutting points reduce and smooth the tooth surfaces by grinding.

- Abrasives must be used with a coolant to reduce the elevated temperatures.

Characteristics

1. Design

- Abrasive particles are held together by means of a binder (base) of variable nature.

- Most commonly a ceramic binder is used, particularly for binding diamond chips.

- Rubber or shellac binder may be used for soft grade stones.

2. Factors influencing the abrasive efficiency of Dental Stones

i. Shape of abrasive particles

- An abrasive should be in irregular shape to prevent a sharp edge.

- Therefore, the more irregular the particles, the greater the abrasive efficiency of the stone.

ii. Hardness of the abrasive material

- The harder the abrasive material relative to the hardness of the work, the more the abrasive efficiency of the stone.

iii. Size of the abrasive particles

- The larger the particles, the deeper the scratches on the surface of the work and the faster the work will be worn away.

3. Types of Dental Stones

- Dental stones are of two types,

  i. *Mounted*
  - the abrading head is permanently welded to the shank and attachment part.
  - are available in short, regular or long lengths; latch or friction grip form.

  ii. *Unmounted*
  - the abrading head is supplied separately and may be mounted on an appropriate mandrel.

- Dental stones are available in plenty of shapes, i.e. cylinder, wheel, cone, inverted cone, tapered, dough nut, round, filamentous, V-shaped, hour glass, etc.

4. Classification

- *Based on the composition of the abrasive particles,*

i. Diamond Stones

- They are the hardest and most efficient abrasive stones for removing tooth enamel.

- Available in either coarse or fine grits and for either high or low speed handpieces.

- They should not be used to cut metals or unfilled acrylic resin.

— Their use is limited to the reduction of tooth substance, backed porcelain and composite resin.

ii. Carbides
— They are of silicon carbides or boron carbides.

— The carbides are sintered with a binder into grinding wheels, discs or stones.

iii. Sand
— Sand and other forms of quartz (cuttle) can be bounded and mounted into different shapes of discs, stones and strips.

iv. Aluminum Oxide
— One of the most efficient abrasives for stones in fine cutting.

v. Garnet
— These particles contain a number of different minerals which possess similar physical properties and crystalline forms.

— Used for finishing and polishing of dental appliances.

vi. Rubber Abrasives
— Are made for polishing of metal.

vii. Crocus discs
— These are paper discs charged with iron oxide.

— They smoothen the margins of castings after the use of sand paper abrasives.

Fundamental rules for the use of Diamond Instruments
1. Require high speed for efficient cutting.
2. Are best used with light pressure.
3. Cut most rapidly when used with water.
4. Cut harder substance more efficiently than soft.
5. For better control, they are used in a dragging movement, but without pressure rather than in a pushing movement.
6. Care must be taken to keep them out of contact with surfaces outside the field of operation.

Fundamental Rules for the use of Tungsten - Carbide Burs
1. Require high speed for efficient cutting.
2. Should be used with the light pressure.
3. Do not run bur in reverse direction.
4. Bur must always be rotating before being brought into contact with the surface to be cut.
5. For better control, bur should be used in dragging motion rather than pushing.

6. Greater care must be taken to guard against contact with surfaces outside the field of operation.

USES AND LIMITATIONS OF ROTARY INSTRUMENTS
1. Rotary instruments are the most efficient tools for the gross removal of tooth structure.
2. Dental stones (especially diamonds) have the highest efficiency in removing enamel (brittle material) whereas carbide burs have the highest efficiency in removing dentin (elastic material).
3. Use of dental stones is confined to the removal of superficial 0.5 - 1 mm of dentin. Burs are efficient for the removal of dentin of 2 mm or more.

LOW SPEEDS
Uses
1. For cleaning teeth.
2. Occasional caries excavation.
3. Finishing and Polishing procedures.

Advantages
1. Better tactile sensation.
2. Less chance for overheating of cut surfaces.

Disadvantages
1. Ineffective
2. Time consuming
3. Requires heavy force application
4. Patient discomfort
5. Burs tend to roll out of the tooth preparation

HIGH SPEEDS
Uses
1. For tooth preparation
2. Removal of old restorations

Advantages
1. Faster removal of tooth structure with less pressure, vibration and heat generation.
2. No. of rotary cutting instruments needed is reduced.
3. Better control and ease of application.
4. Instruments last longer.
5. Patient comfort.
6. Several teeth can be treated in a single appointment.

Disadvantages
1. Improper care during preparation results in the slippage of the instrument and tend to injure adjacent hard and soft tissues.

2. Scarring of adjacent un involved tooth.

3. Excessive removal of un-involved tooth structure.

ULTRASONIC INSTRUMENTS

– The ultrasonic dental unit consists of an ultrasonic generator separated from a magnetostrictive transducer located with in the hand piece, and a water cooling system incorporated into the equipment for controlling heat generation.

– Ultrasonic instruments are generally not used for cavity preparations, they are mostly used for calculus and stain removal from teeth and restoration surfaces.

RESTORING INSTRUMENTS

PARTS

– Each restoring instrument is composed of three parts like hand cutting instruments, i.e. Handle, Shaft and Nib.

TYPES

– These are divided into,

1. Mixing Instruments

   – Spatulas are employed for the purpose of mixing.

   – Spatulas have flat and wide nibs with blunt edges and straight shank.

   – They are made of stainless steel, ivorine or plastic.

2. Plastic Instruments

   – These are used for carrying and handling materials after mixing while the materials are still in their plastic stage.

   – They possess a flat sided nib with blunt edges and corners.

   – They are also available in teflon coated ones which minimizes the material adhesion and facilitates easy cleaning.

3. Condensing Instruments

   – They differ from each other in the surface configuration of the nib face, depending upon the material they are used with, i.e. amalgam requires smooth surfaced faces, gold foil requires serrated surfaced faces.

   – The nibs are available in different shapes, i.e. rounded, triangular, rectangular, diamond, parallelogram, etc.

4. Burnishing Instruments

   – The nibs of the burnishers can be ball shaped egg shaped, apple shaped, beaver tail shaped, conical hour glass shaped, fish tail shaped, bullet shaped, etc.

   – The nibs are of smooth faced.

   – *Sprately burnishers* are special type of burnishers which are used for burnishing of proximal gingival margins of metallic restorations.

   – Burnishers are also available in the form of burs which possess perfectly smooth heads.

5. Carvers

   – Carvers are basically cutting instruments with their blades either bevelled or knife edged.

   – The most commonly used carver is Hollen beck carver which possess double sided, knife edged, pointed edged nibs with curved monangle or binangle shanks. They are very efficient for carving of amalgam and wax.

   – The discoid and cleoid excavators can be used as Amalgam and Gold carvers.

   – There are also special forms of carvers are available with triangular nibs and diamond shaped nibs.

6. Files

   – Are used less commonly.

   – Used for margination of restorations if knives and carvers will not suffice.

   – The nibs are in the form of foot shaped, hatched shaped or parallelogram shaped.

   – The serration on the face of nib makes a file to be pulled or pushed.

7. Knives

   – Nibs possess knife edged faces on one of their side only.

   – The most commonly used knife is Bard - Parker knife and has several shapes.

   – Black's knives have the nibs at right angle to the handle, with the cutting edge facing away from the handle in one set and towards the hand in another set.

   – Wilson's knife has the nib right angle to the shaft, which can be introduced interproximally for proximal and gingival manipulation of restorative materials.

   – Stein's knife has a trapezoidal nib which is mainly used for direct gold contouring and margination.

FINISHING AND POLISHING INSTRUMENTS

– Most of the instruments are of rotary type, i.e. burs, stones, paper carried abrasives, brushes, rubber (wheel cups or cones) cloth or felt, etc.

1. Finishing Burs

– It should be atleast 12 fluted and they are available up to 40 fluted.

– They are made up of Stainless steel (for amalgam) or Tungsten carbide (for composite resins).

– They do not grossly cut the restorative material but removes excess and thus creates smoother surface.

– Burs are available in different shapes, i.e. rounded, apple shaped, cylindrical, inverted cone, etc. and in different sizes.

2. Paper Carried abrasives

– These are usually sand, cuttle, garnet or boron carbide glued to paper discs or strips.

– They are attached to a mandrel and used by hand in a back and forth motion similar to a shoe polishing action.

3. Brushes

– Are available in different forms, i.e. wheels, cylinders, cones, etc.

– They can be attached by a screw in the hand piece, to a mandrel or by their own frictional attachment extension.

– Available in different sizes and used with abrasives or polishing pastes.

4. Cloth

– It is carried on a metal wheel used in the final stages of polishing with or without a polishing medium.

5. Felt

– Used to obtain lustre for metallic restorations with a polishing paste.

– Has different shapes, i.e. wheels, cones and cylinders.

MAINTENANCE OF CUTTING INSTRUMENTS

– Restorative procedures cannot be done adequately without proper maintenance of equipment.

– Sharp cutting instruments are particularly important and present a continual maintenance problem for the dentist. Regardless of what type of cutting procedure is to take place, it is very important to have sharp instruments.

ADVANTAGES OF SHARP INSTRUMENTS

1. Less chances of traumentizing the patient's soft tissues.
2. Decreased operator fatigue.
3. Increased operator efficiency.
4. Accurate control of instrument.

SHARPENING EQUIPMENT

It is of three types,
1. Stationary sharpening stones
2. Mechanical sharpeners
3. Handpiece sharpening stones

1. STATIONARY SHARPENING STONES

– Also called as 'oilstones' because of practice of applying a coating of oil on them as an aid in the sharpening process.

– Most frequently used sharpening equipment consist of a block or stick of abrasive material called 'stones'.

– Sharpening stones are available as Grits, Shapes and Materials.

i. Grits

– These are available in coarse, medium and fine.

– Fine grit stone is suitable for final sharpening of dental instruments.

– Coarse and Medium grits are used for initial reshaping of badly damaged instrument or for sharpening other dental equipment such as bench knives.

ii. Shapes: Stationery stones of various shapes include,
  – Flat
  – Grooved
  – Cylindric
  – Tapered

– Flat stones are preferred for sharpening all instruments with straight cutting edges.

– Cylindric stones are used for sharpening instruments with concave edges.

– Tapered stones permit using a portion of the stone with a curvature matching that of the instrument.

iii. Materials: Sharpening stones are made from,
  – Natural Material, Synthetic material.

- Four types of materials commonly used for sharpening stones are,
  - A. Arkansas Stone
  - B. Silicon Carbide
  - C. Aluminium Oxide
  - D. Diamond

A. Arkansas Stone

- It is a naturally occurring material, i.e. mineral containing microcrystalline quartz.
- These are available in hard and soft varieties.
- The hard stone cut slower and is preferred because the soft stone scratches and grooves easily.
- Stones are lubricated with light machine oil because, this assists in fineness of sharpening, prevents clogging of the stone pores and avoids the creation of heat.
- When stone appears dirty, it is wiped with a clean woolen cloth soaked in oil.
- When the stone is extremely dirty, it may be wiped with a cloth soaked in alcohol.

B. Silicon Carbide (SiC)

- It is widely used as an industrial abrasive.
- It is commonly used material for grinding wheels and sandpapers, as well as for sharpening stones.
- SiC stones are available in many shapes in coarse and medium grits.
- SiC stones are normally of a dark colour, often black or greenish black.
- These stones are moderately porous and require lubrication with light oil.

C. Aluminium Oxide

- It is increasingly used to manufacture sharpening stones.
- Coarse and medium grit stones appear as speckled tan or brownish in colour.
- Fine grit stones are white.
- Water or light oil is used as lubricant.

D. Diamond

- It is hardest available abrasive and most effective for cutting and shaping hard materials.
- It is the only material capable of sharpening carbide as well as steel instruments.
- Diamond hones are small metal blocks with fine diamond particles impregnated on the surface.
- These hones include grooved, rounded and straight surfaces and are adaptable for sharpening instruments with curved blades.

- These hones are nonporous.
- Use of lubricant will extend the size of hones.
- They may be cleaned with a mild detergent and a medium bristle brush.

2. MECHANICAL SHARPENERS

- Rx Honing Machine is an example of a mechanical sharpener.
- This instrument moves a hone in a reciprocating motion at a slow speed, while the instrument is held at the appropriate angulation and supported by a rest.
- Interchangeable aluminium oxide hone of different shapes and coarseness are available to accommodate the various instrument sizes, shapes and degree of dullness.
- This type of sharpener is versatile and can fill almost all instrument sharpening needs.

3. HANDPIECE SHARPENING STONES

- Mounted SiC and aluminium oxide stones for use with both straight and angle handpieces particularly the cylindric instruments with straight sided silhouettes, are more useful for sharpening hand instruments.

PRINCIPLES OF SHARPENING

1. Sharpen the instruments only after they have been cleaned and sterilized.
2. Establish the proper bevel angle (45 degrees) and desired angle of the cutting edge to the blade before placing the instrument against the stone, and maintain these angles throughout sharpening.
3. Use a light stroke or pressure against the stone to minimize frictional heat.
4. Use a rest or guide whenever possible.
5. Remove as little metal from the blade as possible.
6. Lightly hone the unbeveled side of the blade after sharpening to remove the fine bur that may be created.
7. After sharpening sterilize the instrument.
8. Keep the sharpening stones clean and free of metal cuttings.

TECHNIQUES FOR SHARPENING INSTRUMENTS

1. MECHANICAL TECHNIQUES

- It is a quick method of sharpening hand instruments and can be easily mastered with little practice.

- Chisels, hatchets, hoes, angle formers or GMT are sharpened on a reciprocating honing sharpener.
- The blade is placed against the steady rest.
- Proper angle of the cutting edge of the blade is established before starting the motor.
- Light pressure of the instruments against the reciprocating hone is maintained with a firm grasp on the instrument.
- A trace of metal debris on the face of a flat hone along the length of the cutting edge is an indication that the entire cutting edge is contacting the hone.
- For instruments with curved blades, especially the inside curve of blades, handpiece stones are used.
- Here the instrument is held lightly against the stone with a modified pen grasp.

2. STATIONARY STONE TECHNIQUES

- The stationary sharpening stone should be at least 2 inches wide and 5 inches long.
- It should be medium grit for hand cutting instruments.
- Before the stone is used, a thin film of light oil should be placed on working surfaces.
- *Fundamental rules to be followed while using the stationary stone.*

1. Place the stone on a flat surface and do not tilt the stone while sharpening.
2. Grasp the instrument firmly, usually with a modified pen grasp, so that it will not rotate or change angles while being sharpened.
3. To ensure stability during the sharpening strokes, use the ring and little fingers as a rest, and guide along a flat surface or along the stone. This prevents rolling or dipping of the instrument which results in a distorted and uneven bevel.
4. Use a light stroke to prevent the creation of heat and the scratching of the stone.
5. Use different areas of the stone's surface while sharpening as this helps in preventing the formation of the grooves on the stone that impair efficiency and accuracy of the sharpening procedure.

SHARPENING OF INDIVIDUAL INSTRUMENTS

1. Chisels, Hatchets or Hoes

- Grasp the instrument with modified pen grasp.
- Place the blade perpendicular to the stone.
- Tilt the instrument to establish the correct bevel.
- Slide the instrument back and forth along the stone.

- The motivating force should be from the shoulder. So that the relationship of the hand to the plane of the stone is not changed during the stroke.

2. Angle Formers

- It is same as that used for chisels, hatchets except that allowance must be made for the angle of the cutting edge to the blade.

3. Gingival Margin Trimmers

- Require more orientation of the cutting edge to the stone before sharpening.
- Palm and thumb grasp is used when sharpening a trimmer with 95 or 100 centigrade cutting edge angle.
- When single bevel instruments are sharpened, a thin rough edge of distorted metal, called burr or burr edge is collected on the unbeveled side of blade.
- This side of the blade is placed flat on the stone and one short forward stroke is made.

4. Amalgam or Gold Knife

- It has a very thin blade tapering to the sharpened edge.
- In sharpening this instrument, only the edge bevels should be honed.
- To sharpen, the blade is placed on the stone with the junction of the blade and shank immediately over the edge of stone.
- The blade is then titled to form a small acute angle with the surface of stone and the stroke is straight along the stone and towards the edge of the blade.
- This method produces the finest edge and eliminates any burrs on the cutting edge.

5. Spoon Excavators and Discoids

- Spoon is placed on the far end of the stone and held so that the handle is pointing towards the operator.
- As the instrument is pulled along the stone toward the operator, the handle is rotated gradually away from the operator, until it is pointing away from the operator at the end of the stroke.
- The instrument is placed on flat surface or held in hand for this procedure.
- To hone the flat inside surface of the blade, a small cylindric stone is passed back and forth over the surface.
- Other means of sharpening spoon excavators are by grooved stone, mounted discs or stones for use with a straight handpiece.

TEST FOR SHARPNESS

The following methods of testing instruments of sharpness are available,

1. ### The Light Test

    – This test requires you to look directly at the sharpened edge.

    – A shiny edge indicates that the instrument is blunt while a sharp edge will appear as a black line.

    – A sharp edge will not reflect light caused by the fine line that appears as sharpness is achieved.

2. ### The Thumbnail Test

    – Hold the sharpened edge of the instrument at 45° angle to the nail.

    – Using light pressure, push or pull the instrument (as dictated by the function of the instrument).

    – If the instrument slips or glides along the nail, it is still blunt.

    – If the instrument grabs or shaves the nail, a sharp edge has been acquired.

3. ### Another method of testing sharpness is by lightly resting the cutting edge on a hard plastic surface.

    – Light pressure is exerted in testing for sharpness.

    – If it slides the instrument is dull.

    – If the cutting edge digs in during an attempt to slide the instrument forward over the surface the instrument is sharp.

CHAPTER 06

THE OPERATING FIELD

BASIC INSTRUMENT TRAY SETUP

− The order of arranging the instruments in the bracket tray is as follows,

1. **Diagnostic instruments:** Mouth mirror, Probe, Explorer, Tweezer.
2. **Excavating Instruments:** Spoon excavator, Discoid, Cleoid.
3. **Hand Cutting Instruments:** Enamel Hatchet, GMT.
4. **Filling Instruments:** Cement Spatula, Agate Spatula, Plastic filling instrument.
5. **Condensing Instruments:** Round Condenser, Parallelogram condenser.
6. **Burnishing Instruments:** Ball burnishers.
7. **Carving Instruments:** Hollenback, Ward's and Diamond Carvers.
8. **Amalgam Carrier.**
9. **Miscellaneous Instruments:** Scissors, B.P. Blade, Matrix bands and retainers, Cotton holder, Dappendish, etc.

POSITIONING OF THE DENTAL TEAM AND THE PATIENT

A. **OBJECTIVES**

1. Access to the operative field
2. Visibility
3. Comfort
4. Patient Safety

B. **ZONES OF OPERATIVE FIELD**

− Operative field is divided into 4 zones, they are,

1. *Operator's Zone*
   − This is the zone where the operator seats and it has several common positions.
2. *Transfer Zone*
   − Located near the oral cavity where instruments and materials are transferred between the operator and the assistant.
3. *Assistant Zone*
   − It is the zone where the assistant is seated and it allows the assistant to access both the transfer zone and the static zone.
4. *Static Zone*
   − Contains auxiliary equipments and supplies for the operating team.

C. POSITIONING OF THE OPERATOR

- Operator is seated well back on the stool with feet flat on the floor, legs relaxed and relatively together and thighs parallel to the floor.
- The back is straight and supported by the back rest.
- The head and neck are slightly bent toward the patient, so that eyes are directed downward.
- An optimal eye to work distance is regarded as 16 - 18 inches.

D. OPERATOR'S CHAIR POSITION

- Operator seats in the operator's zone and the following are the several positions which are practiced at working field.

For a right handed operator

1. 12 O' Clock : Direct Rear Position

- Operator is located directly behind the patient and looks down over the patient's head.
- Position is primarily used for operating on the lingual surfaces of mandibular anterior teeth.
- *Disadvantage:* Severe bending of the operators back and neck.

2. 11 O' Clock : Right Rear Position

- It is considered to be universal operating position as it provides access to all areas directly or indirectly using a mouth mirror except the more distal areas of the mandibular right quadrant, the cervical areas on the patient's right posterior quadrants.

3. 9 O' Clock : Right Position

- The operator is directly to right of patient.
- It provides access for operating on the facial surfaces of the Maxillary and Mandibular right posterior teeth. Occlusal surfaces of Mandibular right posterior teeth.

4. 7 O' Clock : Right Front Position

- Position provides access to Mandibular anterior teeth, Mandibular posterior teeth and maxillary anterior teeth.

E. POSITIONING OF THE DENTAL ASSISTANT

- The Assistant should be seated at a higher position (such that the assistant's head is 4 to 6 inches higher than the operator's) on his/ her stool, so his/her knees will be in level with the patient's head, with his/her feet resting on the foot rest of his/her chair.
- The assistant should be seated with his/her back straight and with an unobstructed straight line view of the field of operation.

F. POSITIONING OF THE PATIENT

- The Patient is positioned in a semi-supine or supine position so that the operative field is over the operator's lap at the height of the operator's elbow. The patient may aid the operator by slight head rotation toward or away from the operator.
- This supine position enables the operator's forearms to be parallel to the floor when working in the operative field.
- If the patient's legs are positioned higher than the head, postural hypertension may occur, therefore prolonged placement in this position is not recommended.
- When gaining access to the most posterior regions of the mandibular right quadrant for right handed operators (mandibular left for left handed operators) it may be required to lower the chair base and raise the chair back until the operator's forearms are parallel to the floor.

ISOLATION OF THE OPERATING FIELD

- Removal of moisture, excellent vision, access to the site and room for instrumentation are requisites to the preparation of biologically and mechanically sound cavities.

GOALS OF ISOLATION

1. Moisture Control

- Moisture in mouth can render a hinderance towards the operating procedures.
- Moisture control refers to excluding sulcular fluid, saliva and gingival bleeding from operating field.
- Effective method of moisture control is use of rubber dam, suction devices and absorbents.

2. Retraction and Access

- This is to provide maximum exposure of operating field.
- It involves, open mouth and retracting the gingival tissue, tongue, lips and checks.
- Rubber dam, high volume evacuators, absorbents, retraction cords, mouth prop are used.

3. Harm Prevention

- Major priority is minimal harm to patient.
- Excessive saliva and handpiece spray can alarm the patient.
- Small instruments and restorative debris can be swallowed and accidental soft tissue damage can occur.
- Rubber dam, high volume evacuators are used.

METHODS OF ISOLATION

I. To isolate from Moisture
   1. *Indirect Methods*
      i. Relaxed position of the patient
      ii. Local anesthesia
      iii. Drugs (Antisialogogues, antianxiety drugs, Muscle relaxants)
   2. *Direct Methods*
      i. Rubber dam
      ii. Gingival retraction
      iii. Cotton rolls and cellulose wafers
      iv. Throat shields
      v. High volume evacuators and saliva ejectors

II. To isolate from Soft tissues
   i. Retraction of cheek, tongue, lips
   ii. Gingival retraction

1. Local Anesthesia

– It plays an important role in eliminating the discomfort and controlling moisture.

2. Cotton roll isolation and cellulose wafers

– Partial isolation with cotton rolls, absorbent wafers and saliva ejectors provides a rapid and effective control of the operating field.

– *Isolation of Maxillary teeth:* A medium sized cotton roll is placed in facial vestibule.

– *Isolation of Mandibular teeth:* A medium sized cotton roll in the facial vestibule and a larger one between the teeth and tongue.

– Cellulose wafers may be used to retract the cheek and provide additional absorbency.

– Cotton rolls and wafers must be replaced as soon as they become saturated.

– Dry cotton rolls are moistened before they are removed to prevent the pulling of the epithelial covering of the mucosa.

3. Throat Shields

– These are indicated when there is danger of aspirating or swallowing small objects.

– A gauge sponge is unfolded and spread over the tongue and the posterior part of the mouth.

– Used to recover small objects.

4. High volume evacuators and Saliva ejectors

– High volume evacuators are used for suctioning water and debris from the mouth.

Advantages

– Debris is removed from operating site.

– Improves access and visibility.

– No dehydration of Oral Tissues.

– Patient experiences less pain.

– Precious metals are more readily salvaged.

– Quadrant dentistry is facilitated.

– Evacuator tip is placed just distal to the tooth to be prepared.

– Saliva ejector removes saliva that collects on the floor of the mouth.

– Disposable, inexpensive plastic ejectors that can be shaped by bending with the fingers are preferred.

– Svedopter is a helpful device that serves as both a saliva ejector and a tongue retractor.

5. Gingival Tissue Retraction

– Gingival tissue retraction refers to apical and lateral displacement of gingival tissue to aid in proper visibility and accessibility during sub gingival tooth preparation and to aid in proper flow of impression material into the area.

Methods of Gingival tissue retraction

1. Physico Mechanical Method.
2. Chemical Method.
3. Electro Surgical Method.
4. Surgical Method.

1. Physico Mechanical Methods

– This involves mechanically forcing the gingival tissue away from tooth surface, laterally and apically.

– *Methods :* 1. Application of extraheavy weight rubber dam, 2. Replacement of Cotton twigs in the gingival sulculus, 3. Placement of cotton twigs impregnated with zinc oxide eugenol. This pack should be remain for a minimum of 48 hours, 4. Copper bands, 5. Aluminium shell, 6. Temporary acrylic resin copings.

2. Chemical Method

– This method involves carrying various chemicals into gingival sulcus.

– *Chemicals used are*

   1. Vasoconstrictors like Epinephrine and Nor-epinephrine.

   2. Biologic fluid coagulants like Alum, Aluminium Chloride, Aluminium Potassium Sulphate, Tannic acid, etc.

– These chemicals coagulate blood and tissue fluids.

– Astringents like zinc chloride and silver nitrate.

– *Gingival retraction cords*

   Available as :   Braided
                     Twisted
                     Flattened
                     Knitted

– They may be supplied as already impregnated with chemical.

– A suitable length of the cord is tucked into the gingival sulcus using blunt ended instrument around the tooth.

3. Electro Surgical Method

– Here 4 types of action can be produced at the electrode end namely, cutting, coagulation, fulguration and dessication.

– For gingival tissue retraction mostly cutting and rarely coagulation action are employed.

4. Surgical Method

– This involves surgical excision of interfering gingival tissue using a sharp scalpel blade or surgical knife.

– *Method:* Gingivoplasty, Rotary gingival curettage (Gingettage).

Other Methods Include

Mirror and Evacuator tip Retraction

– A secondary function of the mirror and evacuator tip is to retract cheek, lip and tongue.

Mouth Props

– Used in restorative procedures of posterior teeth.

– Maintains adequate mouth opening and permits extended or multiple operations of desired.

– Available as block type or ratchet type.

Drugs

– Drugs like Atropine are used to control salivation.

– Rarely indicated.

RUBBER DAM

– Introduced to dentistry by Dr. Stanford C. Barnum in 1864.

Advantages

1. Maintains dry, clean operating field.

2. Improves the accessibility and visibility.

3. Aids in the reduction of pain (The dry fibrilla in dentin lose their ability to transmit sensations of pain) Aids in a more thorough examination of the teeth.

4. Prevents the aspiration of instruments.

5. Enhances the operators efficiency.

6. Potentially improves the properties of dental materials.

7. Acts as barrier between patient and operator and thus prevents cross infection between them.

Disadvantages

1. The patient can no longer speak easily during surgical procedure.

2. The teeth which has been clamped may be sensitive for some hours after the clamp has been removed.

3. Time consuming for application.

4. Difficulty in applying and removal.

5. Not economic.

6. The rubber is allergic to some patients.

Contra Indications

1. Teeth that are not completely erupted.

2. Procedures on third molars.

3. Extremely malposed teeth.

4. Patients suffering from asthma.

5. Patients allergic to latex.

Rubberdam Kit

– It consists of,

   1. Rubberdam Material

   2. Rubberdam Punch

   3. Rubberdam Stamp

   4. Rubberdam Clamps (Retainer)

   5. Rubberdam Clamp forceps

   6. Rubberdam Lubricant

   7. Rubberdam Napkin

   8. Rubberdam Holder or Frame

   9. Waxed dental floss or tape

   10. Miscellaneous

1. Rubberdam Material

– It is usually latex rubber.

– Available in rolls or precut sheets of sizes 5" x 5" for children and 6" x 6" for adults.

– It is available in variety of thicknesses, i.e. *thin* (0.15 mm), *medium* (0.20 mm), *heavy* (0.25 mm), *extra heavy* (0.30 mm) and *special extra heavy* (0.35 mm)

– It is also available in colors, i.e. *green* (heavy), *blue* (medium) and *black*.

– A Dark coloured one is preferred because it contrast well with the teeth; fragments torn off and left behind are seen easily and removed.

– Rubberdam material is shiny at one side and dull on another side.

– Because dull side is less light reflective, it is placed facing the occlusal side of the isolated teeth.

– Advantages of the thinner sheet are its easy application and the comfort it provides to the patient.

– Advantages of the heavier sheet are its ability to retract soft tissue and its resistance to scuffing and tearing by the dental bur.

– Medium thickness is recommended for molar applications, heavy (or extra heavy) for anterior and bicuspid applications.

2. Anchoring Devices

– For the rubberdam to be securely attached to the area being isolated, there are several devices and methods.

A. Anchoring Clamps

– Each clamp consists of two jaws, one on each side carrying the tooth attachment blades (prongs) and sometimes dam engaging projections (wings), a bow which connects the two jaws and which should be elastically strainable and resistant enough to impart a gripping force on the attaching blades against the teeth.

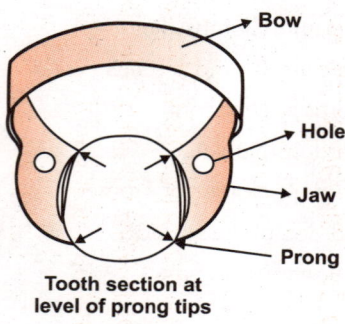

**Tooth section at
level of prong tips**

– According to the type and shape of the tooth attachment blades, clamps can be,

1. Clamps with four point contact blades (with wings) : (The blade portions of the jaw point inwards at each corner, so that all the gripping forces will be applied on these four points only). They contact the axial angles of the tooth and create a very secure attachment with the tooth. It is indicated when the retaining curvature of the tooth surfaces is not present (newly erupting teeth) and in single tooth isolation. The disadvantages are that the clamp has

possible traumatic effect on weakened undermined tooth structure; interference with the placement of matrix bands, retainer and wedges.

2. Clamps with circumferential contact blades (Wingless): The blade portion has no projections and will contact the tooth surface evenly throughout its length. It is less retentive. It is less traumatic. It is used when the axial angles are lost or do not coincide with the corners of the four point contact clamps and when the axial convexity of the tooth surface is sufficient for anchorage.

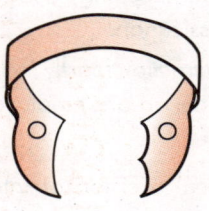 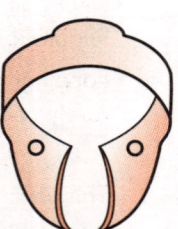

**MOLAR CLAMPS -
WINGLESS**   **MOLAR CLAMPS -
WINGLESS**

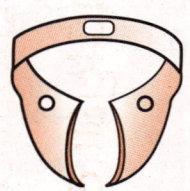 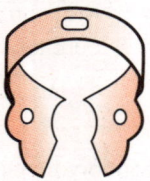

**BICUSPID CLAMPS -
WINGED**   **BICUSPID CLAMPS -
WINGED**

– Wings are provided to give extra retraction of rubberdam from the operating field.

– A good basic set of clamps has the following,

1. BW, JW molar clamps, wingless : used when the clamp is positioned on the tooth before the rubber.

2. K molar clamp, winged : the wings allow the clamp and rubber to be placed simultaneously.

3. GW premolar clamp.

4. EW clamp used on any small tooth.

5. AW molar clamp, wingless used on partially erupted teeth only.

6. Cervical clamp, Ferrier pattern, for use on anterior teeth where retraction of rubber or gingivae is required to allow access to a cervical cavity.

B. *Retracting anchoring clamps*

- These are clamps especially designed to other functions besides anchoring the dam to the tooth.

i. The 212 Clamp series consists of double bowed clamps, specially designed for retracting the facial or lingual gingiva away from class-5 cavity preparations.

ii. The Schultz clamp series resembles the 212 clamp but are split in half facio-lingually making them a gingivally retracting clamp with one bow only. Used especially when a second bow cannot be accommodated due to a lack of space or limited access.

3. Rubberdam Punch

- Used to cut the holes in the rubber which will encompass the teeth to be isolated.

- It has a lever type plunger and a rotatable table containing holes of different diameters.

- Usually the larger holes accommodate molars, medium size holes are for premolars, upper cuspids and sometimes for upper incisors, and the smallest holes are for lower incisors.

- The edges of the holes are very angular. The appropriate hole in the table is moved to coincide with the plunger, and the rubber is placed in between the plunger and the table and appropriate hole is punched.

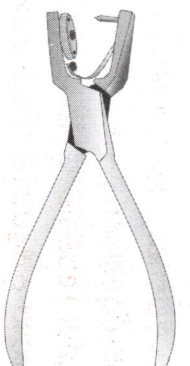

RUBBERDAM PUNCH

4. Rubberdam Stamp

- Used for marking the positions of the holes.

- The inked rubber stamp produces a series of dots on the rubber corresponding to the average positions of the teeth.

- When the dam is in position, it should reach upto a point just below the patients nose, thus covering the mouth but not the nose.

- To achieve this when applying the rubber to the maxillary teeth or mandibular third molars, the position of the upper central incisors should be stamped about 2.5 cm (1 inch) from the top edge of the rubber sheet. For mandibular teeth the holes should be placed further up the sheet to avoid the rubber covering the nose.

5. Rubberdam Clamp Forceps

- This is a modified forceps which retracts the jaws of a clamp away from each other, allowing the clamp to overcome the occlusal diameter of the tooth and to be seated apical to the height of the axial contour.

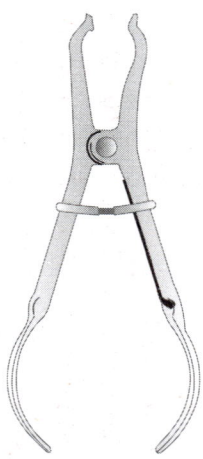

RUBBERDAM FORCEPS

6. Rubberdam Lubricant

- A water soluble lubricant applied on the area of the punched holes facilitates the passing of the dam septa through proximal contacts.

- It is commercially available.

7. Rubberdam Napkins

- These are absorbent paper or cloth towels that can be applied between the rubberdam and the patients face.

Advantages

1. Absorbs saliva and prevents drooling.

2. The additional comfort reduces the stimulated flow.

3. Reduces the allergic reactions by preventing the contact between rubberdam and the skin of the patient.

4. Aids in the prevention of pressure marks often created by tension of the rubberdam across the face.

5. Serves as a drying device for wiping the external tissues of the face during the removal of rubberdam.

6. Prevents the debris from falling beneath the clothing of the patient.

– Overall measurement is 9 inches square, with a 1 inch concavity at the upper border, the concavity extending from 1 inch from either end. The size of the mouth hole for upper arch is 2 inches long, 1 inch wide, and for lower arch is 3 by 1 ⅜ inches.

8. Rubberdam Holder or Frame

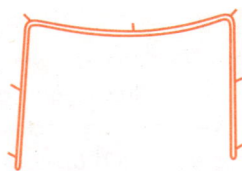

RUBBER DAM FRAME

Objectives

1. To keep the peripheries of the dam out of the mouth.
2. To stretch the applied dam in four directions.
3. To retract the tongue, cheek and lips.
4. To clear the operation field for further procedures.

Classification

– They can be classified as,

A. Strap type

– It depends on the back of the patient's head for anchorage.
– It is more convenient for the operator because they do not obstruct the field of vision in anydirection. Ex : Woodburry holder, Wizzard holder.

B. Hanging frame holders

– Are, U-shaped, elliptical or rectangular metal or plastic frames, with multiple prongs at their peripheries.
– Are most popular holders.
– Advantages are ease of application and allowance for minimal contact of the rubber with the skin.

9. Waxed Dental Floss or Tape

– Used to carry the rubber past a tight contact point; also in adjusting the septal portions of the rubber.

10. Miscellaneous

A. Rubber bands

– Frequently a small piece of rubber band may be used to retract the rubberdam comfortably and hold the gingival region to the contact point, in lieu of additional clamps.

B. Beavertail Burnisher

– Used to tuck unturned ends of the rubber under the free margin of the gingival.

C. Zinc Oxide Ointment

– A little soothing ointment placed on the corners of the mouth by a cotton roll applicator prevents cracking of the lips from long dryness.

D. Black Impression compound

– Can be made into cylinders of varying sizes which are used to secure the clamps to the teeth, ensuring no movement during the operation.

E. 70% alcohol

– Used for cleaning the dam and teeth after application.

Placement of Holes

– The holes are placed to conform to the curvature of the arch and are spaced according to the distances between the teeth.
– Holes are punched only when they are positioned and marked on the rubber.
– To assure the uniformity of rubber borders after application, two landmarks can be used ; For Maxillary applications, the incisors should lie one inch from the upper border, for Mandibular applications, the most posterior hole is slightly right or left of the center of the rubber.
– Distances between the holes should be comparable to spaces between the centers of each tooth.
– The circumference of the arch is reflected in the location of the holes to space the holes so that the rubber will snugly engage each tooth without puckering.
– If the holes are placed too closely together or incorrectly aligned, they will fit over the teeth but will be stretched to the side, permitting saliva to leak by.
– If the holes are too far apart, excess rubber stock remains and is puckered between the teeth.
– *A liberal number of teeth should always be included in a dam application. An anterior application should include a minimum of seven teeth. Posterior application should usually reach from the first or second molar to the opposite cuspid.*
– Generally clamp is attached one tooth distal to the tooth receiving treatment.
– Holes must be sharp and clean cut. Holes with ragged edges will cause the rubber to tear when tightly stretched.

Procedure of Application

1. Preparation

– *Armamentarium*

1. Basic four instruments: mirror, explorer, cotton pliers, plastic instruments.

2. Rubberdam kit

3. Saliva ejector

4. Scissors

− Gross bits of calculus and other debris are removed, contact points are checked by the passage of dental tape and sharp edges of enamel that might cut the rubber are removed.

− *For Tight and Broad Contacts :* Open the contact slightly with pressure from a beavertail burnisher wedged for a moment just gingival to the contact point as the septal rubber dam passes.

− *For sharp cavity edges :* Smooth with chisels or hatchets or cavity is reopened and outline form is re-established.

− *For sharp or rough restoration margins:* Trim to contour with gold knife, disks or strips.

− *For foreign material between teeth :* Remove with ligature, explorer, and warm water.

2. Punch Holes

− Select the size of rubber dam needed.

− The distance of one hole to the next is equal to the distance of the center of the next tooth at the gingival third. This is the position of the rubberdam when completely placed.

− *Note :* When preparing class 2, 3 or 4 cavities, the rule on distance between the tooth centers should be modified on that septum where the cavity lies.

− Follow the arch form of the teeth (especially the irregularities of tooth position) in punching holes. A hole may be punched in the upper left hand corner for identification of that corner during the placement of the upper (first) snap of the rubber dam holder on to the left border of the rubberdam.

Rubberdam for Upper Teeth

1. First holes punched are for central incisors, 1 inch from the superior border (center) of the rubberdam. *Modifications :* A. For a narrow upperlip, especially in a women or child, the holes should be a little less than 1 inch from the superior border, B. For a long upper lip or in the presence of mustache, the distance is little more than 1 inch.

2. Upper teeth to be included in the rubber dam ordinarily should be according to the following plan (FDI notation) for class 1, 2, 3 and 4 cavities.

Cavity Teeth	Extend from ____ to ____
12, 11, 11 or 22	14 − 24
13 or 23 mesial	14 − 24
13 distal	16 − 24
23 distal	14 − 26
15 and 14	16 − 21
24 and 25	11 − 26
16 mesioocclusal	17 or 16 − 21
26 mesioocclusal	11 − 26 or 27
16 mesioocclusal	17 − 21
26 mesioocclusal	11 − 27
17 mesioocclusal	18 or 17 − 21
27 mesioocclusal	11 − 27 or 28
18 or 17 distoocclusal	18 − 21
28 or 27 distoocclusal	11 − 28

3. *Size of holes to punch :* The punch has 5 holes, from the smallest (No.1) to the largest (No.5). No. 2 and 4 are sufficient for all purposes. No.2 is for anterior teeth and bicuspids ; No. 4 is for molars. One size larger should be used for the tooth to receive the clamp.

4. The lines of holes should follow irregularities in teeth. The arch of the holes should not follow the incisal edges of the anterior teeth but should correspond to the position of the teeth at their cervical lines.

Rubberdam for Lower Teeth

1. The first hole punched is the one through which the holding clamp is to be placed.

   A. *First Molar:* The rubber dam should be imaginarily divided into three equal portions by two vertical lines extending from the superior to the inferior (chin) border. At a point 3 inches from the superior border of the rubber dam and 1/4 inch toward the center of the rubberdam from one of the lateral lines, is the point for punching the hole for the first molar.

B. *Second Molar :* The hole is punched about 1/8 inch chin wise from that of the first molar and slightly toward the center of the dam.

C. *Third Molar :* The hole is punched about 1/4 inch chin wise from that of the first molar and slightly towards the center of the dam.

D. *Second bicuspid :* Use anterior rubberdam. The hole is punched about 1/8 inch nosewise or of that for a first molar.

E. *First bicuspid :* Use anterior rubberdam. The hole is punched about 1/4 inch nosewise from the first molar point.

2. Lower teeth to be included in the rubberdam should follow the following plan for class 1, 2, 3 and 4 Cavities.

Cavity Teeth	Extend from _____ to _____
32, 31, 41 or 42	34 – 44
33 or 43 mesial	34 – 44
33 distal	36 – 42 or 32
43 distal	42 or 32 – 46
34 mesioocclusal	36 – 42 or 32
44 mesioocclusal	42 or 32 – 46
34 distoocclusal or 35	36 – 44
44 distoocclusal or 45	44 – 46
36 mesioocclusal	37 or 36 – 34
46 mesioocclusal	44 – 46 or 47
36 distoocclusal	37 – 34
46 distoocclusal	44 – 37
37 mesioocclusal	38 or 37 – 34
47 mesioocclusal	44 – 47 or 48
37 distoocclusal or 38	38 – 34
47 distoocclusal or 48	44 - 48

3. Size of the hole may be confined to No. 2 and 4.
4. Follow the irregularities as mentioned above.
5. When punching holes for the teeth to be included in the rubberdam it is helpful to punch an additional hole in that corner of the dam which will be at the upper left position when adjusted. This is for identification since in the punching and preliminary placement, the entire dam may be twisted.

Rubberdam punching for the class - 5 (gingival) cavity:

1. Include only those teeth in the rubberdam to permit the modelling compound which holds the special cervical clamp in place to rest on teeth and not on the rubber dam.

2. Punch the holes in the correct position for selected teeth except the hole for the tooth having the class 5 cavity. This should be punched outside the arch.

3. Placement of Rubberdam

   – A dental floss is used to check the interproximal contacts and remove debris from the teeth to be isolated.

   – After assessing the form and tooth alignment, now punch the holes.

   – Lubricate the dam on both sides. Lips and corners of the mouth are also lubricated to prevent irritation.

   – Select the retainer and test the retainer's retention and stability by lifting gently in an occlusal direction. An improperly fitting retainer will rock or be easily dislodged.

   – Positioning the dam over the retainer: Before placing the dam, the floss tie is threaded through the anchor hole.

     – Now stretch anchor hole of the dam over the retainer and then under the jaws.

     – The septal dam must always pass through its respective contact in single thickness.

     – If in case it does not pass through, dental tape can be used.

   – Rubber dam is grasped and pulled through the napkin and position it on the patient's face.

   – Unfold the dam and, hold the frame in place, attach the dam to the metal projections on the left and right side simultaneously.

   – Attaching the neck strap is optional.

   – If there is a tooth distal to the retainer, the distal edge of the posterior anchor hole should be passed through the contact to ensure a seal around the anchor tooth.

   – If the stability of retainer is questionable, low fusing modelling compound may be applied.

   – Dam is passed over the anterior anchor tooth, anchoring the anterior portion of the rubber dam.

- By stretching the septal dam faciogingivally and linguogingivally one can pass the septa through as many contacts as possible without a dental tape.

- Waxed dental tape can be used to pass the dam through the remaining contacts.

- Now invert the dam into the gingival sulcus to complete the seal around the tooth and to prevent leakage.

- Facio lingually the inversion is completed using an explorer or a beaver-tail burnisher, by moving the explorer around the neck of the tooth facially and lingually.

- Confirm the properly applied rubber dam.

- In case of proximal surface preparation a wedge is placed interproximally as final step in rubber dam application.

4. Removal of Rubber dam

- Before removal, suction away any debris thus preventing it from falling into the floor of mouth.

- Stretch the dam facially, pulling the septal rubber away from the tooth.

- Clipping each septum with blunt tipped scissor, free the dam from interproximal spaces.

- Engage the retainer with retainer forceps and remove the retainer.

- Once the retainer is removed, remove the dam and frame simultaneously.

- Wipe the lips, rinse the mouth and massage the tissues to enhance circulation around on the anchored teeth.

- Examine the dam to determine that no portion of the dam has remained between or around the teeth.

INFECTION CONTROL

- Infection control is compulsory in dentistry.

- Dentist either can get the infection from the patient or he can spread the infection from one patient to another patient or from himself to the patient.

- *OSHA:* Occupational Safety and Health Act was passed by U.S. Congress in 1970.

- *SOPS :* Standard Operating Procedures is a term used in former OSHA regulations.

Regulations of OSHA

1. Provision for Hepatitis B vaccination.

2. Universal precautions such as,

- Careful handling of sharp instruments.

- Use of devices to reduce contamination risks (High volume suction, Rubberdam and Protective sharp containers).

3. Personal protective equipment : Gloves, Mask, Gown.

4. House Keeping is term related to clean up instruments, operatory equipment, floors, walls and management of waste, sterilization procedures.

5. Implement engineering controls to reduce the production of contaminated spatter, mist, aerosol Ex : Rubberdam, High volume suction.

6. Implementation of work practice controls to minimize the splashing, spatter or contact of bare hands with contaminated surfaces Ex : When using the brush to scrub instruments hold the instruments well down in the sink and brush away from yourself.

7. Never contact telephones, switches, door handles with soiled gloves.

8. Safe handling of needles.

9. Provision of proper washing facilities-washing hands after removing gloves.

10. Maintenance of proper sterilization of instruments.

11. Removal of blood contaminated waste properly and disposed thoroughly.

12. Provision of laundering of protective garments used for universal precautions.

Disinfection of Surfaces and Equipment in the Dental Office

- The surfaces and equipment which do not permit sterilization should be treated with disinfectant prior to seating the patient and in between patients. Ex : Operating light handles, chair controls, tray arms and release levers, 3 way syringe handles.

- Detergent solutions assist in removing dried blood.

- Alcohol, 90% isopropyl or 70% ethyl alcohol aids in solubilizing dried blood and saliva.

- 70% isopropyl alcohol has become an effective agent for surface decontamination in dental office.

Methods to Reduce Cross Infection

1. *Safety glasses :* to protect eyes from splatter and aerosols and to avoid injury.

2. *Masks* should be worn for protection against aerosols and any blood or saliva emnating from the oral cavity.

3. *Gloves* should be worn routinely due to risks in treating patients who may themselves be unaware that they are carriers of infectious disease.

Methods of Sterilization

1. Auto claving, steam pressure sterilization.
2. Chemical vapour pressure sterilization.
3. Dry heat.
4. Ethylene oxide sterilization.

1. Auto Claving

- In this apparatus the material is exposed to 121°C for 15 - 20 min at 15 lb pressure / sq. inch.
- It is used to sterilize—Culture media, Rubber goods, Syringes, Gowns, Instruments.

Sterilization of Burs in Autoclaving

- Burs are placed in 2% Sodium nitrate containing bottles, either glass beakers or metal beakers are kept in autoclave for sterilization.

2. Chemical Vapour Pressure Sterilization

- Sterilization by chemical vapour under pressure, i.e. 131°C - 20 lbs pressure sq. inch - 30 min.
- *Uses :* Sterilization of Corrosion sensitive burs, metallic instruments, pliers.

3. Dry Heat Sterilization

- *Red heat:* It is directly by holding on flame used for needles, forceps, inoculating wires.
- *Hot air oven:* carbon steel instruments and burs.
- *Incineration:* Hospital dressings are burnt.

4. Ethylene oxide sterilization

- Used to sterilize complex instruments and delicate materials.
- Ethylene oxide gas at high temperature below 100° C for several hours.

5. Sterilization of Hand Pieces and related rotary instruments

- Scrubbing with disinfectant
- Steam sterilization
- Chemical vapour pressure
- Cleaning with soap
- Wiping with alcohol

6. Sterilization of impressions

- Washing the impression with disinfectant solution, such as 3% phenol, ethyl alcohol, and formaldehyde.

CHAPTER 07

CONTACTS AND CONTOURS

– The site of actual contact between two teeth on the mesial and distal surfaces and is erroneously called a *contact point*.

– Contact areas are not present on the distal surfaces of third molars of permanent teeth and distal surfaces of second molars in deciduous teeth (which have no teeth distal to them).

– A positive relationship should exist between the contacts to resist food impaction and to protect the gingival tissue. It can be tested by passing dental floss between the teeth and observing the resistance when the floss is moved from the gingiva between the two enamel surfaces.

– The contact area in the posterior teeth is located nearer at the facial surface which causes a larger lingual embrasure.

– The contact area in anterior teeth is located nearer at the lingual surface, which causes a larger facial embrasure.

– The contact areas are usually parallel to the incisal edges of the teeth and to a line drawn through the posterior facial cusp tips.

– Contact areas are classified as rounded, broad and flat.

– The flat contact or the square shaped tooth is more difficult to clean and thus more prone to caries.

– Whenever possible a rounded contact with an open embrasure in positive relationship should be produced in the proximal restoration.

Purpose of Ideal contacts

1. To prevent food impaction.
2. To conserve healthy gingival tissue.
3. To make the areas self cleansable.
4. To help ensure permanence of proximal restorations.
5. To maintain normal mesio-distal relationship of the teeth in the dental arch.
6. To improve esthetic appearance, especially on anterior teeth.

Purpose of breaking contact point

1. To make the areas self cleansable (after restoration)
2. To place matrix band
3. To eliminate caries

EMBRASURES (SPILLWAYS)

– When two teeth in the same arch are in contact, their curvatures adjacent to the contact areas form spillway spaces called *embrasures*.

– The spaces that widen out from the area of contact labially or buccally and lingually are called *labial or buccal and lingual inter proximal embrasures* respectively.

– Above the contact areas incisally and occlusally, the spaces which are bounded by the marginal ridges as they join the cusps and incisal ridges, are called the *incisal or occlusal embrasures.*

– The *gingival embrasure or interproximal* space is a triangular space formed by the contact areas of two teeth and the supporting bone. The base of the triangle is located on the bone.

Purpose

1. It makes a spill way for the escape of food during mastication.

2. It prevents food from being forced through the contact area.

3. Reduce the load of occlusal forces.

4. Permit a slight amount of stimulation to the gingiva.

HEIGHT OF CONTOUR

– The area of greatest circumference on the facial and lingual surfaces of the tooth is called the height of contour.

– It protects the gingival tissues by preventing food impaction of the facial and lingual gingiva.

– On the posterior teeth the contour is located in the gingival third of the facial surface and in the middle one-third of the lingual surface.

– These contours divert food over the free gingival margin and they should be placed in the restoration for protection of the periodontium.

MARGINAL RIDGES

– Are those rounded borders of the enamel that form the mesial and distal margins of the occlusal surfaces of premolars and molars and the mesial and distal margins of the lingual surfaces of the incisors and canines.

MAMELON

– It is any one of the three rounded protruberances found on the incisal ridges of newly erupted incisor teeth.

– Each mamelon represents a lobe or the primary section of the formation in the development of crown to which it belongs to.

– They are worn out with usage or they may be missing by birth (as incase of Syphilis, where the central lobe or mamelon will be missing congenitally).

OVERHANG

– The projection of a restoration beyond the cavosurface angle, particularly that which overlays the tooth surface; also the projection of a restoration outward from the normal tooth surface.

CONSEQUENCES OF FAULTY REPRODUCTION OF CONTACTS AND CONTOURS

1. Contact Size

– A contact that is too broad bucco lingually or occluso gingivally changes the anatomy of the interdental col, which results in the development of periodontal disease, the areas less able to clean.

– A contact that is too narrow bucco lingually or occluso gingivally changes the anatomy of the tooth, which results in food impaction and periodontal disease.

– A contact area placed too occlusally results in a flattened marginal ridge at the occlusal embrasures.

– A contact area placed too buccally or lingually results in a flattened restoration at buccal or lingual embrasures.

– A contact area placed too gingivally results in increased depth of occlusal embrasures and impingement on the interdental col.

– An open (loose) contact results in the continuity of the embrasures with each other and with the interdental papilla.

2. Contact Configuration

– A flat contact area results in a contact area that is too broad buccally, lingually, occlusally, and / or gingivally.

– A contact area with excessive convexity results in diminishing of the extent of the contact area.

3. Contour

i. *Facial and lingual convexities*

– Over convex curvatures result in accumulation of cariogenic and plaque ingredients and depriving of the free and attached gingiva from the massaging, stimulating, keratinizing effect of the food.

ii. *Facial and lingual concavities*

– Deficiency in concavities occlusal to the height of contour results in premature contacts during mandibular movements and excessive concavities result in extrusion, rotation and tilting of cuspal elements.

- Deficiency in concavities apical to the height of contour results in restoration over hangs and excessive concavities result in areas which are difficult to clean.

iii. Areas of proximal contour

- Faulty reproduction of these areas result in restoration overhangs, underhangs, food impaction and impingment on the adjacent periodontal structures.

4. Marginal Ridges

- Improper restoration of the marginal ridges results in:
- Forces direct toward the proximal surface of the adjacent teeth.
- Forces tend to drive the two teeth away from each other.
- Food impaction.

SEPARATION OF THE TEETH

PURPOSE OF SEPARATION

1. To examine the proximal surfaces in the detection of caries.
2. To restore to original positions those teeth which have drifted.
3. To gain access for cavity preparations on anterior teeth.
4. For proper restoration of anatomic proximal contours.
5. For polishing the interproximal restorations.
6. To create a sufficient space for the placement of matrix band interproximally.

METHODS OF SEPARATION

1. Slow or delayed or previous separation.
2. Rapid or immediate separation.

1. SLOW SEPARATION

- Separation should not exceed more than 0.5 mm.

Advantages

1. Comparative absence of soreness of teeth.
2. Less danger to the periodontium.
3. Ability to force away temporarily with gutta percha, swollen tissue from the gingival margins of cavities.

Disadvantages

1. Time consuming.
2. Repeated application of separating material.

Methods

1. Separating wires
2. Oversized Resin temporaries
3. Orthodontic appliances
4. Gutta percha
5. Use of wood or rubber

2. RAPID SEPARATION

- This is a mechanical type of separation which creates either proximal separation at the point of the separator's introduction and / or improved closeness of the proximal surface opposite the point of the separator's introduction.
- It can be used as preparatory to slow tooth movement or to maintain a space gained by slow tooth movement.
- Separation should not exceed 0.2 - 0.5 mm.

Advantages

1. Quickness.
2. Ability to prevent movement of the teeth during the procedure.

Disadvantages

1. Danger of the rupturing of the periodontal ligament.
2. Pain of too rapid separation.

Methods

A. Wedge Method

- Separation is accomplished by the insertion of a pointed wedge shaped device between the teeth.
- The more the wedge moves facially or lingually, the greater will be the separation.

Example

1. Elliot separator

Application

- Adjust the two opposing wedges of the separator interproximally so that they are positioned gingival to the contact area.
- Move the knob clockwise so that wedges move towards each other establishing desired separation.

2. Wood or plastic wedges

B. Traction Method

- This uses mechanical devices which engage the proximal surfaces of the teeth to be separated by means of holding arms.

Example

1. Non interfering True separator

- Indicated when continuous stabilized separation is required.
- Advantages are (1) separation can be increased or decreased after stabilization and (2) is non interfering.

2. Ferrier double bow separator

- With this device, the separation is stabilized throughout the operation.
- Advantage is that the separation is shared by the contact teeth and not at the expense of one tooth as with the previous type of instrument.

Advantages of mechanical separators

1. For examination of interproximal spaces.
2. For use as preparatory to slow separation.
3. For preparation of cavities.
4. For removal of foreign bodies.
5. To maintain the space gained by slow separation.
6. For insertion and polishing of restorations.

MATRICES

- A dental matrix may be defined as *a properly shaped piece of metal, or other material, used to support and give form to the restoration during its introduction and hardening.*
- Matrix is formed of two parts, i.e. the *band*, which is a piece of metal or polymeric material used to support and give form to the restorative material during its introduction and hardening and the *retainer*, which is a device by which the band can be retained in its designated position and shape.
- The retainer could be a mechanical device, a wire, dental floss and or compound.

SPECIFICATIONS OF A MATRIX

- It should,
  1. be easy for application.
  2. be easy to remove.
  3. be rigid.
  4. confine the restorative material within the cavity preparation.
  5. be biocompatible.
  6. be economic.

FUNCTIONS

1. Acts as a temporary wall of resistance during the restoration.
2. Gives shape to the restoration.
3. Maintains the form of the restoration during hardening or setting.
4. Assists in holding back the gingiva and rubberdam during restoration.

MATRIX BAND MATERIALS

- Matrix bands are made of stainless steel, copper and celluloid.

MATRIX BAND THICKNESS

- Ranges from to 0.0015" to 0.002".

HEIGHT OF THE MATRIX BAND

- Occlusally should be 1-2 mm above the marginal ridge.
- Gingivally 1 mm below the gingival margin.

CLASSIFICATION

I. Based on the material

1. *Metallic matrix:* made up of stainless steel. Ex: Ivory No: 1 and 8.
2. *Non metallic matrix:* made up of plastic like material. Ex: Myeloid strip.

II. Based on the retainer

1. *With retainer (mechanical):* needs retainer to keep the matrix in its place. Ex: Ivory No. 1 and 8.
2. *Without retainer (anatomical):* do not need retainer. Ex: Automatrix, T-band, Soldered band, compound supported matrix.

III. Matrices are also classified as

1. Circumferential: Ex: Tofflemaire, Ivory No. 8.
2. Unilateral: Ex: Ivory No. 1, Automatrix.
3. Mechanical retainer supported.
4. Compound supported/wedge supported.
5. Precontoured band.
6. Uncontoured band.

MATRICES FOR INDIVIDUAL CAVITY PREPARATIONS

I. Matrices for class - 1 cavity, designs 4, 5, 6, 7 and 8 preparations

- Double banded Tofflemire matrix.

II. Matrices for class - 2 cavity

1. Single - banded Tofflemire matrix (Designs 1, 2, 3, 6, 7 and 8).

2. Ivory matrix No: 1 (unilateral class - 2)

3. Ivory matrix No: 8 (Designs 1, 2 and 3)

4. Black's matrices (Designs 1, 2 and 3)

5. Soldered band or seamless copper band matrix (Designs 6, 7 and 8)

6. The anatomical matrix (Designs 1, 2, 3, 6, 7, and 8)

7. Roll - in band matrix (auto - matrix)

8. S - shaped matrix band (Designs 4, 5, and 7)

9. T - shaped matrix band.

III. Matrices for amalgam restorations on the distal of the cuspid

1. S - shaped matrix.

2. Tofflemire matrix.

IV. Matrices for class - 3 direct tooth coloured restorations

1. For Silicate cements - celluloid strips, mylar strips.

2. For Resins - cellophane strips, mylar strips.

3. T - shaped matrix band.

V. Matrices for class - 4 direct tooth coloured restorations

1. Plastic strip for inciso - proximal cavities.

2. Aluminium foil incisal corner matrix.

3. Transparent crown form matrices.

4. Anatomic matrix.

5. Modified S - shaped band.

VI. Matrices for class - 5 amalgam restorations

1. Window matrix.

2. S - shaped matrix.

VII. Matrices for class - 5 direct tooth coloured restorations

1. Anatomic matrix for non-light cured materials.

2. Aluminium or copper collars for non-light cured materials.

3. Anatomic matrix for light and non-light cured materials.

1. UNIVERSAL / TOFFLEMIRE MATRIX

– It is a circumferential matrix.

– Available as straight and contrangled (both facially and lingually).

– Ideally used for MOD cavity and can also be used for class - 2cavity preparation.

Advantages

1. Can be placed facially or lingually.

2. Stable band and retainer.

3. Bands of variable occlusal, gingival heights are available.

4. Small bands are available for primary dentition.

5. Provides superior contact and contour.

6. Helps in holding the cotton rolls in place.

7. Permits easy removal.

Disadvantage

– Unnecessary space creating on the other side if used in unilateral class - 2 preparation.

2. IVORY NO. 1

– It is a unilateral matrix.

– Available for premolars and molars.

– The jaws of the retainer should engage the gingival embrasure area.

– Gingival edge has shorter length that allows the retainer to draw the band tight at the gingival margin.

3. IVORY NO. 8

– Indicated in class - 2 with buccal or palatal extension; class - 2 with no adjacent tooth; MOD and complex cavities.

– Tofflemire is preferred over Ivory No. 8.

4. BLACK'S MATRICES

– Of all the different designs for matrices presented by Black, only two are mainly used.

– The first is the simplest form and which is recommended for the majority of the small and medium-sized cavities.

– The second form is used for grossly destructed teeth.

5. AUTOMATRIX: (Roll-in-band matrix)

– It is a retainerless matrix system with four types of bands that are designed to fit all teeth regardless of circumference.

– **Height:** 4.7- 7.9 mm.

– **Indication:** for extensive class - 2 preparation and cuspal restoration.

Advantages

1. Convenience

2. Improved visibility (retainer is not present)

3. Auto lock loop can be positioned facially or lingually.

4. Decreased time of application.

Disadvantages

1. Cannot be precontoured.
2. Difficult to develop physiological proximal contour.

6. COMPOUND SUPPORTED MATRIX

- Particularly valuable when the amalgam is condensed by mallet force, for example, in the use of the Hollenback pneumatic condenser.
- *Application :* A piece of 0.003 inch stainless steel is placed between the teeth. A wedge is placed at the gingival area both buccally and lingually. After wedging, modelling compound is placed both sides around the exposed portion of the wedge.
- Used in two surface proximal restorations.

7. SOLDERED BAND

- Also called as seamless copper band matrix.
- Indicated in badly broken down teeth, especially for pin - retained amalgam restorations with large buccal and lingual extensions.
- This band is made by taking a measurement of the neck of the tooth and soldering a band of metal to fit.

8. T - SHAPED MATRIX BAND

- These are premade T - shaped stainless steel matrix bands.
- The long arm of the T is bent or curled to encompass the tooth circumferentially and to overlap the short horizontal arm of T. This section is then bent over the long arm, loosely holding it in place.

9. WINDOW MATRIX

- It can be formed using either a Tofflemire matrix or copper band matrix.
- A band is selected and a window is cut in the band slightly smaller than the outside of the cavity. Wedges are placed mesially and distally to stabilize the band.

WEDGES

- Wedge *is a wooden or plastic device placed interproximally which approximates the band on to the tooth and prevents gingival overhang of restoration.*
- In cross-section, the base of the triangle will be in contact with the interdental papillae, gingival to the gingival margin of the proximal cavity.

- The two sides of the triangle should coincide with the corresponding two sides (i.e. mesial and distal) of the gingival embrasure.
- The apex of the triangle should coincide with the gingival start of the contact area.

FUNCTIONS

1. To prevent the gingival overhanging of the restorative material.
2. To adapt closely the matrix band to the tooth.
3. To protect gingival interdental papilla.
4. To protect proximal periodontal tissues.
5. To create some separation to compensate for the thickness of the matrix band and minor drifting of the teeth.
6. To establish atraumatic retraction of the rubberdam.
7. To immobilize the matrix band.

TYPES OF WEDGES

1. Wooden
2. Resin (plastic)

Advantages of Wooden Wedge

1. Can be easily cut and trimmed.
2. Absorb water intraorally and swells thus improves inter proximal retention.

Advantages of Plastic Wedges

- Can be moulded and bent according to the shape of the interdental papilla.

WEDGING TECHNIQUE

- Break off 1 - 2 cm of round tooth pick.
- Grasp the broken end of tooth pick with a No. 110 plier.
- Insert the pointed tip from the facial or lingual embrasure whichever is larger, slightly gingival to gingival cavosurface margin.
- Lubricate the wedge in water before wedging.

CLASSIFICATION OF WEDGES

I. Based on the material,

 (1) Plastic
 (2) Wooden

II. Based on the shape,

 (1) Round
 (2) Triangular (anatomical wedge)

III. Based on either modified or unmodified wedges,

1. Modified wedge: prevents the distortion of matrix contour, used for very wide spacing between teeth. Ex: A custom made tungblade wedge.

2. *Unmodified wedge:* usually inserted into the interdental space from the lingual side because the lingual embrasures are larger.

   - **Triangular wedge** is indicated for class - 2 with deep gingival margin because it has its greatest width at its base.

   - **Round wedge** is indicated for class - 2 with shallow gingival margin because its wedging action is nearer to the gingival margin.

WEDGING TECHNIQUES: (OR TYPES OF WEDGING)

1. Piggy back wedging
2. Double wedging
3. Wedge wedging

1. Piggy back wedging

   - **Indication:** in cases where there is recession of the inter proximal gingiva and gingival recession.

   - **Technique:** If the first wedge is placed significantly apical to the gingival margin, a second wedge usually smaller than the first one may be piggy back on the first wedge to adequately wedge the matrix band against tooth margins.

2. Double wedging

   - **Indication:** Occasionally permitted if proximal box is wide faciolingually.

   - **Technique:** Insert two wedges one from facial embrasure and otherone from lingual embrasure.

3. Wedge wedging

   - Used if the concavity on the proximal surface is gingival to the contact area extending into the root.

   - Also used to wedge the matrix band tight against such a margin, a second pointed wedge is inserted between the first wedge and the band.

CHAPTER 08

DENTAL AMALGAM RESTORATIONS

Requirements

- 90° or greater amalgam margin (max of 100°), i.e. butt joint form to be produced due to its poor edge strength.
- Adequate depth (thickness of amalgam).
- Adequate mechanical retention form (undercut form).

CLASS-1 CAVITY PREPARATION

A. INITIAL TOOTH PREPARATION

1. *Outline form*

- The Class 1 amalgam tooth preparation should include only the faulty, defective occlusal pits and fissures.
- Cavity margins occulsally should be located on smooth surfaces, inclined planes of cusps, marginal ridges and crossing ridges.
- Begin, the tooth preparation by entering the deepest faulty pit with a `punch cut' using a No. 245, round carbide bur.
- Bur should be positioned parallel to the long axis of the tooth.
- Entering the distal pit first provides increased visibility for mesial extension.
- For a Class 1 preparation, a faciolingual width of not more than 1 to 1.5 mm or 1/4th of intercuspal distance and a depth of 1.5 to 2 mm is ideal, and the depth measured at the central fissure.
- Extension of the cavity is made using a plain straight fissure carbide bur.
- Cavity is extended along the central fissure toward the mesial pit following the DEJ creating a flat pulpal floor.

2. *Primary Resistance form*

- Flat pulpal floor in sound tooth structure to resist forces directed in long axis of the tooth.
- Occlusal buccopulpal and linguopulpal line angles are rounded.
- Minimal extension of external wall.
- Strong, ideal enamel margins.
- Adequate depth.

3. *Primary Retention form*

- Parallelism or right occlusal converge of two or more opposing external walls.

4. *Convenience form*
   - Shape and form of the cavity gives the accessibility during the restoration.

B. FINAL TOOTH PREPARATION
   - Removal of the remaining enamel pit-and-fissure in the pulpal floor.
   - The floor of the cavity is deepened to eliminate the fault and to remove the caries.
   - Infected dentin is best removed by discoid type spoon excavator or a slow revolving round carbide bur.
   - When removing the infected dentin, stop the excavation when the tooth structure feels hard or firm.
   - External walls are finished, providing an approximate of 90 to 100 degree cavosurface angle.
   - Prepared tooth is inspected and cleaned before restoration.
   - Tooth is rinsed with air water syringe.

DESIGNS OF CLASS I CAVITY PREPARATION

1. Class - 1, Design - 1
   - *Involves occlusal surfaces of molars and premolars.*
   - *Indications*
   1. Penetration of caries does not exceeding 0.5 mm to 1mm into dentin.
   2. Decay not involving more than 1/4th of the intercuspal distance.
   3. Patients with good oral hygiene and low caries index.

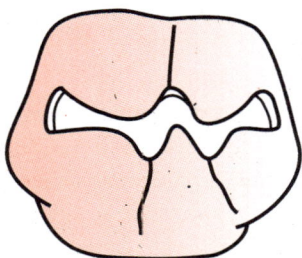

CLASS - 1, DESIGN - 1

2. Class - 1, Design - 2
   - *Involves occlusal surfaces of molars and premolars.*
   - *Indications*
   1. Penetration of caries exceeding 1mm into dentin.
   2. Decay involving more than 1/4th of the intercuspal distance.

3. Patients with high plaque and caries indices.
4. Teeth with intact cusps

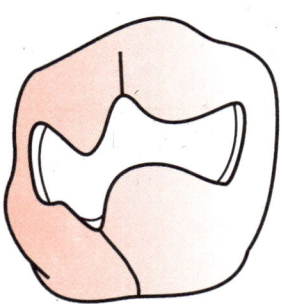

CLASS - 1, DESIGN - 2

3. Class - 1, Design - 3
   - Involves the occlusal one-to two-third of the facial and lingual surfaces of molars and on the lingual surfaces of upper anterior teeth (usually the lateral incisors).

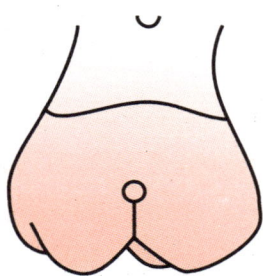

CLASS - 1, DESIGN - 3

4. Class - 1, Design - 4
   - Involves molars in addition to involvement of occlusal surfaces, the grooves of facial and or lingual surfaces are also involved.

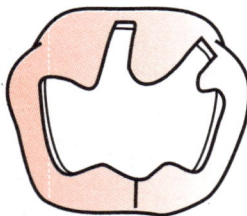

CLASS - 1, DESIGN - 4

5. Class - 1, Design - 5
   - Involvement is confined to molar teeth, where in addition to involving part of the occlusal surface, most or all of the facial and lingual surfaces are also involved.

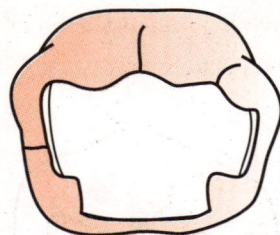

CLASS - 1, DESIGN - 5

6. **Class - 1, Design - 6**
   - Involves a part of the occlusal surfaces of molars or premolars and a portion of the facial, proximal or lingual surface in the form of a table of an entire cusp (marginal ridge) or a section of a cusp (marginal ridge).

7. **Class - 1, Design - 7**
   - Involves the occlusal, facial and / or lingual surfaces of molars and premolars.

8. **Class - 1, Design - 8**
   - Involves molars and premolars, it is used on the occlusal and sometimes on the occlusal and / or facial lingual surfaces. Also used on the lingual surfaces of anterior teeth.

CLASS - 2 CAVITY PREPARATION

Factors affecting the success of Class 2 Amalgam Restoration

1. Tooth preparation
2. Proper matrix selection and adaptation of matrix.
3. Isolation of the operating field.
4. Proper manipulation of restorative material.

A. Initial tooth preparation

1. Occlusal outline form
   - Occlusal outline is similar to that of class I amalgam tooth preparation.
   - Begin the tooth preparation by entering into the pit nearest involved proximal surface punch cut using no. 245 bur.
   - Bur should be positioned parallel to the long axis of the tooth, create facial, lingual and distal walls with slight occlusal convergence.
   - Initial depth is 1.5 - 2 mm or 1/2 to 2/3 of the cutting length of No. 245 bur. Depth is measured from central fissure.
   - Dovetail is created at the opposite end of the proximal involvement.

   - Width of the cavity is 1/4th of the intercuspal distance.

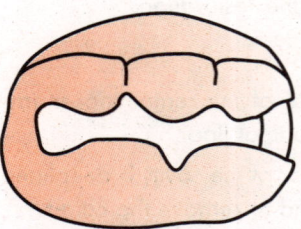

OCCLUSAL OUTLINE FORM

2. Proximal outline from
   - Visualize and locate the facial and lingual walls of the proximal box relatively to the contact area.

Objectives of extension of proximal margins
   - to include all caries.
   - to create 90° cavosurface margin.
   - to establish 0.5 mm clearance with the adjacent proximal surface facially, lingually and gingivally.

Proximal ditch cut
   - Position the bur over the pulpal floor next to the remaining marginal ridge, cut the ditch gingivally along the exposed DEJ.
   - 2/3rd of the expense of the dentin (0.5 to 0.6mm)
   - 1/3rd at the expense of the enamel (0.2 to 0.3mm)
   - Pressure is directed gingivally and the bur move facially and lingually.
   - *Gingival seat is located 1-2mm below the contact area.*
   - *Axial depth of gingival seat is about 0.6 to 0.8mm in dentin.*
   - Proximal ditch cut may be diverged gingivally to make the facial lingual extension gingivally greater than occlusal and this is done by using no. 245 inverted cone bur.
   - Removing the remaining undermined enamel with enamel hatchet in a scrapping motion on facioproximal, linguoproximal and gingival wall.

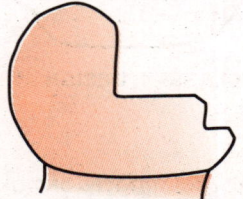

PROXIMAL OUTLINE FORM

3. Primary Resistance form
   - Flat and perpendicular pulpal and gingival walls to resist forces directed with long axis of the tooth.

— Restricting the extension of walls to allow strong cusp ridges to remain with sufficient dentin support.

— Restricting the occlusal step.

— Reverse curve at the junction of occlusal step and proximal box gives strength to amalgam and tooth.

— *Internal line angles are rounded.*

— *Axiopulpal line angle is rounded.*

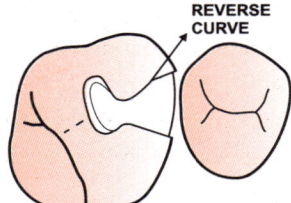

4. *Primary Retention form*

— Occlusal convergence of facial and lingual proximal wall.

— Dovetail design on the occlusal step.

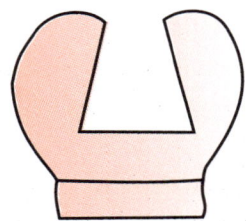

5. *Convenience form*

— It is achieved by extension of mesial, distal, facial, lingual walls and also facio proximal, linguo proximal and gingival walls.

B. FINAL TOOTH PREPARATION

— Removal of any remaining defective enamel and infected carious dentin.

— Removal of old restoration.

— Infected carious dentin is removed with slow speed round bur or discoid type spoon excavator.

1. *Pulp Protection*

— Base applied is - Zinc poly carboxylate or Zinc phosphate.

2. *Secondary Resistance and Retention form*

— Restricting of extension of external walls.

— *Bevelling the axiopulpal line angle.*

— Induction of retentive locks located occlusal to the axiopulpal line angle prove more resistance.

— Proximal retentive locks in the axiofacial and axiolingal line angles.

— Induction of grooves in the proximal box.

— The occlusal convergence of the facial and lingual wall and the dovetail design provide sufficient retention form.

— Introduction of proximal locks by using No. 169L bur.

3. *Procedure for finishing external walls*

— Preparation walls should be free of unsupported enamel rods and marginal irregularities.

— 90° degree cavosurface angle at the proximal margin.

— Use GMT to establish a slight cavosurface bevel at the gingival margin.

— Prepared tooth is cleaned and inspected before restoration.

— Disinfectants are used for cleaning tooth preparation.

DESIGNS OF CLASS - 2 CAVITY PREPARATION

1. Class 2, Design - 1 (Conventional Design)

— *Involves proximal and occlusal surfaces.*

— Indications

1. Moderate to large size proximal lesion with the involvement of occlusal surface.

2. Proximal lesion undermining an adjacent marginal ridge or not accessible through any other means but involvement of the occlusal surfaces.

3. A class - 2 in stress bearing areas.

4. An oral environment where local cariogenic conditions contraindicate a modern design.

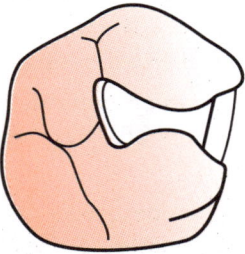

CLASS - 2, DESIGN - 1

2. Class - 2, Design - 2 (Modern Design)

— *Involves proximal and occlusal surfaces.*

— Indications

1. A moderate to small sized proximal lesions.

2. A class - 2 in a stress bearing area.

3. An occlusal lesion undermining one or both marginal ridges and not exceeding a width of 1/4 of the intercuspal distance.

3. **Class - 2, Design - 3 (Conservative Design)**

   – *Involves primarily the proximal surface and a very limited part of the occlusal surface not extending beyond the adjacent triangular fossa.*

   – Indications

1. The decay is restricted to the proximal surface only and the occlusal surface is completely sound.

2. When the restoration is expected to be subjected to minimal loading.

3. There are sound pronounced occlusal crossing ridges and the inclined planes of the adjacent cusps are smooth and are devoid of any crossing fissures.

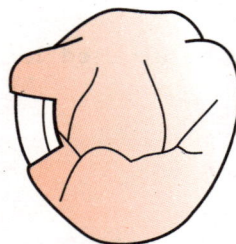

CLASS - 3, DESIGN - 3

4. **Class - 2, Design - 4 (Simple Design)**

   – *Involves proximal surfaces only.*

   – Indications

1. Decay is restricted to contacting or proximal surfaces without undermining the corresponding marginal ridges.

2. When there is diastema or the adjacent tooth is missing and facilitating direct access.

3. The affected tooth is rotated or inclined so that the contacting surface is not the anatomical proximal one, again facilitating access.

4. The proximal lesion is located very gingivally at or apical to the CEJ, accompanied by gingival recession.

5. The proximal lesion occurs on tapered teeth with wide gingival embrasures facilitating facial or lingual access to the lesion.

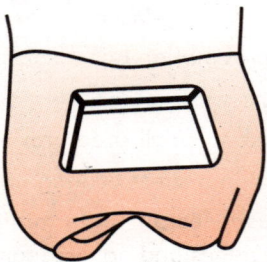

CLASS - 2, DESIGN - 4

5. **Class - 2, Design - 5**

   – *Involves part of the proximal surface with a very limited access area on the facial and lingual areas.*

   – Indications

1. Small to medium sized proximal lesions.

2. Restoration is expected to be subjected to normal displacing forces.

3. Marginal ridge is intact and adequately supported apically and occlusally.

4. Lesion does not involve the contact area nor does it undermine enamel in the contact area.

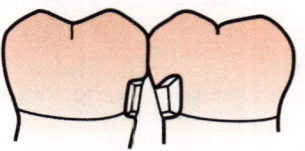

CLASS - 2, DESIGN - 5

6. **Class - 2, Design - 6**

   – *Involves the occlusal, proximal and part of the facial and / or lingual surfaces.*

   – Indications

1. Cusp is completely missing or undermined.

2. The cusp length is double or more its width either throughout or at certain portions of the cusp.

3. When a foundation for cast restoration is required.

4. Teeth with a doubtful prognosis both endodontically and periodontally.

5. A cast restoration is not indicated.

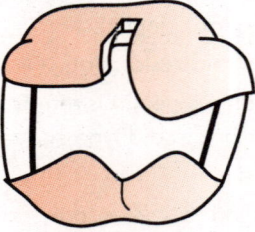

CLASS - 2, DESIGN - 6

7. **Class - 2, Design - 7 (Combination of Class - 2 with Class - 5)**

   Shape A : The junction between the class - 2 and Class - 2 via the proximal, crossing the axial angles.

   – *Involves the occlusal, proximal and part or all of the gingival third of the facial and or lingual surfaces with the intervening part of the axial angle.*

– Indications

1. A location apical to the contact area, an occluso-proximal lesion joins a senile decay.

2. Class - 5 lesion undermines enamel or directly involves tooth structure of the adjacent axial angles in a tooth having a proximo occlusal lesion.

3. Surface defects or decalcifications at the axial angle of the tooth are continuous with a proximo occlusal cavity preparation or lesion apical to the contact area.

Shape B : The junction between the class - 2 and Class - 5 is through the occlusal via the buccal and or lingual grooves.

– *Involves the proximal, occlusal, facial and or lingual surfaces.*

– Indications

1. A class - 5 lesion connecting with an occluso proximal lesion via a facial or lingual fissured groove.

2. Surface defects or decalcifications on the facial or lingual surface connecting a class - 5 lesion with an occluso proximal lesion.

3. A class - 5 lesion which is continuous with a Class - 1, Design 4 which inturn is continuous with an occluso proximal lesion.

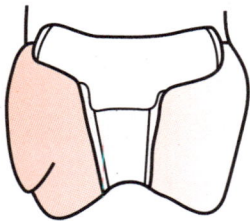

CLASS 2, DESIGN - 7

8. Class - 2, Design - 8

– *Involves two or more surfaces of an endodontically treated tooth that does not require post retention.*

– Indications

1. The remaining tooth structure, after endodontics can support and retain an amalgam restorations.

2. The tooth has a sufficient pulp chamber to accommodate, retaining, self resisting amalgam bulk, i.e. a minimum 2 mm thickness in three dimensions.

3. The post endodontic pulp chamber has at least two opposing intact walls.

4. The tooth contains sufficiently large root canals to accommodate, retaining, resisting amalgam bulk at its occlusal 1/3rd.

5. A foundation is needed for a reinforcing restoration.

MODIFICATIONS IN TOOTH PREPARATION FOR CLASS - 2 CAVITY

1. Rotated Teeth

– Tooth preparation for rotated teeth follows the same principles as normally aligned teeth.

– The outline form for a tooth preparation on the rotated mandibular second premolar differ from normal, i.e. proximal box is displaced facially as the proximal caries involves the mesiofacial line angle of the tooth crown.

– In case the tooth is rotated to 90 degrees, then the preparation requires an isthmus that includes the cuspal eminence.

– If in case the lesion is small, then slot preparation is required.

2. Unusual Outline Form

– The outline form should conform to the restoration, requirement of the restoration.

Example

1. Usually a dovetail is not required in the occlusal step of a single proximal surface preparation unless a fissure, emanating from the occlusal step is involved.

2 In an occlusal fissure, i.e. segmented by coalesced enamel, if the preparations are separated by approximately 0.5 mm or more of sound tooth structure then it should be restored with individual amalgam restoration.

3. Adjoining Restorations

– When two restorations adjoin, care must be taken that the outline of the second restoration does not weaken the amalgam margin of the first.

– The preparation requires, that the intersecting margins of the two restoration be at right angles.

4. Abutment Teeth for Removable Partial Denture

– When the tooth is an abutment for a planned removable partial denture, the occlusoproximal outline form adjacent to edentulous area needs additional extension for the rest seat.

– If the rest seat is to be within the amalgam margins then 0.5 mm of amalgam between the rest seat and the margins is recommended.

– If the rest seat involves both amalgam and enamel no modification of the outline form of the tooth preparation is indicated.

5. Tunnelling / Amalgam Tunnel Tooth Restorations

 – This preparation joins an occlusal lesion with a proximal lesion by means of a prepared tunnel under the involved marginal ridge.

 – Marginal ridge remains essentially intact.

 – Developing appropriately formed preparation walls and excavating caries may be compromised by lack of access and visibility.

6. Amalgam Box-only Tooth Restorations

 – Box only tooth preparations are advocated for posterior teeth in which a proximal surface requires restoration but the occusal surface is not faulty.

 – Proximal box is prepared and specific retention form is provided.

 – An occlusal step is included.

 – These restorations are more conservative as less tooth structure is removed.

REVERSE CURVE

 – *The external outline of the occlusal surface where the isthmus joins the buccal proximal flare is often in the form of a convex or a straight line. When the position of the isthmus and the proximal external outline becomes substantially offset buccal-lingually, a reverse curve taking the form of a concave curve is used as a means of conserving sound tooth tissue.*

 – *Significance :* Preserves the triangular ridge of the affected cusp.

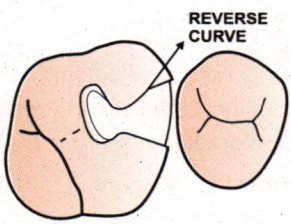

CLASS - 3 CAVITY PREPARATION

 – This is the basic design for the distal aspect of cuspids.
 – A lingual access preparation is recommended.

A. INITIAL TOOTH PREPARATION

 – Outline form is similar to the conventional class - 3 composite preparation.

 – No. 2 bur is used for initial entry on distolingual marginal ridge and bur penetrates the carious lesion beneath contact area.

 – Bur is positioned perpendicular to lingual surface of the tooth.

 – Initial axial depth is 0.5 to 0.6 mm into the DEJ.

 – The cavosurface angle should be 90 degree at all margins.

 – Internal line angles are rounded.

B. FINAL TOOTH PREPARATION

 – Removal of remaining infected dentin.

 – Finishing of external walls.

 – Secondary retention form is provided by gingival groove in the axiofacio gingival point angle and it is positioned in the dentin of 0.2 mm between the groove and the DEJ.

 – Alternatively retention is obtained by Incisal cove and Lingual dovetail.

 – Axiopupal line angle is bevelled using gingival margin trimmer.

 – Remove any unsupported enamel, smoothen the enamel walls and margins and refine cavosurface angles.

 – Completed tooth preparation is carefully inspected and cleaned.

CLASS - 5 CAVITY PREPARATION

A. INITIAL TOOTH PREPARATION

 – Enter the carious lesion using a tapered surface bur of suitable size.

 – Use the edge of the end of the bur to penetrate the area.

 – Bur is maintained to ensure that all the external walls are perpendicular to the external tooth surface.

 – Initial axial depth is 0.5 mm inside the DEJ.

 – And if the root surface is involved, the axial depth, is approximately 0.75 mm.

 – For tooth preparation, which is extended inciso gingivally, the axial wall should be more convex.

 – Round bur is used to define internal line angles.

B. FINAL TOOTH PREPARATION

 – Remove the remaining infected dentin with No. 2 or No. 4 round bur.

- Remove the old restoration.
- Use a No. 1/4 bur to prepare two retention grooves, one on incisoaxial line angle and other, on gingivoaxial line angle.
- Or alternatively four retention coves may be prepared, one in each of the four axial point angles.
- Depth of grooves : 0.25 mm.
- In case of inadequate accessibility an angle former chisel can be used to prepare the retention form.
- Clean the preparation.
- Inspect for completeness.

FAILURES OF AMALGAM RESTORATIONS

- The causes are,

1. **Wrong selection of cases**
   - Amalgam restoration is not suitable for very large caries involving multiple surfaces.

2. **Improper cavity preparations**
   - It affects the resistance and retention of amalgam restoration leading to fracture or dislodgement of restoration.

3. **Delayed expansion**
   - Due to moisture contamination the Zinc content of amalgam reacts to release hydrogen gas and causes pressure effects and pain.

4. **Inadequate cleaning of the cavity**

5. **Inadequate pulp protection**
- Results in microleakage causing secondary caries and pain.

6. **Inadequate matrix application**
- Causes improper interproximal contours, overhanging restoration which further leads to food impaction and periodontal disease.

7. **Improper manipulation of materials**
   i. *Improper selection of amalgam*
   ii. *Improper Hg / Alloy Ratio*
      - Decreased strength
      - Increased creep
      - Increased expansion of Amalgam
      - Decreased corrosion resistance

iii. *Improper trituration*
iv. *Improper condensation*
   - High condensation: Amalgam constriction
   - Low condensation: Amalgam expansion
   - Low Condensation Pressure :
     - Decreased strength
     - Increased creep rate
     - Decreased corrosion resistance

8. **Improper or Non carved amalgam are susceptible to fracture.**

9. **Failure to polish decreases corrosion resistance.**

FINISHING AND POLISHING OF AMALGAM RESTORATIONS

- Finishing of amalgam restoration is necessary to correct a marginal discrepancy or improve the contour.
- Amalgam polishing is done usually after 24 hours of insertion because crystallization is not complete within 24 hours.

1. **Occlusal Surfaces**
   - Any irregularities are removed with Green stones. Stones are tapered or inverted cone.

   Initial polishing
   A. Unwebbed rubber cup and soft cup brush with a slurry of silex is used.
   B. Finishing burs of different sizes and shapes.

2. **Proximal Surfaces**
   - Overhangs are eliminated with No. 12 BP blade or Gold foil knives or spoon excavators.

   Finishing and polishing
   - Narrow, fine water resistant finishing strips and / or dental tape are placed beneath the contact and passed back and forth.

3. **Buccal and Lingual proximal margins**
   - Finished with adequately fixed extra fine water proof disk.

4. **Final Polishing**
   - Of the occlusal surface and accessible area of proximal surface : with a fine grit rubber polishing point or with the rubber cup with flour of pumice followed by a high luster agent such as precipitated chalk.

CHAPTER 09

COMPLEX AMALGAM RESTORATIONS

PIN RETAINED AMALGAM RESTORATIONS

– Pin retained amalgam restorations are defined as any restoration requiring placement of one or more pins for providing adequate retention.

INDICATIONS

1. It is mainly indicated to restore badly broken young permanent teeth where there is insufficient amount of dentin present to get retention form, by means of grooves or slots but sufficient amount of dentin present for placement of pins.
2. It can be used as a transitional restoration prior to endodontic, periodontic, orthodontic treatments.
3. Pin retention is required in foundations for partial or full veneer cast restoration or metalo-ceramic restorations.
4. As an auxiliary or reciprocal retention.

CONTRAINDICATIONS

1. In extremely large pulp chamber (due to insufficient amount of dentin for placement of pins).
2. Subgingivally deep calculus.

ADVANTAGES

1. More conservation of tooth structure.
2. Less time consuming.
3. Economic.

DISADVANTAGES

1. Since pins help only in retention but will does reinforce amalgam, it cannot be used in very high stress bearing area.
2. Difficult to achieve proper contact and contour.
3. Risk of possibility of perforation of pulp, or periodontal ligament space unless skillfully done.
4. Microleakage.
5. Decreased tensile strength of silver.

GUIDELINES FOR THE PLACEMENT OF PINS

– Pin should be located close to the line angles of tooth.
– Pin hole should be at least 0-5 mm from the Dentinoenamel junction.
– The optimum interpin distance is 5 mm.
– Pins should be placed so that their axes are not parallel.
– Pins should be placed 0.5 mm from the vertical wall of the tooth.

- The fewest number of pins which will provide adequate retention should be used.
- The choice of pin size should be made on the basis of the amount of tooth structure remaining and need for retention.
- Increase in diameter increases retention.
- Pin retention increases with increased embedment in dentin.
- The optimum length of a pin is 2 mm.
- The number of pins placed varies with amount of tooth structure lost.
- Ex: For molar - 1 pin per missing cusp.
  For premolars - 2 pins per missing cusp.

TYPES OF PINS

- Classified on the basis of *retentive mechanism,*
  1. Cemented pins
  2. Friction lock (Frictional grip pins)
  3. Self threading / self shearing pins

1. CEMENTED PINS

- In this type, *pin channel is larger in diameter than the pin.*
- Available in two sizes,

Pin channel diameter	Pin diameter
(1) 0.027″	0.025″
(2) 0.021″	0.020″

Indications

1. Ideal for all pin retained restorations (as it creates least crazing and stresses in the tooth).
2. Only technique to be used for endodontically treated teeth.
3. Only techniques to be used when the pin location is very close to DEJ (0.5-1.0 mm distance is enough).
4. Only technique for using U- and L- shaped pins in Class-4 restorations and foundations.
5. Used when limited bulk of dentin is available for pin placement.
6. Ideal technique for a sclerosed, tertiary, calcified barrier or any other highly mineralized or dehydrated dentin.
7. Only technique for the cross-linking of two parts of the same tooth.

Disadvantages

1. Cementing medium is necessary for its retention.

2. Least retentive.
3. Requires additional step, in technique for the cementation.
   - Pin holes are placed at a depth of 3 to 4 mm.
   - Reinforced ZOE or GIC is used for the cementation of pin.

2. FRICTION LOCK PINS

- *The pin channel is slightly narrower in diameter than the pin.*
- Available in one size,

Pin channel diameter	Pin diameter
0.021″	0.022″

Indications

- Least used of all pin techniques because of the following requirements,
1. Should be used in vital teeth only.
2. At least 4 mm bulk of dentin should be present around the pin (in all three dimensions).
3. Pin should be located at least 2.5 mm from the DEJ.
4. Should be used only in the accessible areas of the mouth (so that the seating force will be parallel to the long axis of the pin).

Disadvantages

1. Maximum stresses are exhibited.
2. Strict indications
   - Pin holes are placed at a depth of 2-3 mm.
   - It is retained by frictional resistance and resiliency of dentin.
   - These are 2-3 times more retentive than cemented pins.

3. SELF THREADED PINS

- *The pin channel diameter is narrower than the pin.*
- Available as,

Pin channel diameter	Pin diameter
0.027″	0.031″
0.021″	0.023″
0.018″	0.020″
0.013″	0.015″

Indications

- It is the most applicable and feasible technique.
1. Used for vital teeth.
2. The dentin to be engaged for the pin (whether it is primary or secondary) should be properly hydrated.
3. Pin location should be at least 1.5 mm from DEJ.
4. When a minimal number of pins are needed.
5. When the maximum retention is needed.

Disadvantages

Dentinal trauma may be caused as the threads cut into the tooth structure.

- Pin holes are placed at a depth of 1.3 - 2 mm
- They rely on the mechanical grasp of the threads into dentin.
- They are 2-3 times more retentive than the cemented pins.

PIN-CHANNEL PREPARATION

- Three basic instruments are used for the preparation.

1. *The Twist drill*

- It is an end cutting, revolving instrument with two blades, bibevelled in longitudinal section.
- It should be used at ultra low speed (300 - 500 RPM).
- Should be used in direct cutting acts and do not use in lateral cuttings as it widens the pin channel and lead to drill fracture.
- Should be finished in one or two thrusts.
- Never use the drill in enamel as they do not cut enamel and become dull.

2. *No.1, 2 or 3 round burs :* Are used to establish a leading hole in the center of which pin channel drilling is started. This avoids the skidding of the twist drill.

3. *Measuring probes or depth gauge* are used to verify the depth of the pin channel.

Danger areas for Pin Placement

1. Mesial surface of upper 1st premolar.
2. Mesiobuccal line angles of upper and lower first molar.

Failure of Pin-retained Restorations

- Failure may occur,
  1. Within the restoration : restoration fracture.
  2. At the interface between the pin and the restorative material : pin restoration separation.
  3. Within the Pin: Pin fracture.

4. At the interface between Pin and dentin Pin dentin separation.
5. Within the dentin : dentin fracture.

Failure locations for different types of pins

1. In case of cemented pins, failure usually occurs at the cement dentin interface.
2. In case of Friction grip pins, failure always occurs at the pin dentin interface.
3. In case of small threaded pins, failure usually occurs within pin themselves.
4. In case of large threaded (regular) pin, failure usually occurs in the dentin itself.

Pin Hole Perforations

- Whenever a pin hole is placed, the tooth is examined for possible perforations.
- The tooth is dried and an endodontic paper point should be placed in the pin hole.
- If a perforation exists paper point will become moistened.
- If no perforation the paper point should be dry.
- Pulpal perforation is treated by placing a calcium hydroxide intermediary base into the pin hole.
- Periodontal perforations are sealed using amalgam.

Enlarged Pinholes

- If the pin fails to engage itself and the threads do not hold the pin, then the pin hole is too large.
- To overcome this one can,
  - Drill the hole deeper and reinsert a fresh pin.
  - Redrill a larger hole and use a larger pin.
  - Cement the existing pin in place.

MECHANICS OF PIN-RETAINED RESTORATIONS

A. Stressing Capability of Pins

1. *Type of pins*

- Maximum stresses are associated with friction grip pins.
- Little or no stresses with cemented pins.
- Intermediate stresses with Threaded pins when compared to other pins.

2. *Diameter of pins*

- The greater the diameter of the pin, the greater will be the stress induction.

3. *Depth of the pin*

- The greater the depth of the pin channel, the greater will be stress induction.

4. *Bulk of dentin*

   — The greater the amount of dentin pulpally or toward the surface from the pin, the lesser will be the stress induction.

5. *Types of dentin*

   — Primary dentin of young teeth is least affected by stress induction due to its high elastic and plastic limit.

   — The greater the mineralization and dehydration of the dentin, the lesser will be the dentinal tolerance to the stresses.

   — *The order of stress tolerance of different types of dentin in the decreasing order is primary dentin, secondary dentin, sclerosed dentin, tertiary dentin and calcific barrier.*

   — Stress tolerance is greatly decreased when the dentin looses its vitality.

   — Accordingly, threaded or frictional grip pins are not used in endodontically treated teeth and in the dentinal areas with dead tract formation. So cemented pins are routinely used in this situation.

   — Friction grip and threaded pins are not used in the areas of tertiary dentin, sclerosed dentin and calcific barrier. Cemented pins are preferred for this.

6. *The inter-pin distance*

   — The lesser the distance between the pins, the greater will be the concentration of stresses.

7. *Number of pins*

   — The lesser the number of pins per tooth, the less will be the stresses.

B. Retention of Pins

1. *Types of pins*

   — Cemented pins are least retentive.

   — Friction grip pins are 2-3 times more retentive than cemented pins.

   — Self-threading pins are 5-6 times more retentive than cemented pins.

2. *Shape of the pin channel relative to the pin*

   — Greater the coincidence between these two shapes the better will be the retention.

3. *Number of pins*

   — Pin location and its proximity relative to displacing forces (not the total no. of pins per tooth) affects the retention.

   — Pins placed closer than 2 mm to each other in a tooth results in the loss of retention.

4. *Surface texture of pins*

   — Pins with surface serrations or threading have good retention.

5. *Type of Dentin*

   — The decreasing order of pin retention of different types of dentin is primary dentin> tubular secondary dentin> scleorosed dentin> calcific barrier> dehydrated dentin (non vital dentin).

6. *Bulk of the dentin around the pin*

   — Greater the amount of dentin separating pins from the pulp, tooth and root surface, the greater will be the retention.

7. *Types of cement : (For cemented pins)*

   — The decreasing order of retention for different types of cement is copper-phosphate cement> $Zn PO_4$ > polycarboxylate > ZOE.

SLOT RETAINED AMALGAM RESTORATIONS

— *Slot is a retention groove in dentin whose length is in a horizontal plane.*

— Slots are particularly indicated in short clinical crowns and in cusps that have been reduced 2 to 3 mm for amalgam. Compared to pin placement more tooth structure is removed in preparing slots.

— Slots are less likely to create microfractures in the dentin and to perforate the tooth or penetrate into the pulp.

Tooth Preparation

— Slot length depends on the extent of the tooth preparation.

— Slots are usually placed on the facial, lingual, mesial and distal aspects of the preparation.

— The slot may be continuous or segmented, depending on the amount of missing tooth structure and whether pins were used.

— Slots are generally 0.5 to 1 mm in depth and the width of the No. 33 1/2 bur. Their length is usually 2 to 4 mm, depending on the distance between the remaining vertical walls. No. 33 1/2 bur is used to place a slot in the gingival floor 0.5 mm axial of the DEJ.

— Slots can be used in combination with pins to generate additional retention and resistance forms.

AMALGAPIN

- Introduced by Shavell in 1980 for complex amalgam restorations.
- A round end bur is used for placing 2 to 3 mm deep holes.
- Amalgam is then condensed into the holes and the remainder of the restoration is condensed and carved.

- These amalgapin chambers are much larger by volume than the pinholes.
- The shear strength of the amalgapin is weaker than an amalgam with self threaded pins.

Indication

- Weak gingival areas.

Disadvantage

- Associated with greater tooth substance removal.

CHAPTER 10

ESTHETIC RESTORATIONS

ESTHETIC RESTORATIVE MATERIALS

1. FUSED PORCELAIN
- Refer 'DENTAL CERAMICS'.

2. SILICATE CEMENT
- First translucent material, introduced in 1878 by Fletcher in England.
- Recommended for small restorations in anterior teeth of patients with high caries activity.
- Liner or base required to protect pulp tissue from irritation due to initial low pH of material.

Advantages
- Tooth matching ability
- Ease of manipulation
- Anticariogenic
- Good insulator

Disadvantages
- Discolouration
- Loss of contour

3. ACRYLIC RESINS
- Developed in Germany in 1930.

Uses
- As a restoration, most successful in protected areas of teeth where temperature change, abrasion and stress are minimal.
- Esthetic veneer on facial surface of class - 3 and class - 4 metal restorations.
- Temporary restorations in operative and fixed prosthodontic indirect restoration procedures.

Disadvantages
- Poor wear resistance.
- Low strength and would flow under load.
- Discolouration at the margins because of polymerization shrinkage and microleakage.

4. GLASS IONOMERS

1. Conventional glass ionomers
- Developed first by Wilson and Kent in 1972.

Advantages
- Anticariogenic effect
- Favourable co-efficient of thermal expansion
- Tooth coloured
- Chemical adhesion
- Less soluble compared to silicate cement

Disadvantages

   – Low resistance to wear.

   – Low strength compared to composite or amalgam.

2. **Resin Modified Glass Ionomers**

   – Refer 'DENTAL CEMENTS'.

3. **Compomers (Poly acid modified composites)**

   – Refer 'DENTAL CEMENTS'.

5. COMPOSITES

COMPOSITES

– Introduced by Bowen in 1962.

COMPOSITION

1. **Resin matrix :** a plastic resin material that forms a continuous phase and binds the filler particles Ex: BIS-GMA, TEGDMA.

2. **Fillers :** reinforcing particles and/or fibers that are dispersed in the matrix Ex: Silica.

   Purpose

   1. Increases strength, hardness and wear resistance.
   2. Reduces polymerization shrinkage.
   3. Reduces thermal expansion and contraction.
   4. Improves workability.
   5. Reduces water sorption, softening and staining.
   6. Increased radiopacity.

3. **Coupling agent :** Bonding agent that promotes adhesion between filler and resin matrix Ex. organosilanes, zirconates, titanates, etc.

4. **Activator :** Generates free radicals ; chemical activator is tertiary amine; external energy activation is by heat, light or microwave.

5. **Initiator :** Initiates the polymerization Ex: Benzylperoxide.

6. **Inhibitor :** Minimizes or prevent spontaneous or accidental polymerization of monomers. Ex: Butylated Hydroxy Toluene (BHT).

7. **Opacifiers :** Ex: Titanium dioxide, Aluminium oxide.

INDICATIONS

1. Class - 1, 2, 3, 4, 5 and 6 restorations.
2. Pit and fissure sealants.
3. Esthetic enhancement procedures, i.e. veneers, tooth contour modifications, diastema closures, etc.
4. Core buildups.
5. Splinting purpose.
6. Cements (for indirect restorations).
7. Temporary restorations.

CONTRAINDICATIONS

1. Grossly destructed tooth
2. Areas difficult to isolate

ADVANTAGES

1. Esthetics
2. Conservation of tooth structure
3. Bonded to tooth structure
4. Good retention
5. Minimal interfacial staining
6. Repairable
7. Insulative

DISADVANTAGES

1. polymerization shrinkage
2. technique sensitive
3. difficult to finish and polish
4. difficult to establish proximal, axial contours and embrasures
5. greater occlusal wear
6. time consuming
7. not economic

CLASSIFICATION

I. Based on filler particle size and size distribution

Sl. No.	Type	Size
1.	Traditional (large particle)	1–50 μm
2.	Hybrid (large particle)	0.04–20 μm
3.	Hybrid (mid filer)	0.04–10 μm
4.	Hybrid (minifiller/small particle filled)	0.04–2 μm
5.	Packable hybrid	Midfiller/minifiller hybrid with lower than fraction.
6.	Flowable hybrid	Midfiller hybrid with finer particle size distribution.
7.	Homogenous microfill	0.04 μm
8.	Heterogeneous microfill	0.04 μm

II. Based on curing mechanism
1. Chemically activated
2. Light activated
   i. U.V. Light
   ii. Visible light

1. CONVENTIONAL/TRADITIONAL/MACRO FILLED COMPOSITES

– *Contain 75% to 80% inorganic filler by weight.*

– *Average particle size is 8 μm.*

Disadvantages

– Rough surface texture.

– Resin matrix wears at faster rate than filler particles.

– More susceptible to discolouration from extrinsic staining.

– Higher amount of initial wear at occlusal contacts.

2. MICROFILLED COMPOSITES: (Polishable Composites)

– Designed in 1970 to replace rough surface characteristic of conventional composites with a smooth lustrous surface similar to tooth enamel.

– *Particle size is 0.01 to 0.04 μm.*

– *Inorganic filler 35 to 60% by weight.*

– Soft or friable glass such as strontium and / or barium-composite is made radio opaque.

Advantages

– Produces smoothest restorative surface.

– Low modulus of elasticity allow microfill composite restorations to flex during tooth flexure thus better protecting bonding interface.

– Clinically very wear resistant.

Disadvantages

– Inferior physical and mechanical properties.

3. HYBRID COMPOSITES

Definition

– *A particle-filled resin that contains a graded blend of small and colloidal silica filler particles to achieve an optimal balance among the properties of strength, polymerization shrinkage, wear resistance and polishability.*

– *Filler content : 75 to 85% by weight.*

– *Average particle size : 0.4 to 1.0 μm.*

Classification and uses

– *Based on filler size,*

1. *Hybrid (large filler)*

   – For high stress areas requiring improved polishability (class - 1, 2, 3 and 4).

2. *Hybrid (Mid filler)*

   – For high stress areas requiring improved polishability (class - 3 and 4).

3. *Hybrid [minifiller/small particle filled (SPF)]*

   – For moderate stress areas requiring optimal polishability (Class - 3 and 4).

Advantages

1. Smooth surface
2. Good strength
3. Can be used for stress-bearing and posterior restorations

Disadvantages

– inferior mechanical properties than SPF composites.

4. FLOWABLE COMPOSITES

Definition

– *A hybrid composite with reduced filler level and a more narrow particle size distribution that increases flow and promotes intimate adaptation to prepared tooth surfaces.*

– *Filler content : 40 to 60% by weight.*

– *Average particle size : 0.6 to 1.0 μm.*

Uses

1. Preventive resin restorations
2. Cavity liners
3. Restoration repairs
4. Cervical restorations
5. Small class I restorations
6. Low stress bearing restorations

Advantages

1. Easy to use
2. Favourable wettability
3. Good handling properties

Disadvantages

1. Lower filler content
2. Inferior physical properties
3. Higher polymerization shrinkage
4. Lower wear resistance

5. PACKABLE COMPOSITES

Definition

- A hybrid resin composite designed for use in posterior areas, where a stiffer consistency facilitates condensation in posterior teeth.
- Filler content : 65-81% by weight.
- Size :fibrous form.

Uses

- For use in class - 1, 2 and 4 cavity preparations.

Advantages

1. High depth of cure
2. Low polymerization shrinkage
3. Radiopacity
4. Low wear rate

Disadvantages

1. increased viscosity
2. resistance to packing

COMPOSITES FOR POSTERIOR RESTORATIONS

- These are available in two forms,
    1. Direct posterior composites
    2. Indirect posterior composites

1. DIRECT POSTERIOR COMPOSITES

Indications

1. Esthetics
2. Need for conservation of tooth structure
3. To minimize thermal conduction

Contraindications

1. Not to be used for cuspal coverage.
2. Large restorations exceeding one-third the buccolingual width of the tooth.
3. Patients with parafunctional habits.

Types of composites used

1. Traditional composites
2. Hybrid composites
3. Microfilled composites
4. Packable composites

2. INDIRECT POSTERIOR COMPOSITES

- Indirect composites for fabrication of onlays are polymerized outside the oral environment and luted to the tooth with a compatible resin cement.

Methods of Resin Inlay fabrication

1. Direct fabrication

- Application of the separating medium to the prepared tooth.
- The restorative resin pattern is then formed, light cured and removed from the preparation.
- The rough inlay is then exposed to additional light for approximately 4 to 6 min or heat activated at approximately 100°C for 7 min.
- Then the preparation is etched.
- Now the inlay is cemented into the place with a dual cure resin and it is then polished.

2. Indirect fabrication

- Indirect inlay resin requires an impression and is fabricated in the laboratory.
- In addition to conventional light and heat curing, laboratory processing may employ heat (150° C) and pressure (0.6 mpa for 10 min) for the fabrication.

POLYMERIZATION OF COMPOSITES

Methods of Polymerization

A. Self cured composites

- Contains catalyst and base.
- Since components are mixed, there is greater chance for air inclusion in mixture and therefore greater internal porosity.
- Working time to insert self cured material is restricted by speed of chemical reaction.
- Requires increased finishing time.
- Less colour stable because of eventual breakdown of polymerization initiating chemical ingredients, tertiary amines.
- Direction of polymerization shrinkage of self cured materials is generally centralized (towards center of mass). This may help maintain marginal adaptation to prevent microleakage.

B. Light cured materials

- Provide increased working time.
- Require less finishing time.
- Exhibit greater colour stability and less internal porosity.
- Effects of polymerization shrinkage can be partially compensated by an incremental insertion technique and positioning light source close to material.
- Light curing mechanisms.

- Quartz / tungsten / halogen
- Light curing units
- Plasma arc curing
- Argon laser curing
- Blue light emitting diodes—Less polymerization shrinkage more efficient, cooler, portable.

Polymerization Shrinkage

- Composites shrink while hardening, it is referred to as polymerization shrinkage.
- Polymerization shrinkage usually does not cause significant problems with restorations cured in preparations having all enamel margins.
- However, when a tooth preparation has extended onto a root surface, polymerization shrinkage can cause a gap formation at the junction of composite and root surface.
- The V - shaped gap occurs because of the force of polymerisation of composite is greater than the initial bond strength of composite to dentin of the root.
- The V - shaped gap is probably composed of composite on restoration side and hybridized dentin on root side.

ACID ETCHING

- It was conceived by Michael Buonocore in 1950's.

Purpose

1. Increases the mechanical retention of the restoration.
2. Better wetting of the resin.
3. Increases surface area which inturn increases the potential for bonding.

Indications

1. Support of Class - 1 and 2 posterior restorations.
2. Class - 3 restorations.
3. Class - 4 incisal angles of anterior teeth.
4. Class - 5 in occlusal or incisal enamel as added retention.

Mechanism of Action

- The acid leaves a clean enamel surface which permits the increased wetting of the surface by resin.
- The acid attacks the enamel surface leaving microscopic surface irregularities with peaks and valleys in the enamel which allow for mechanical interlocking.

Procedure

1. *Dentin and Pulp Protection*

- Prior to the application of acid for etching, the dentin must be protected by placing a liner. If a liner is not placed, the acid causes irritation to the pulp.

- For this purpose light activated glass ionomer is the preferred liner.

2. *Method*

- Phosphoric acid may be brush applied or injected in viscous gel form.
- Brush is recommended because, 1. the fine tip confines the acid to the enamel periphery. 2. the soft bristles prevent a heavy rubbing or scrubbing mode of acid application which may result in decreased retention caused by the fracture of interstitial enamel surrounding the micropores.

3. *Time*

- The acid should be applied for a period of 15 to 20 seconds.
- Prolonged etching does not improve the bond.
- The application time should be increased to 1 minute for fluorosed or deciduous enamel because both are relatively resistant to the etching procedure.

4. *Acid concentration*

- 30%-40% concentration is most reliable, effective.

5. *Type of Acid*

i. Aqueous solutions are easy to apply but difficult to control because of their free flow nature.

ii. High viscosity gels can be readily controlled clinically; particularly used in the treatment of cervical erosion lesions by means of dentin bonding materials and in posterior composite restorations.

6. *Post etch cleaning*

- After acid etching, the enamel surface should be thoroughly cleaned by means of a copious water lavage for atleast 15 or 30 seconds.
- Failure in thorough cleaning results in bond failure.

7. *Drying the enamel surface*

- Drying should never be accomplished with a dual air water syringe because this cause micro contamination of enamel surface with microdroplets of water.
- Warm air drying is preferred though chemical drying agents are also in use.
- After drying the enamel surface should present a chalky white opaque appearance and this is the critical state because it is most sensitive to contamination.
- If contamination occurs, it should be cleaned by the application of phosphoric acid for a period of 15 to 20 seconds.

Special Considerations

1. Teeth of patients rinsed on a fluoride water supply possess enamel that is resistant to decalcification and often require reapplication of the acid etching procedure.

2. Immature enamel in a child is more rapidly etched than mature enamel in the adult patient.

CONDITIONING OF THE CAVITY

Purpose

– Removes the smear layer.

– Opens the dentinal tubules, increases dentin permeability and decalcification of the intertubular and peritubular dentin, exposing collagen fibres there by formation of smear plugs which increases bonding.

Conditioning agents

1. Orthophosphoric acid (37%) for composites.
2. Polyacrylic acid (10%) for GIC.
3. Citric acid (50%) for root conditioning.
4. Pumice wash.

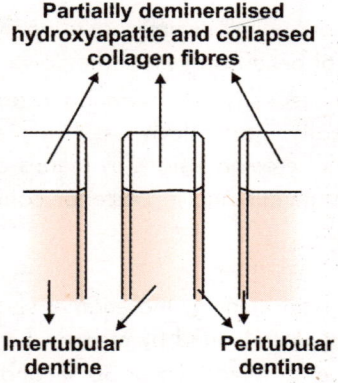

Partiallly demineralised hydroxyapatite and collapsed collagen fibres

Intertubular dentine   **Peritubular dentine**

DENTAL ADHESION

CONCEPTS OF ADHESION

Adhesion

– "The state in which two surfaces are held together by interfacial forces which may consist of valence forces or interlocking forces or both". (Definition given by the American Society for Testing and Materials (ASTM) SP No. D 907).

Adherend

– Materials substrate that is bonded to another material by means of an adhesive.

Adhesive

– A substance that promotes adhesion of one substance or material to another.

Mechanism of Adhesion

– There are four different mechanism of adhesion, i.e.

1. *Mechanical Adhesion:* Interlocking of the adhesive with irregularities in the surface of the substrate or adherend. Ex: Amalgam restoration.

2. *Adsorption Adhesion:* Chemical bonding between the adhesive and the adhesion. Ex: GIC.

3. *Diffusion Adhesion:* Interlocking between mobile molecules. Ex: Adhesion of two polymers.

4. *Electrostatic Adhesion:* An electrical double layer at the interface of a metal with a polymer.

Classification

– Based on the type of atomic interactions.

1. *Physical bonding :* It involves vander wall or electrostatic interactions. Bonding occurs if surfaces are smooth and dissimilar.

2. *Chemical bonding :* Bonding occurs between adhesive and adherend. Ex : Glass Ionomer Cement.

3. *Mechanical bonding :* It is due to the interface that involves undercuts and other irregularities that form interlocking of materials. Ex : Amalgam restoration Occlusal convergence.

4. *Micromechanical bonding :* Mechanical roughness produces a microscopically interlocked adhesive and adherend, this situation is called Micromechanical adhesion/Micromechanical retention. Ex : Composites.

Requirements for Good Adhesion

– Good wetting (close contact).

– The surface tension of the adhesive must be lower than the surface energy of the enamel and dentin.

ENAMEL BONDING AGENTS

– The bond agent is usually a low viscosity, unfilled BIS - GMA resin.

– The theory is that the use of such an intermediate resin will ensure maximum tag formation and therefore better bond strength of the composite restoration to the enamel.

– The exact additive effect of the bond agent is not yet defined.

SMEAR LAYER

– *It is an amorphous microcrystalline layer of cutting debris on freshly cut dentinal tooth surface.*

– It is a few micrometers thick.

- Composed of Denatured collagen, Hydroxyapatite and other cutting debris.
- Smear layer serves as natural bandage on freshly cut dentinal surface and it occludes with dentinal tubules. forming smear plug.
- It acts as good protective layer or barrier and has weak attachment to the dentin.
- During Glass Ionomer Cement restoration, smear layer has to be removed as it tends to inhibit effective ionic exchange and bonding of the Glass Ionomer to the underlying tooth surface.
- Agents for removal of smear layer : Citric acid, EDTA, Tannic acid.
- Most effectively used is Polyacrylic acid.

Smear plug

- *The micro structure which forms when the cutting debris is forced into the dentinal tubules.*

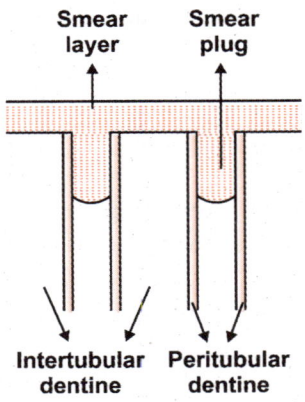

HYBRID LAYER

- *An intermediate layer of resin, collagen, and dentin produced by acid etching of dentin and resin infiltration into the conditioned dentin.*

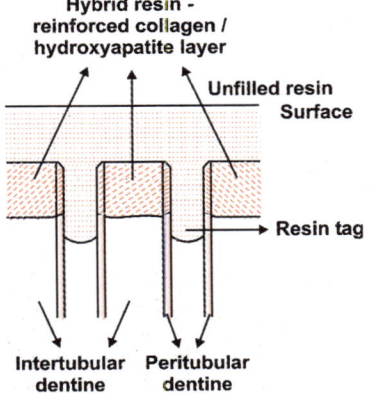

CLASSIFICATION OF DENTIN BONDING AGENTS

I. **Based on Generation: (*DEEWEY'S classification*)**
1. I - Generation
2. II - Generation
3. III - Generation
4. IV - Generation
5. V - Generation
6. VI - Generation

II. **Based on Composition**
1. Oxalates
2. Phosphates
3. Isocyanides
4. 4 - META
5. Glutaraldehyde

III. **Based on Smear Layer**
1. Removed
2. Retained
3. Modified

DEEWEY'S CLASSIFICATION

I. Generation : NPG - GMA
- *Mechanism of Adhesion :* Phosphate group of GMA chelates with the calcium ion in tooth which is bonded chemically to the tooth structure.
- But carbon B Analysis shows no chemical bond.
- *Bond strength :* 2-3 Mpa and which is poor.

II. Generation : Phosphate ester 4 HEMA
- *Mechanism of Adhesion :* By Polar attraction between negatively charged phosphate groups and positively charged calcium ion in the tooth.
- *Bond strength :* 4 - 6 Mpa.
- Ex : Scotch Bond, Clearfil, Universal Bond.

III. Generation
- In this modification of the smear layer, component used - PENTA.
- Here some system of acid etching was used which had hydrophobic monomer resulting in no penetration into dentinal tubules and resulted in modified smear layer.
- Ex : Gluma, Scotch bond tooth.
- *Bond Strength :* 10 Mpa.

IV. Generation
- It is a 2 component system.

1. *Primer*

   – It acts as water chaser and enhances adhesive penetration.

2. *Adhesive*

   – It is acetone based.

   – Hydrophobic - BISGMA

   – Hydrophillic - HEMA

   – Acid etching was done, removed the smear layer thus increased dentinal permeability.

   – *Bond strength : 17 - 24 Mpa.*

V. Generation

– It is a single component with primer and adhesive together.

– Thus less clinical steps are required.

– *Bond strength : 17 - 30 Mpa.*

– Ex : Prime Bond, Single bond, Sintac Sprint.

VI. Generation

– These are self etching primers.

– The primer includes phosphorated resin which includes etching and bond simultaneously.

– No separate etching is required.

– It reduces rinsing, over wetting, overdrying which has negative influence on bond strength.

– Ex : PROMPT L - TOP.

PULPAL PROTECTION

– Pulpal protection is an attempt to create an environment within the pulp that lessen the immediate insult of preparation and restoration of the tooth.

– Application of liners and bases serve as a barriers to an irritating chemical; Aids in the attainment of healthy pulpal response.

Pulpal Protection Beneath Composite Resin

– A cavity prepared to minimum depth can be treated by application of thin paste like consistency of glass ionomer to the exposed dentin as a cavity liner.

– The lining cement is placed against the axial wall of the cavity.

– If a prepared cavity extends into a dentin to an extent that a pulp exposure is evident or less than 0.5mm thickness of dentin, then a thin layer of calcium hydroxide is placed as medicament.

– Upon this, liner of glass ionomer is placed.

– Other Cements used are light activated Calcium hydroxide, Polycarboxylate cements.

– **Note:** *Zinc oxide eugenol cement and cavity varnish are contraindicated beneath filled and unfilled resin.*

– In zinc oxide eugenol cement, eugenol interferes with the polymerzation of resin system and leaves the resin soft at the interface between resin and cement.

– A varnish is not acceptable as the monomer portion of resin dissolves the varnish, thus removes the protective barrier.

TOOTH PREPARATIONS

Initial clinical procedure

1. Administration of local anesthesia.

2. Preparation of the operating site by cleaning the site with slurry of pumice.

3. Shade selection

   – Shade of tooth should be determined before teeth are subjected to any prolonged drying because dehydrated teeth become lighter in shade as result of decrease in translucency.

   – The incisal third (mostly enamel) is lighter and more translucent than cervical third (mostly dentin) where as middle third is blend of incisal and cervical colours.

   – VITA shade guide (Vitazahn fabrik, Germany) is a universally accepted shade guide.

   – Natural light is preferred for selection of shades.

   – If no windows are present, colour corrected operating lights or ceilings lights can be used.

   – If dental operating light is used, it should be moved away to decrease intensity. Thus allowing effects of shadows to be seen.

   – In choosing appropriate shade, hold entire shade guide near teeth to determine general colour. Now select and hold a specific shade tab beside the area of tooth to be restored.

   – The shade tab should be partially covered with patient's lip or operators thumb to create natural effect of shadows.

   – Make the selection as rapidly as possible.

   – Final shade selection can also be verified by patient with use of hand mirror.

   – To be more certain of proper shade selection, a small amount of material of selected shade can be placed directly on tooth in close proximity to area to be restored and cured.

   – If the shade is correct an explorer is used to remove the cured material from tooth surface.

4. Isolation of operating site by Rubber dam application or using cotton rolls with or without retraction cord.

5. Other pre-operative considerations

    – When restoring posterior proximal surfaces, a pre-operative wedge should be placed firmly into the gingival embrassure.

    – Pre-operative wedging assists in re-establishing a proximal contact with a composite restoration.

    – Pre-operative assessment of occlusion should be made.

CLASS - III CAVITY PREPARATION
1. CONVENTIONAL PREPARATION

Indication : Restoration of root surfaces.

Procedure

I. Initial Cavity Preparation

   1. Outline form

    – A no 1/2, 1 or 2 round bur or diamond bur is used to prepare outline form on root surface.

    – The bur is placed parallel to the plane of proximal surface following the dentino- enamel junction.

    – *Initial depth* of 0.75 mm is obtained.

   2. Retention form and Resistance form

    – It is attained within the external outline of the proximal surface by preparing the cervical and incisal walls converging toward the opening of the cavity.

    – Extend the external walls to sound tooth structure.

    – Prepare external walls perpendicular to root surface thus forming a 90° cavosurface angle.

II. Final Cavity Preparation

    – Removal of infected dentin using round burs or small spoon excavators or both.

    – Remaining old restorative material on axial wall should be removed if following conditions exist.

    – Amalgam restoration.

    – Radiographic evidence of caries under old restoration.

    – Preoperatively the pulp was symptomatic.

    – Periphery of remaining restorative material is not intact.

    – Use of underlying dentin to effect a stronger bond for retention purposes.

    – If above conditions doesn't exist leave the remaining restorative material to serve as a base.

– Retention groove is located 0.25 mm from root surface and is parallel to root surface.

– For maximum retention continuous groove is prepared.

– For less retention - groove is either omitted or placed only in gingivoaxial and / or inciso axial line angles.

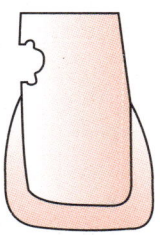

2. BEVELED CONVENTIONAL CLASS-III TOOTH Preparation

– *Indications:* Replacing existing defective restoration in the crown portion of tooth, Large carious dentin.

– It is characterized by external walls that are perpendicular to enamel surface, with enamel margins beveled.

A. Lingual Access

Advantages

1. Facial enamel is conserved for esthetics.

2. Some unsupported enamel but not friable may be left on facial wall.

3. Colour matching not critical.

4. Discolouration of restoration is less visible.

Procedure

1. *Outline form:* Use a round carbide bur or diamond stone ; size depending on extent of caries or defective restoration.

2. *Extend external wall to sound tooth structure*, while extending the cavity do not

   i. Include proximal contact area.

   ii. Extend onto facial surface.

   iii. Extend subgingivally.

3. *Axial wall depth initially 0.2 mm into DEJ.*

   – Axial wall should be outwardly convex.

   – Axial wall should be 0.5 mm into dentin if retention groove is required.

   – When restoration extends to root surfaces axial wall depth should be 0.75 mm at the gingivoaxial angle.

4. Prepare enamel walls perpendicular to external tooth surface.

5. Removal of infected dentin using round bur or small spoon excavators or both.

6. Preparation of retention grooves if required along gingivo axial line angle and incisoaxial line angle.

7. Bevel or flare of cavosurface margin is prepared with flame shaped or round diamond instrument, resulting in an angle approximately 45° to external tooth surface.

8. *Bevel width* : 0.25 to 0.5 mm.

9. Preparation is cleaned of visible debris.

B. Labial Access (Facial Access)
Indications

1. Caries present on facial surface such that facial access conserves tooth structure.

2. Lingually inclined teeth.

3. Extensive caries extending on to facial surface.

4. Faulty restoration originally placed from facial approach and needs to be replaced.

   – Cavity preparation is similar to lingual access.

   – Direct vision is used.

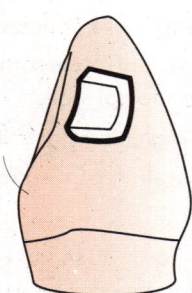

3. MODIFIED CLASS - III TOOTH PREPARATION
Indication

– Small and moderate lesions.

– It is designed to be as conservative as possible.

– Preparation design includes fault or defect and is prepared from lingual approach.

– External walls have no specific shapes or forms, other than external angles of 90° or greater.

– Design of preparation appears to be scooped or concave.

– *Initial axial wall depth* - 0.2 mm into dentin.

– Cavity is as conservative as possible by scooping out defective tooth structure.

– Bevel or flare is placed for large lesions.

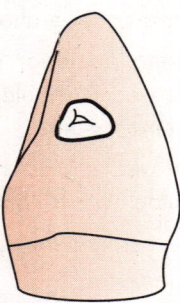

CLASS - IV CAVITY PREPARATION

– Prepare the outline form using an appropriate size round carbide bur or diamond instrument at high speed with an air water coolant.

– Remove all weakened enamel and establish initial axial wall depth at 0.5 mm into dentin.

– Prepare the walls parallel and perpendicular to long axis of the tooth.

– Excavate any remaining infected dentin.

1. CONVENTIONAL CLASS - IV

– Cavosurface is 90° angulated.

– Retention groove is placed.

2. BEVELLED CONVENTIONAL CLASS - IV

– Cavosurface margin is beveled and bevel is prepared at a 45° angle to external tooth surface.

– Width of the bevel is 0.25 - 2 mm.

– For additional retention : increase the width of enamel bevels.

– Place retention under cuts.

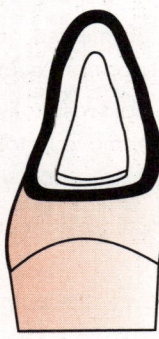

3. MODIFIED CLASS - IV

– *Objective* : Remove as little tooth structure as possible.

– Cavosurface margins are beveled or flared.

– *Initial axial depth* : 0.2 mm into DEJ.

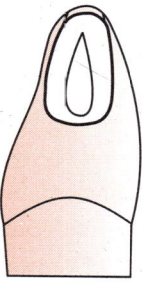

CLASS - V CAVITY PREPARATION

Initial Preparation

- Extension of the cavity on to sound tooth structure with tapered fissure carbide bur.
- *Axial depth* of 0.75 mm.
- Axial wall should follow original contour of facial surface, which is convex outward mesiodistally and sometimes occlusogingivally.

Final Preparation

- Removal of remaining infected dentin or old restorative material on axial wall.
- Applying calcium hydroxide liner if necessary.
- Preparing retention groove with No. 1/4 bur along the full length of gingivoaxial and inciso axial line angle.
- These grooves are 0.25 mm in depth into external walls.

1. CONVENTIONAL CLASS - V

- *Features :* 90° cavosurface angle.
- Uniform depth of axial line angle.
- Sometimes retention groove is placed.

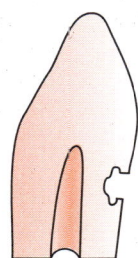

2. BEVELLED CONVENTIONAL CLASS - V

- *Features :* 90° cavosurface margin (Subsequently will be bevelled).
- *Uniform axial wall depth :* 0.2 mm to 0.5 mm.
- Bevel enamel margin with a width of 0.25-0.5 mm in final preparation.
- Retention grooves are placed.

3. MODIFIED CLASS - V

- Lesion is scooped out eliminating all enamel lesion.
- Preparation extends into dentin and not more than 0.2 mm into dentin.
- No effort is made to prepare 90° cavosurface margins.

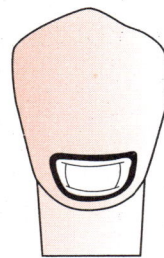

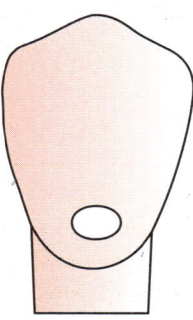

CLASS - I AND II CAVITY PREPARATIONS

Procedure

- Similar to Silver Amalgam cavity preparation with few differences.
- The differences between these preparations are
    1. Intercuspal width of preparation is one fifth the intercuspal distance in direct tooth coloured materials.
    2. Internal line and point angles are externally rounded in composites.
    3. Walls and / or pulpal and gingival floors could be in enamel in tooth coloured restorations.
    4. Walls and floors can accommodate dentinal grooves.
    5. Undermined enamel can be retained.
    6. These preparations do not require a reverse curve at the occluso proximal junction.
    7. For thinned cuspal elements circumferential skirting is indicated and this is not done in amalgam preparation.
    8. Dentinal portions should always be mortise shaped.

9. Peripheral portions of enamel walls to be etched should be beveled.

10. Saucer shaped Class - 2 preparations for tooth coloured materials.

FINISHING AND POLISHING OF COMPOSITES

Significance

1. A smooth surface texture minimizes the staining and accumulation of plaque.

2. It reduces the marginal excess and establish a physiologically acceptable contour.

3. Occlusal relationships can be refined.

4. Smooth surface helps in easy removal of plaque during oral hygiene practice.

5. In anterior teeth, better esthetics are obtained.

Procedure

1. Facial areas

- *Removal of excess and contouring :* A flame shaped carbide finishing bur or polishing diamond is used with medium speed with light intermittent brush strokes and an air coolant.

- *Final finishing and polishing :* Rubber polishing point, Aluminium oxide, Polishing paste, Disc systems are used for contouring and polishing.

- Discs are used from coarse to fine grit rotated at low speed.

- *Final polishing:* With a fine grit disc or suitable rubber points or cups

2. Lingual areas

- *Excess removal and Smooth surface contouring:* Round or oval 12 - bladed carbide finishing bur or diamond at medium speed with light intermittent pressure with an air coolant.

- *Final finishing :* White stones in various shapes and sizes.

3. Proximal areas and Embrassure areas

- *Floss :* It is used to assess the proximal surface contours and margins.

- Floss is positioned below the gingival margin and 'shoe shined' as it is pulled occlusally.

- If floss catches or frays additional finishing is indicated.

Removal of excess

A. With a sharp gold finishing knife or Amalgam knife, No.12 surgical blade mounted in Bard parker handle.

- These instruments are moved from tooth to restoration or along margins using light shaving strokes.

B. Special carbide finishing burs (Esthetic trimmers) and carbide hand instruments (Carvers) are used to remove excess and opening embrasure areas.

C. Abrasive finishing strips for contouring and finishing of proximal surfaces. These strips are curved over restoration and tooth in fashion similar to that used with shoe shine cloth.

4. Occlusion Evaluation

- Evaluation of occlusion is done by placing a piece of articulating paper and asking the patient to bite lightly and slide the mandibular teeth over restored area.

- If excess composite is present, remove only a small amount at a time with alumina impregnated rubber points.

GLASS IONOMER CEMENT RESTORATIONS

Indications

1. Root surface caries in Class - V locations.

2. Slot like preparations in either class - II or Class - III cervical locations (Not involving proximal contact).

3. Notched cervical defects of idiopathic erosion or abrasion origin.

4. As temporary treatment of anterior teeth where caries is not controlled.

Instrumentation and Cavity Preparation

- Rubber dam
- Mouth mirror
- Explorer
- Cotton pliers
- Matrix material
- No. 330, 1/4, 1/2, 1 and 2 burs
- Curved chisel
- Monangle hoe
- GMT
- Wooden wedge

Procedure

- Application of rubber dam for isolation. Cavity design is similar to that for resins.

- The cavity outlines are extended only to facilitate removal of grossly weakened tooth structure.

– The burs and instruments used to make the preparation are identical to those used for resin preparations.

– If the pulp is less than 2.0 mm from the preparation, a fast setting calcium hydroxide preparation is placed in the deep portion.

– Most conventional GI systems require etching dentinal surfaces to remove smear layer, there by effecting improved adhesion of glass ionomer to dentin.

– To etch dentin, mild acid such as 10% polyacrylic acid is placed in preparation for approximately 20 secs followed by rinsing and removal of excess water leaving dentin moist.

– Additionally, some RMGI's and all compomers use an intermediary bonding agent to facilitate bonding.

– Original GIC's require careful mixing of powder and liquid within 30 sec to optimize powder incorporation.

– If conventional type of GIC is used, place a thin coat of light cured resin bonding agent on surface immediately after placement to prevent dehydration and cracking.

– If RMGI is used, cure for minimum time of 40 secs.

– RMGI can be contoured and polished immediately after light curing.

– For conventional type, final contouring and finishing is done after 24 hours, as it requires 24 hours for polymerization.

– Contouring and finishing done with micron finishing diamonds used with petroleum lubricant or flexible abrasive discs are used.

– A fine grit Al_2O_3 polishing paste applied with prophylaxis cup is used to impart a smooth surface.

VENEERS

Definition

– It is a layer of tooth coloured material which is applied to a tooth to restore localized or generalized defects and intrinsic discolourations.

Materials for Veneers

– Chairside composite, processed composite, porcelain and pressed ceramic, etc.

Indications

1. Teeth with facial surfaces that are malformed, discoloured, abraded, eroded.

2. Teeth with faulty restorations.

Types of Veneers

I. Based on the extent of coverage

1. *Partial Veneers*

– Indicated for the restoration of localized defects or areas of intrinsic discolouration.

2. *Full Veneers*

– Indicated for the restoration of generalized defects or areas of intrinsic staining involving the major portion of the facial surface of the tooth.

II. Based on the method of fabrication

1. Direct Technique
2. Indirect Technique

1. DIRECT TECHNIQUE

Indications

1. When a small number of teeth are involved.
2. When the entire facial surface is not defective.

Advantages

1. Single appointment.
2. Useful for single discoloured tooth.
3. Useful in young patients.
4. Useful when the limited time period is available.
5. Economic.

Disadvantages

1. Time consuming
2. Labour intensive

2. INDIRECT TECHNIQUE

Indication

– Used when the multiple teeth are to be veneered.

Advantages

1. Less sensitive to operator technique.
2. When multiple teeth are to be veneered.
3. Lasts longer.

Disadvantages

1. Tooth preparation is necessary.
2. Expensive
– To achieve esthetic and physiologically sound tooth, an intraenamel preparation and location of the gingival margin of the preparation are important.

1. Intraenamel Preparation

– It is the roughening of the surface in under contoured areas of the tooth.

Significance

1. To provide space for veneering material.
2. To remove the fluoride rich layer of enamel which is more resistant to acid etching.
3. To create a rough surface for improved bonding.
4. To create a definite finish line (important for placing indirectly fabricated veneers).

2. Location of the Gingival Margin

– If the defect or discolouration does not extend subgingivally, then the margin of the veneer should not extend subgingivally.

BASIC PREPARATION DESIGN FOR VENEERS

1. Partial Veneers

– The veneers does not extend subgingivally and does not involve incisal angle.

2. Full Veneers

– There are two basic preparation designs are exist, i.e.
  1. A window preparation.
  2. An incisal lapping preparation

1. *Window Preparation*

– Recommended for most of the direct and indirect composite veneers.

Indications

1. To preserve the functional lingual and incisal surfaces of the maxillary anterior teeth.
2. For indirectly fabricated porcelain veneers if the patient exhibits significant occlusal function (as evident by wear facets on the lingual and incisal surfaces).
3. To prepare maxillary canines in a patient with canine guided lateral guidance.

Advantages

1. Better preservation of functional surfaces of enamel.
2. Reduces the potential for accelerated wear of the opposing tooth.

2. *Incisal Lapping Preparation*

Indications

1. When the veneering tooth needs lengthening.

2. When the incisal defects are present.
3. Used for porcelain veneers.

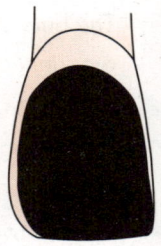

Advantages

1. Accurate cementation.
2. Improved esthetics along incisal edge.

I. DIRECT VENEER TECHNIQUE

1. Direct Partial Veneers

– Small localized intrinsic discolourations or defects that are surrounded by healthy enamel are ideally treated with direct partial veneers.
– These defects can be restored in one appointment with a light cured composite.
– Preliminary steps include,
  1. Cleaning
  2. Shade selection
  3. Isolation with rubber dam
– Outline form is dictated solely by extent of defect.
– Use a coarse elliptical or round diamond bur with adequate water or coolant to prepare the tooth to a depth of about 0.5 mm to 0.75 mm.
– After preparation, etching and restoration of the defective areas is done.
– If the entire defect or stain is removed then a microfilled composite is recommended for restoring the preparation.

2. Direct Full Veneers

– Extensive enamel hypoplasia involving all of the maxillary anterior teeth is treated by direct full veneers.
– Preliminary steps are,
  1. Cleaning
  2. Shade Selection
  3. Isolation with rubber dam
– Prepare both incisors with a coarse, rounded ended diamond instrument.
– The window preparation is typically made to a depth roughly equivalent to half the thickness of the facial enamel ranging from approximately 0.5 mm to 0.75 mm midfacially.
– Tapering down to a depth of about 0.2 to 0.5 mm along the gingival margin.
– A heavy chamfer at the level of the gingival

crest provides a definite preparation margin.

- The preparation for direct veneer normally is terminated just facial to the proximal contact.
- The teeth should be restored one at a time.
- After etching, rinsing and drying, apply and polymerize the resin-bonding agent.
- Place composite in increments.
- After the first veneer is finished restore the second tooth in a similar manner.

II. INDIRECT VENEER TECHNIQUE

- The window preparation is made with a tapered, round end diamond instrument.
- Depth is 0.5 mm to 0.75 mm midfacially diminishing to a depth of 0.3 to 0.5 mm along the gingival margin depending on thickness of enamel.
- The interproximal margins should be extended into the facial and gingival embrasures without engaging the undercut.
- If a small amount of dentin is exposed then a thin coat of dentin bonding agents is applied and cured.
- An elastomeric impression is made of the preparation.
- A stone working cast is made from impression with individually removable discs to facilitate access to interproximal areas.
- Once the veneers are fabricated, the patient is recalled and fit of each veneer is evaluated on individual tooth.
- Now the teeth to be veneered are cleaned with a pumice slurry.
- A thin layer of resin bonding agent is applied to the tooth side of the veneer, with a microbrush or small sponge.
- A light cured resin bonding medium is recommended for bonding the veneer to the tooth.

Materials Used

1. Processed composite
2. Feldspathic porcelain
3. Cast or pressed ceramic.
- Feldspathic porcelain is most popular because of its superior strength, durability and esthetics.

1. Processed Composite

Advantages

1. Improved physical and mechanical properties.
2. Superior Shading.
3. Better control of facial contours.

Disadvantages

1. Limited bond strength
2. No longevity

2. Etched Porcelain / Feldspathic Porcelain

Advantages

1. High bond strength
2. Highly esthetic
3. Stain resistant
4. Periodontal compatibility

3. Pressed Ceramic

- Excellent Esthetics
- More Translucent Nature

DIASTEMA CLOSURE

Materials

1. If the diastema spaces are small and occlusal factors normal, light cured, microfilled materials are indicated.
2. If the diastema spaces are large and predominate occlusal factors, heavy filled, light cured hybrid or macrofilled materials are indicated.

Technique

1. Proper shade selection.
2. Application of rubber dam.
3. The proximal enamel surfaces adjacent to the diastema space are lightly disced up to and including the proximo labial line angles.
4. The enamel must be thoroughly cleaned with a pumice and water mixture and then fully rinsed from the teeth.
5. After phosphoric acid etching, washing and drying of the proximal enamel surfaces, a thin layer of bonding resin is applied and cured.
6. A thin crown form matrix is trimmed and fitted to the proximal area.
7. The crown form matrix is removed, filled with composite, placed, stabilized, light cured and finished.

MISCELLANEOUS

ABFRACTION / IDIOPATHIC EROSION
Definition

- "The loss of tooth surface at the cervical areas of teeth caused by tensile and compressive forces during tooth flexure, which begins as microfracture of thin enamel tooth structure occlusal to CEJ and produces a notched defect when combined with abrasive tooth brushing."

Etiology

– Has been found in association with parafunctional habits such as clenching or bruxism.

Clinical Features

– Seen in adults.

– Seen as a wedge - shaped notching at the cervical areas of involved teeth.

Treatment

– Restoration of the defective area.

– Adjustment of the bite for the evenly distribution of chewing forces.

GOLDEN PROPORTION

– It results from the division of a straight line in such a way that the shorter part is to the longer part as the longer part is to the whole.

– Each ratio equals to 0.618.

$$\frac{S}{L} = \frac{L}{(S+L)} = 0.618$$

– Linear progressions and surface division by the same number are common in nature both geometrically and arithmetically.

– *The geometrical progressions can be obtained by multiplying each term by 1.618 or dividing by 0.618:*

$1.000 \times 1.618 = 1.618$ **or** $1.000 : 0.618 = 1.618$
$1.618 \times 1.618 = 2.618$ **or** $1.618 : 0.618 = 2.618$
$2.618 \times 1.618 = 4.236$ **or** $2.618 : 0.618 = 4.236$

– *In the arithmetic progression, each term is the sum of the preceding two terms:*

$0.618 + 1.000 = 1.618$
$1.000 + 1.618 = 2.618$
$1.618 + 2.618 = 4.236$

– As can be seen here, the progression using the Golden number is unique because three different methods produce the same results.

– Obviously, the Golden proportion is not the only parameter that defines harmony and therefore beauty.

– However, numerous studies and experiments have demonstrated that this surface division creates an esthetic appeal, independently from ethnic or civilization factors.

Golden Proportions in Facial and Dental Elements

– The nasal height (A) is related to the maxillary height (B) as 1.000 : 0.618. The sum of nasal height and maxillary height (A + B) are related to the mandibular height (C) as 1.618 : 1.000.

– The mandibular height (C) is related to the maxillary height (B) as 1.000 : 0.618.

– The orofacial height (A + B) is related to the nasal height (A) as 1.618 : 1.000.

– Note that each ratio is 1.618.

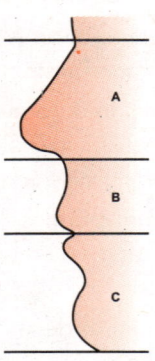

Dental Proportions

– The width of the central incisor is in golden proportion to the width of the lateral incisor (from the labial view), which inturn is in golden proportion to the part of the canine that is visible from the front.

– The dark space between the corners of the mouth and the outer surface of the canines during a smile (line 1.0) is called Negative space. The Negative space is in Golden Proportion with one half of the width of the upper anterior segment (line 1.618).

– Even though the negative space escapes the attention of the public, it cannot be ignored.

– It creates a balance between cohesive and segregative forces in a smile and provides a harmonious relationship between the smile and other facial features.

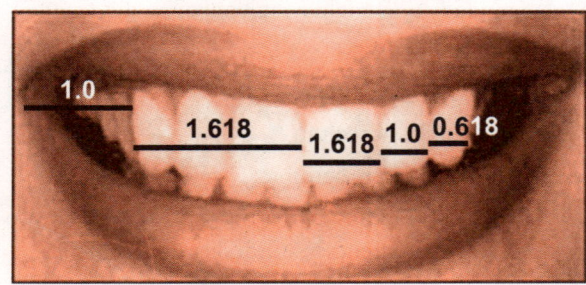

SANDWICH TECHNIQUE

– Also called as *Bilayered Restoration.*

– *It consists of placing the glass ionomer cement as an intermediate layer between the tooth structure and a resin based composite.*

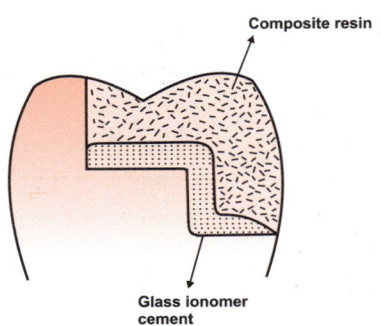

Composite resin

Glass ionomer
cement

Advantages

1. Chemical bonding of GIC to tooth structure.
2. Fluoride releasing ability of GIC to minimize caries.
3. Esthetic quality of composite.
4. Durability of composite.
5. Better seal with increased retention.

Technique

— It involves the placement of glass ionomer in the cavity at a thickness of about 1 mm.

— The materials is placed like a conventional lining for a class - 5 or class - 2 cavity except that it is extended out to the aproximal margin in case of the class - 2 cavity, and to the gingival margin for the class - 5 cavity.

— Then the surface of the glass ionomer is etched and dried.

— Apply the composite resin.

— Bonding between the resin and glass ionomer surface is through penetration of resin into the surface irregularities of the etched cement surface.

— Setting of the resin is by mechanical interlocking.

DIFFERENCES BETWEEN CLASS - 2 CAVITY PREPARATION FOR AMALGAM AND COMPOSITE RESTORATIONS

Features	Amalgam	Composite
1. Outline form:	— include defects. — may extend to break proximal contact — includes adjacent suspicious area	— same — same — does not include
2. Pulpal depth:	— uniform 1.5 mm	— usually not uniform
3. Axial depth:	— uniform 0.2 – 0.5 mm into DEJ	— usually not uniform
4. Cavosurface margin:	— 90 degree	— 90 or more than 90 degrees
5. Bevels:	— only gingival	— given
6. Texture of the prepared walls:	— smoother	— rougr
7. Primary retention form:	— occlusal convergence	— none (bonding/roughness)
8. Secondary retention form:	— grooves, slots, locks, pins, bonding	— bonding; grooves for very large or root – surface preparation.
9. Resistance form:	— flat floors, rounded angles, box-shaped form, floors are perpendicular to occlusal forces	— same for large preparations; No special form for small to moderate size preparations.

CHAPTER 11

DIRECT FILLING GOLD (DFG)

INDICATIONS

1. Occlusal, buccal and lingual pit and fissure cavities on teeth (Class - I).
2. Gingival third cavities on bicuspids, cuspids and incisors where access and esthetics permit (Class - V).
3. Incipient interproximal lesions of the anterior teeth (Class - V).
4. Cuspal and incisal areas of all teeth.
5. Limited numbers of interproximal cavities on bicuspids and mesial of first molars (Class - II).
6. Small eroded areas on the facial surface of premolars, canines and on incisors.
7. Small, less conspicuous circular and irregular areas such as hypoplasias, white spots or defective pits.
8. DFG is used to repair defective inlay or crown margins and vent holes in crowns.

CONTRAINDICATIONS

1. Inaccessibility
2. Isolation of difficult areas
3. Grossly destructed tooth
4. Un co-operative patients
5. Extensive periodontal involvement
6. Esthetically important areas
7. Undesirable occlusal stress

ADVANTAGES

1. It can last as long as the tooth if restored properly.
2. No tarnish and corrosion.
3. Insoluble in the oral fluids.
4. Perfect adaptability to cavity walls if restored properly.
5. Great density, crushing resistance and edge strength.
6. No cementing medium is necessary for retention.
7. Capability of receiving and maintaining a high polish.
8. Perfect weldability in a cold state.
9. Low tendency to molecular change.

DISADVANTAGES

1. Inharmoneous colour
2. High thermal conductivity
3. Difficulty of manipulation

FORMS / TYPES OF DFG

1. Foil (or fibrous gold)
   i. Sheet
      a. Cohesive
      b. Non-cohesive

ii. Ropes

iii. Cylinders

iv. Laminated foil

v. Platinized foil

2. Electrolytic precipitate (or crystalline gold)

   i. Matgold

   ii. Mat Foil (Mat gold + gold foil)

   iii. Gold calcium alloy

3. Granulated gold (encapsulated powdered gold)

I. GOLD FOIL

– Oldest form of gold and is the most durable.

– Standard No. 4 gold foil is supplied in 4 x 4 inch (100 x 100 mm) sheets that weigh 4 grains (0.259 g) and are about 0.51 µm thick. The numbering system refers to the weight of a standard sheet and reflects the thickness. Thus, No. 3 foil weighs 3 grains (0.194 g) and is about 0.38 µm thick.

– Gold foil is supplied in the following forms,

   i. *Plain gold foil:* which is the product of the cold working procedure without any modifications.

   ii. *Corrugated gold foil:* which is manufactured by placing a thin leaf of paper between two sheets of gold foil and after which the whole unit is ignited. As the paper leaves are burnt out, they shrivel and impart a corrugated shape to the gold foil. It is more cohesive than plain ones; it is the outcome of great Chicago Fire in 1871.

   iii. *Platinum gold foil:* which is produced by sandwiching platinum foil between two leaves of gold foil; platinum increases the hardness of the finished restoration. Therefore it is used in areas of excessive stress such as the incisal edge of anterior teeth.

   iv. *Laminated gold foil:* which has directional properties, i.e. resistant to stresses in one direction better than the other. It is to combine two or three leaves of gold, each from different ingots which have been cold worked in different directions. So they can be resistant in different directions when combined together.

   v. *Gold foil cylinder:* which is produced by rolling cut segments of No. 4 foils into a desired width, usually 3.2 mm, 4.8 mm and 6.4 mm using a modified No. 22 tapestry needle.

Cohesive and Non-cohesive Gold

– Although the forms of DFG can be supplied in both the cohesive and the non cohesive forms only the sheet foil is typically furnished in either of these two forms.

Cohesive Gold

– *The gold foil which is free of surface contaminants is called 'Cohesive Gold'.*

– Gases like oxygen are absorbed at the surface of the gold, thus prevents bonding of gold during compaction.

– Only if gold surface is free from impurities it can be welded at room temperature.

Non - Cohesive Gold

– Ammonia treated foil is called non-cohesive gold.

– *Intentional coating :* Is treating of gold with 18 percent of ammonia.

– This acts as a protective film to prevent adsorption of non-volatile gases and premature cohesion of pellets in their container.

– Non-cohesive gold can also have adsorbed agents like iron salt or an acidic gas on its surface.

– This volatile film is readily removed by heating at 350°C there by restoring the cohesive character of the foil.

– Non-cohesive gold is rarely used nowadays.

– But may be used to buildup the bulk of a direct gold restoration.

II. ELECTROLYTIC PRECIPITATE

A. *Mat gold :* It is a crystalline, electrolytically precipitated gold form that is formed into strips. It is used to form the core of the restoration because of its ease in compaction. It is used in combination technique along with regular cohesive gold.

B. *Mat Foil :* It is manufactured by sandwitching a ribbon of mat gold between two regular cohesive gold sheets.

C. *Gold - Calcium alloy (Alloyed Electrolytic Precipitate):* Newest form, Electralloy R V is alloyed with calcium. The calcium content is 0.1%. Its purpose is to produce stronger restorations by dispersion strengthening. The alloy is sandwiched between two layers of gold foil.

III. POWDERED GOLD : (SPONGY GOLD)

– It is a blend of atomized and precipitated powder embedded in a wax like organic matrix. From this material various sized pellets are cut and encased in gold foil wrappers and packed prior to use. The matrix is burnt away to leave only pure gold.

CHARACTERISTICS OF GOLD

1. *Fibrous gold foil :* It is best suitable for restricted cavity preparations such as small pits and narrow fissures and also used to veneer other forms of cohesive gold.

2. *Mat foil :* Is used as a bulk filler for single surface restorations such as class - I and class - V. It is not used on the surface of a restoration since it has a tendency to become pitted afterwards when some minor abrasion takes place.

3. *Encapsulated Powdered gold :* Used as a bulk filler and for the restoration surface. It is used for the restoration of all classes of cavities where cohesive gold may be indicated.

4. *Alloyed filling gold :* Is used for restoring all classes of cavities where cohesive gold is used most frequently. It is used for class - I, II, III and V cavity restorations.

MANIPULATION OF DFG

– It consists of two stages, i.e.

  1. Annealing / Heat treatment / Degassing.

  2. Condensation / Compaction.

1. ANNEALING

– *Cleansing of the gold surface by heating is referred to as `annealing'.*

– *Purpose :* Annealing removes all of the volatile contaminants, thereby restoring or assuring the cohesive characteristics of the gold.

– There are of two methods for the purpose of annealing, i.e.

A. Bulk method

– Accomplished by using an electric or gas source of heat.

– The required number of pellets of gold is placed on the surface of the annealer. A mica slab is held over an open glass flame until the gold shows a dull red colour. Then the slab is removed from the heat and foil is ready for use.

– *Precaution :* DFG should never be annealed directly in an open gas flame.

Advantage : Convenient method.

Disadvantages

1. Danger of over annealing.

2. Waste formation due to the contamination of unused gold.

3. Inability to select a suitable desired piece from annealed gold.

B. Piece Method

– It is the most practical method.

– Annealing is accomplished using a simple alcohol lamp and a gold foil carrier.

– Acetone - Free alcohol must be used to avoid contamination.

– The wick of the lamp should be about 1/4 inch long and be pointed.

– Gold is picked up with the point of the carrier and brought to the `hot' cone of the flame and heated until to a dull red colour.

– *Precaution :* Pliers should not be used for the piece method to avoid uneven heating.

Advantages

1. Elimination of the chance of contamination between annealing and compaction.

2. Lack of waste

3. Ability to select a piece of desired size.

2. CONDENSATION / COMPACTION

– *Condensation is the procedure used to harden the gold inside the preparation.*

A. Objectives

1. To wedge initial pieces between dentinal walls - especially at starting points.

2. To weld together the pieces of gold.

3. To adapt the gold intimately to the walls and margins of the prepared cavity.

4. To gain a uniform compactness by eliminating voids between the gold pieces.

5. To develop strength within the restoration.

B. Modes of Condensation

  i. *Hand Instrument Condensation :* Can be used only as a first step in a two - step condensation process as the condensation energy produced by this method is not sufficient to fill the cavity.

  ii. *Pneumatic Condensation :* Involves the use of vibrating condensers which work by using compressed air. Though this is the efficient method, but cannot be controllable.

  iii. *Electronic condensation :* It is the most efficient and controlled way of condensation.

  iv. *Hand condenser and mallet :* Oldest method of condensation.

C. Gold Condensers

– They are of the following types

  i. *Round condensers (Bayonet condenser):* Used in initial restoration phase and to establish `ties' in the inner parts of the restoration.

  ii. *Foot condensers :* Used mainly for cavosurface condensation, surface hardening of the restoration and for bulk build-up.

iii. *Parallelogram and Hatchet Condensers:* Used for preliminary condensation and to create the bulk of restoration.

D. Procedure / Principles of condensation

- After the pellet or piece is placed in the tooth, it is compacted to develop hardness and to produce adaptation of the material to the cavity wall.

- When the gold is condensed slip planes develop between the anatomic structure and restoration and the resultant stress produces the hardness.

- Thorough condensation results in a dense, non porous gold restoration.

- Regardless of the type of condensation employed the force should be at least 15 lb /sq. inch.

1. Line of force / Angle of force

- *It is the direction of force exerted by the condenser.*

- It follows and is parallel to an extension of the long axis of the shaft of the instrument regardless of the deflection or angle of the working point.

- *According to Black, the line of force must be directed at an angle of 45° to cavity walls and floors, i.e. should bisect line angles and trisect point angles formed by the cavity walls.*

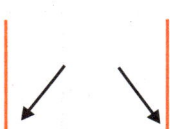 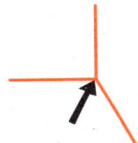

- *Forces of condensation must be directed at 90° to previously condensed gold to avoid shear components which can displace or loosen the already condensed pieces of gold.*

- A building shelf is produced with the first layer of powdered gold for proximal restorations and a gold bank is developed from then on.

2. Bridging

- *When an improper building shelf is produced a bridging occurs, i.e. the gold bulges and produces a convexity in the material, preventing the condenser from reaching the cavity wall, causing porosity.*

- Bridging prevents the proper lines of force from being applied and thus resulting in poor adaptation.

- Bridging is prevented by uniform placement of the material and adequate condensation using the proper lines of force.

- The most important rule is to keep the gold banked against the walls until the cavosurface margin is reached thus creating a concavity.

3. Stepping of the condenser

- *Refers to the overlapping (by one fourth of its diameter) of the previous area of the condenser's stroke both in individual steps and in lines of steps.*

- Stepping can be done in two ways either;

  a. In rows parallel to the wall being approached moving toward this wall, row by row and wedging the last row between the already condensed gold and the wall.

  b. In rows perpendicular to the wall being approached.

- Stepping always start at a point on one side and proceed in a straight line to another point on the opposite side then back to the original side on a different straight line. This ensures that the condenser has covered the entire surface of that piece of gold.

Significance

1. Ensures that each portion of the gold increment has been welded and cold worked.

2. No voids

3. Maximal adaptation

4. Denser restoration

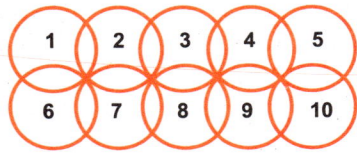

4. Pellet placement

- *It refers to the exact location at which each pellet of gold foil is placed in order to ensure correct building of the gold.*

- Each pellet should be placed where needed to be condensed, not moved around after original placement. If it is moved it becomes harsh and difficult to handle.

- Accurate placing is essential to correct gold building.

- *Convenient points or starting points are refined retention forms placed in the corners of the tooth preparation to accept the first pellets and can be placed in the preparation to facilitate starting the gold. They are usually pyramidal* or triangular and prevent slippage of the pellet or mass of mat or powdered gold. They are often used in proximal class III restoration because these preparations do not have four confining walls.

Condensation of Mat Gold or Mat foil

- Condensation of Mat gold is different from that of regular cohesive gold.

- The metal is condensed by hand and spread thoroughly into the retention forms.

- Mat golds are spongy and thick and require a rocking motion for adaptation.

- If the gold is too thick, the surface strain hardens, preventing the condensation forces from properly forcing the material against the tooth.

- Therefore, if the layer is too thick, the mat gold must be 'broken up' to prevent bridging and for obtaining proper adaptation and condensation.

- Even though adaptation is difficult (because of thickness), mat golds are easy to start in the cavity because they are spongy.

- *Mat golds can be used on axial walls of Class - V and III restorations and pulpal walls of Class - I and II restorations.*

Condensation of Powdered gold

- Powdered gold is manipulated in same way as the mat gold.

- More pressure is required for the hardening of encapsulated powdered gold because of varying sizes and density of pellets.

- There are special condensers with special working points are available.

- The powdered pellets are placed in the cavity and the envelops are ruptured with the face of the condenser.

- The gold is placed in the deepest part of the prepared cavity, and it is spread into the retention forms and line angles. Then pressure is exerted with a rocking motion for gradual hardening.

- The advantage of powdered golds over the mat golds is that they will produce a less porous surface, which does not require a veneer of gold foil.

STEPS FOR INSERTION OF DFG

1. **Three step build - up**

   i. *Tie formation :* It is the connecting of two opposing point angles or starting points filled with gold with a transverse bar of gold. It forms the foundation for the restoration.

   ii. *Banking of walls :* It is the covering of each wall from its floor or axial wall to the cavosurface margin with the direct gold. A wall should be banked in such a way that, it will not obstruct tie formation or banking of other walls in the cavity.

   iii. *Shoulder formation :* It is the connecting of two opposing walls with the direct gold to complete the build-up.

2. **Paving of the Restoration**

   - It is the individual covering of every area of cavosurface margin portion with excess cohesive gold foil. A foot condenser is used for this purpose.

3. **Surface hardening**

   - Done to fulfill the rest of the condensation objectives and to strain harden the surface gold.

4. **Burnishing**

   - Should be done from gold to tooth surface. It enhances surface hardening, adapts restoration to the margins and eliminates voids.

5. **Margination**

   - Done with sharp instruments like knives and files moving from the gold surface to the tooth surface to eliminate excess material.

6. **Burnishing**

   - It follows margination to close marginal discrepancies and to strain harden the surface.

7. **Contouring**

   - Done to create the proper anatomy of the restoration to coincide with that of the tooth. Done with knives, files or finishing burs.

8. **Additional Burnishing**

   - Done to fulfill previously mentioned objectives.

9. **Finishing and Polishing**

   - Done by using precipitated chalk or tin oxide powder on soft bristle brushes or rubber cups.

10. **Final Burnishing**

    - Done to ensure closure of marginal voids and other surface discrepancies.

PRINCIPLES OF TOOTH PREPARATION FOR DIRECT GOLD RESTORATIONS

1. **Outline form**

   - Margins must not be ragged.

   - Margins should be established on sound areas of the tooth, which can be finished and polished.

   - Outline form must include all structural defects.

   - It should be pleasing esthetically.

– *Failure to give proper outline form results in an unsightly restoration.*

2. **Resistance form**

– Pulpal floor should be flat and perpendicular to occlusal forces.

– All the enamel must be supported by sound dentin.

– *Poor resistance form can result in the fracture of the tooth.*

3. **Retention form**

– Can be established by parallelism of some walls and by strategically placing converging walls.

– Walls must be smooth and flat (to provide resistance to loosening).

– Internal line angles must be sharp (to resist movement).

– *Poor retention form results in loosened restoration.*

4. **Convenience form**

– It requires suitable access and a rubberdam isolation.

– Sharp internal line and point angles are created to allow convenient "starting" gold foil as compaction begins.

– Rounded form is allowed when E - Z Gold is used to begin the restorative phase.

– *Improper convenience form can make the tooth preparation unrestorable.*

5. **Final cavity preparation**

– Removal of remaining carious dentin, final planing of cavosurface margins and debridement complete the tooth preparation for direct gold.

TOOTH PREPARATIONS

I. CLASS - I CAVITY

A. SIMPLE CLASS - I IN MOLARS AND PREMOLARS

1. General Outline form

– *Outline form* is similar to Class - I cavity preparation for amalgam with three modifications.

A. Instead of rounded corners, they have *angular corners* at *triangular and linear fossa* areas.

B. The extension in the facial and lingual grooves in molars will end in a *spear like form* (i.e. a pointed termination rather than rounded).

C. *More angular outline form* than amalgam preparation.

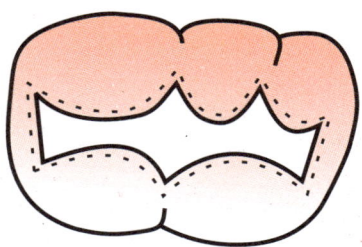

2. Location of the Margins

– The *facial and lingual* margins should be located on the inclined planes of the corresponding cusps or marginal ridges.

– The *mesial and distal* margins are located on the inclined planes of the corresponding ridge, very close to the adjacent pits.

– *Width of the cavity should not exceed 1/5th of the intercuspal distance.*

3. Internal Anatomy

– Definite, very angular line and point angles.

– Flat pulpal floor.

– Cavosurface margin should be partially bevelled; Bevel is at 45° to the direction of the enamel rods and should include at least 1/4th of the enamel wall. Its purpose is to protect the enamel margins from the condensation pressure and to allow the coverage of enamel margins with the *gold.*

B. COMPOUND OR COMPLEX CLASS - I CAVITY

– These are class - I cavity preparations with facial and / or lingual extensions.

1. General Outline Form

– It is same as simple class - I cavity.

– Facial and lingual extensions are parallelogram in shape.

2. Location of the Margins

– *Facial and lingual* margins will be located on the inclined planes of the corresponding cusps or marginal ridges so that the width of the cavity will not exceed 1/5th the intercuspal distance.

– The *mesial and distal* margins are located on the inclined planes of the corresponding ridge very close to the adjacent pits.

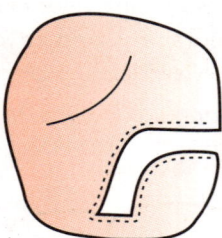

3. *Internal Anatomy*

— Have starting points at the mesial and distal axio gingival corners of the facial and lingual extensions.

— Cavosurface margin should be partially bevelled.

— The bevel is at 45° to the direction of the enamel rods and includes atleast 1/4th of the enamel wall.

— The junction between the dentinal portion of the cavity walls and floors are angular.

— The junction between the partial bevels on the cavosurface margins should be rounded.

C. SIMPLE CLASS - I CAVITY ON THE LINGUAL SURFACE OF UPPER ANTERIOR TEETH AND AT THE FACIAL AND LINGUAL PIT AREAS OF UPPER AND LOWER MOLARS

— *General outline form is tear drop shape or triangular, with the base of the triangle facing gingivally.*

— *Location of the margins can be anywhere, as the entire area is self cleansable.*

— *Internal Anatomy as a flat axial wall, following the same angulation as the adjacent surface and surrounding walls in three planes, i.e. an internal, undercut, dentinal plane; a straight second plane formed of enamel and a dentin; a third plane which is the partial bevel.*

— The junction of the components of the outer plane are rounded and of the internal plane are in angular fashion.

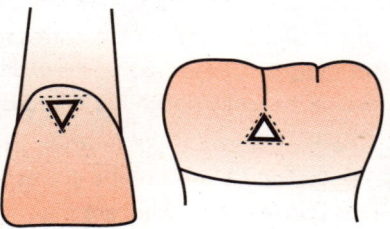

Instrumentation

1. Bur of # 168 size.
2. Angle former to sharpen internal anatomy during final shaping.
3. Smallest Wedelstaedt chisel to prepare enamel bevel.
4. A spear bur to create starting points.

II. CLASS-II CAVITY

— There are three types of designs for Class - II cavity preparation, i.e.

A. CONVENTIONAL DESIGN

1. *General Outline form*

— The *occlusal outline form* is same as simple Class - I cavity preparation in molars and premolars.

— The *proximal outline form* is a one sided inverted truncated cone. The inverted truncation is at the expense of the functional cusp side.

2. *Location of the Margins*

— The margins of occlusal portion are located same as in the simple class - I of molars and premolars.

— The margin of isthmus portion is located on the inclined planes of the remaining parts of the marginal ridge and the adjacent cusps.

— *The width of the cavity should not exceed 1/5th the intercuspal distance.*

— *Gingival margin should just clears the contact area.*

— *Facial and lingual margins should only include the contact area and the area of near approach.*

3. *Internal Anatomy*

i. *Mesio - distal Cross Section*

— Gingival floor is perfectly flat, perpendicular to the long axis of the tooth and formed completely of dentin.

— If the gingival margin is located on the gingival third of the proximal surface, the gingival floor will be in two planed, i.e. an inner, dentinal plane at right angles to the long axis of the tooth and an outer enamel dentinal plane in the direction of the enamel rods.

— If the gingival margin is located at the middle third of the proximal surface, (as in young, incompletely erupted teeth), the gingival floor will be formed of one plane made of enamel and dentin.

— All line angles except the axio pulpal should be very sharp.

— The cavosurface margins are bevelled to 45°C.

ii. Facio - lingual Cross section

A. At the Gingival one-third :
The axial wall will be convex, following the curvature of the proximal surface; *the facial and lingual walls* have four planes, i.e. an *inner dentinal plane* making very sharp and acute angle with the axial wall; *a transitional plane* formed completely of dentin; *an enamel dentinal plane* in the direction of enamel rods, facio proximally and linguo proximally and *a partial bevel plane* completely in enamel.

B. At the middle third

— Each of the facial and lingual walls will have the same planes.

— The inner plane (first) makes a less acute angulation with the axial wall.

C. At the level of pulpal floor :
It has three planes, i.e. an inner dentinal plane at right angles to the axial wall; an outer enamel dentinal plane in the direction of enamel rods facio or linguo proximally and a partial bevel plane.

D. Within the occlusal part :
Facial and lingual walls are in reverse S-shape and has a partial bevel on the proximal extent of the cavity walls.

— These cross sections indicate the existence of triangular retention area at the expense of the dentinal portion of the facial and lingual walls of the proximal part of the cavity preparation.

— The base of the triangle is at the gingival floor level and the tip of the triangle is at the pulpal floor level.

— These triangular areas are also acts as the starting points for formation of gold ties along the axio gingival line angle.

B. CONSERVATIVE DESIGN

1. General Outline form

— The design is similar to that of Class - II, design 3 for amalgam restoration.

2. Location of the Margins

— It is similar to the design for amalgam restorations.

3. Internal anatomy

A. Mesio - distal Cross Section

— The axial wall is very slanted and formed of dentin and enamel.

— Towards the occlusal, the enamel is partially bevelled.

— The gingival floor is in four planes, i.e. an internal, reverse bevel plane - making an acute angle with the axial wall and formed completely of dentin; a transitional plane formed completely of dentin and slightly flat; an outer enamel dentinal plane following the direction of the enamel rods and a partial bevel on enamel only.

B. Facio - lingual Cross Section

— In viewing the same four cross sections of conventional design, the first and second sections are replica of conventional design.

— The third cross section is just short of the occlusal enamel, shows the termination of the facial and lingual triangular areas.

C. SIMPLE DESIGN

1. General Outline form

— It is similar to that for amalgam, except that it has more angular junction between the different margins.

2. Location of the Margins

— The margins can be placed anywhere on the surface and the whole surface is self cleansable.

3. Internal Anatomy

A. Occluso - gingival Cross Section

— The *occlusal wall* is formed of 3 planes, i.e. one plane in the form of dentin, and at right angle to the axial wall; second planed formed of enamel and dentin, inclining occluso proximally and third one in the enamel wall, in the form of bevel.

— *Gingival floor* will appear in four planes, i.e. *inner plane* is formed of dentin and is in the form of reverse bevel making an acute angle with the axial wall; *transitional plane* formed of dentin; *third plane* is formed of dentin and enamel and *final plane* is partial enamel bevel.

B. Facio - lingual Cross Section

— *Axial wall* is slightly rounded.

— *Facial and lingual walls* have the same anatomy, i.e. each wall will have three planes. A *dentinal plane* at right angle to axial wall; an *outer enamel dentinal plane* follows the direction of enamel rods and a *third plane* in the form of partial enamel bevel at the middle third.

III. CLASS-III CAVITY

– There are three types of designs for Class-III cavity preparation, i.e.

A. FERRIER DESIGN

Indications

1. Used when bulky labial, lingual, and incisal walls remain after the removal of carious and undermined tooth structure.

2. Used if the labial extension of the carious lesion facilitates minimal extension of the cavity preparation labially.

3. More indicated for the distal proximal surfaces of anterior teeth than for the mesial proximal surfaces.

1. General Outline form

– *Triangular* in shape, involving about two-thirds to one half of the proximal surface.

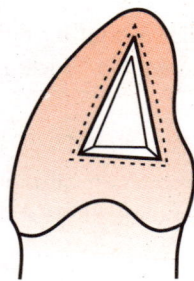

2. Location of the Margins

– As it is a labial and lingual access cavity, the labial and lingual margins should be located within the corresponding embrasures.

– *Facial margin* should be parallel to the calcification lobes.

– *Labial margin* should be minimally extended in the labial embrasure, especially for mesial cavity preparations.

– *Lingual margin* should not encroach on the marginal ridge.

– *Gingival margin* should be located 1/2 to 1mm apical to the free healthy gingiva, following a straight line labio lingually.

– *Incisal margin* usually located in the contact area.

3. Internal Anatomy

i. *Labio - lingual Cross Section :* Axial wall is rounded, but do not follow the convexity of the proximal surface. The *labial and lingual walls* will each have either two or three planes. For Ex : If there are three planes, they are an *inner dentinal plane* at right angle to the tangent of the axial wall; an *outer enamel dentinal plane* in the direction of the enamel rods labio proximally and linguo proximally and a *peripheral partial enamel bevel plane*.

ii. *Inciso - gingival Cross Section :* Incisal wall is formed of three or four planes, i.e. an inner dentinal plane, which is the part of the boxed incisal retention form; a transition plane formed completely of dentin; an outer enamelo dentinal plane following the direction of enamel rods and a partial enamel bevel plane. *Axial wall* appears ranging from flat to slightly rounded. *Gingival wall* is formed of four planes, i.e. an inner reverse bevelled dentinal plane; a transitional plane, an outer enamel plane in the direction of the enamel rods and a peripheral partial enamel bevel plane.

iii. All line and point angles should be sharp except at the junction of line angles of the cavity preparation proper and those of the retention forms which should be rounded.

Instrumentation

1. No. 1/2 round bur is used for the creation of depth, i.e. 0.02 mm from DEJ.

2. Use the base of an inverted cone bur (No. 33¼) to form lingual wall in inciso gingival strokes.

3. With the same bur, formulate gingival wall in labio lingual strokes.

4. Use the side of the same bur to form labial wall in inciso - gingival movements.

5. A Wedelstaedt chisel is used to cut triangle on the labial wall. An angle former is used to cut triangles on the lingual and axial walls.

6. Spear bur is used to create incisal retention.

7. A bi-bevelled hatchet is used to box up the incisal retention form.

8. Angle former is used to place the gingival short partial bevel.

9. Wedelstaedt chisel is used to place the short partial bevel on labial and lingual cavosurface margins.

B. THE LOMA - LINDA DESIGN

– This design is indicated when a combination of powdered gold build-up with a cohesive gold foil veneer is used.

Indications

1. Used when the access is lingual due to the care for esthetics and or to the caries extent.
2. When the lingual marginal ridge is lost or undermined.

1. *General Outline form*

– The *Proximal portion* of the design will be in triangular shape with rounded corners. The *Lingual portion* has an incisal or gingival `turn' according to the access.

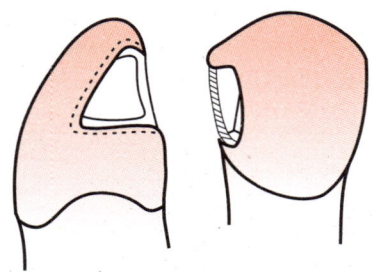

2. *Location of Margins*

– *Gingival margins* are similar to the Ferrier design.

– *Lingual margin* is located far enough into the lingual surface to include the marginal ridge and to facilitate access to the internal parts of the cavity preparation.

3. *Internal Anatomy*

i. *Inciso - gingival Cross Section :* Same as the inciso - gingival cross section of the Ferrier design.

ii. *Labio - lingual Cross Section :* If the labial wall margin is located in contact area, the *labial wall* will be formed of two planes, i.e. an *enamelo - dentinal plane* at right angle to the axial wall in the direction of enamel rods and a *partial enamel bevel plane.* If it is located in the labial embrasure, the labial wall will be same as the Ferrier design. The *lingual wall* is much shorter than the labial wall which has two planes, i.e. *one in the direction of enamel rods and the other is partial enamel bevel.*

iii. The point angles have two cylindrical retention grooves gingivally. They will be directed labio - gingivo - axially and linguo - gingivo - axially extending about 1.5-2 mm into the dentin. The incisal retention mode is in cylindrical form and is directed inciso - labio - axially. The line and point angles and the junction of different retention features should be bulkier and more rounded than in the Ferrier design.

Instrumentation

1. No. 1/2 round bur is used to remove the tooth structure with in the outline form from lingual access.
2. With the base of the No. 33 bur, labial and gingival walls are created in inciso gingival and labio lingual strokes respectively.
3. With the side of the same bur lingual wall is created.
4. A retention point of 1mm deep is created at the gingivo labio axial point with No. 1/4 round bur directing labially, gingivally and axially.
5. Another retention point is created at gingivo - linguo axial point by directing the bur gingivally, lingually and axially.
6. Incisal retention point is created with the same bur directing incisally, labially and axially.
7. Forming labial and lingual wall planes and rounding of the axial wall is done by using Loma-Linda hatchet or an angle former by inciso gingival movements.
8. Sharpening of gingivo axial line angle and making it in the form of a groove at gingival floor is done with angle former.
9. Accentuate the labio - axial and linguo - axial line angle and merge them with the gingival and incisal point retention.
10. Box up the incisal retention form with bi-beveled hatchet.
11. Wedelstaedt chisel is used to place the short partial enamel bevel on the margins.

C. INGRAHAM DESIGN

Indication

– Indicated primarily for incipient proximal lesions in anterior teeth where esthetics are the main concern.

1. *General outline form*

– *Simple parallelogram* in shape.

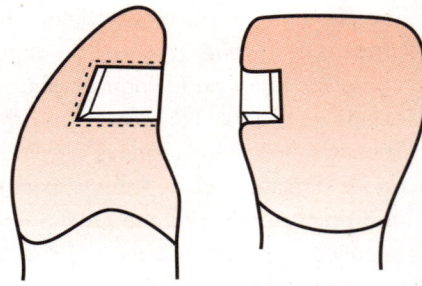

2. Locations of the margins

- *Labial margin* will be in the contact area.

- *Gingival margin* just clears the contact area in the gingival embrasure.

- *Incisal margin* will be within the contact area.

- *Lingual margin* is on the lingual surface past the marginal ridge, and or axial angle of the tooth.

3. Internal Anatomy

i. Inciso - gingival Cross Section

- *Gingival wall* will have three planes, i.e. *an internal dentinal plane* inclining apically, an *outer enamelo-dentinal plane* in the direction of enamel rods and a *peripheral partial enamel plane bevel; axial wall* is perfectly flat; *incisal wall* is same as gingival wall but in the reversed direction.

- At the *middle of the cavity*; has the same anatomy except that the internal dentinal planes create a less acute angle with the axial wall at incisally and gingivally.

- At the *lingual third of the cavity*; each of the incisal and gingival wall have two planes, i.e. one flat enamel dentinal plane at right angles to the flat axial wall and a peripheral partial enamel bevel plane.

ii. Labio - lingual Cross Section

- The *axial wall* is perfectly flat, lies right angle to the labial wall and opens directly to the lingual surface.

- The *labial wall* is formed of three planes, i.e. an *inner dentinal plane* at right angle to axial wall, an *outer enamel dentinal plane* in the direction of the enamel rods and a *marginal enamel bevel plane*.

- Lingually, the axial wall ends with a partial bevel.

Instrumentation

1. Tooth structure is removed by using a No. 168 bur from lingual access in inciso gingival movements.

2. Use 8-9 hatchet to flatten the gingival and incisal walls in direct cutting strokes.

3. Use the hatchet to flatten the labial wall to place it in proper angulation in lateral cutting strokes directing inciso gingivally.

4. Incisal retention mode is created by a spear bur at the inciso-labio-axial point angle by moving it in lingual direction.

5. Gingival retention mode is created by the same spear bur at the gingivo labio axial point angle.

6. Margin trimmer is used to accentuate the incisal and gingival retention.

7. Sharp the labio-axial, gingivo - axial and the inciso-axial line angle with the gingival margin trimmer (GMT).

8. Create the short partial bevel on the labial and lingual margins with the GMT.

IV. CLASS - V CAVITY

- There are four types of designs are there for class V cavity preparation.

A. FERRIER DESIGN

1. General outline form

- *Trapezoidal* in shape, with the short arm gingivally and the long arm occlusally.

- *Advantages of trapezoidal form*

  i. Most convenient and conservative form for the gingival third lesions.

  ii. Most esthetic

  iii. Provide prompt paving and margination of the restoration.

  iv. Assures safe condensation.

  v. Facilitates bulkiest retention forms.

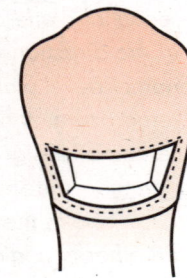

2. Location of the Margins

- According to Ferrier, the *gingival margin* should be half way into the gingival crevice. The *mesial and distal margins* should be partly covered by the gingiva in its ascending path to the interproximal col and partly at, but not involving the axial line angle of the tooth; the *occlusal margin* is at, but not including the height of contour. It should be parallel to the gingival margin and both should be parallel to the occlusal plane.

3. Internal Anatomy

i. *Mesio - distal Cross Section :* Has a convex *axial wall* with the same curvature as the facial or lingual surface. The *mesial and distal* wall has 2 planes, i.e. one plane is divergent and makes an obtuse angle with the axial wall formed of enamel and dentin, the other plane is in the form of a partial enamel bevel.

ii. *Gingivo-occlusal Cross Section :* *Gingival Wall* will be in the gingival third of the facial or lingual surface and is formed of four planes, i.e.

1. An *inner dentinal plane* resembling a reverse bevel making an acute angle with the axial wall.

2. A *transition plane* formed of dentin.

3. A *third plane* in the direction of the enamel rods inclining gingivo facially or lingually.

4. A *fourth plane* in the form of a partial enamel bevel. The occlusal wall may have the same four planes. The only exception is that the outer planes will be inclining occlusofacially or lingually.

B. PROXIMAL PAN HANDLE EXTENSION DESIGN

1. General outline form

- It consists of two portions, i.e. 1. *Facial or lingual* part whose outline is exactly same as the Ferrier design. 2. *Proximal part* is in the shape of *parallelogram* as an extension from the facial (or lingual) in the proximal direction.

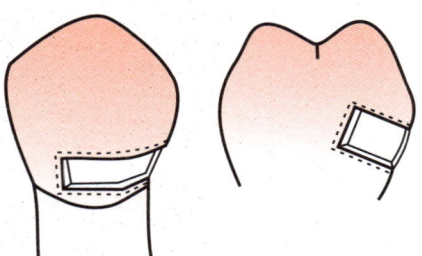

2. Location of the Margins

- The margins of *facial and lingual* portions are located same as in the Ferrier design.

- The proximal portion will have a gingival, occlusal and facial (or lingual) margin.

- All margins should be located in the gingival embrasure, and can extend proximally to the opposite facial or lingual embrasures.

3. Internal Anatomy

- The facial or lingual portion will have the same internal anatomy as Ferrier design.

- The proximal portion has a flat axial wall.

- The gingival floor is same as the gingival floor of the facial or lingual portion.

- The *occlusal wall* is formed of two planes, i.e. a *flat internal plane* formed of enamel and dentin in the direction of enamel rods and a proximal *partial enamel bevel plane*.

- The *facial or lingual wall* is formed of two planes on proximal side, i.e. an *inner dentin enamel plane* at right angles to the axial wall in the direction of enamel rods and a *partial enamel bevel plane*.

- The junction of the two axial walls should be rounded and the other line and point angles should be angular.

- The junctions of the peripheral partial enamel bevels should be rounded.

C. UNI OR BILATERAL 'MOUSTACHE' EXTENSIONS DESIGN

Indication

- Indicated to restore surface defects occlusal to the height of contour which are continuous with a gingival third lesion.

1. General Outline form

- As the name implies, the design appears as a *unilateral or bilateral moustache shape*.

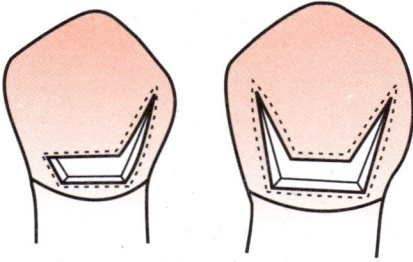

2. *Location of margins and Internal Anatomy*

   – Margins are similar to the Ferrier Design.

   – The additional extension portions have straight mesial and distal walls which end at a point occlusally.

   – The *mesial and distal walls* possess the same partial enamel bevel as the rest of the cavity preparation.

D. PARTIAL MOON (CRESCENT) SHAPE DESIGN

Indications

1. Very apical location and gingival inclination of the height of the contour.

2. Danger of the restoration affecting the esthetics.

3. Mostly indicated in upper and lower cuspids and in upper first molars.

1. *General Outline Form*

   – *Semi - lunar* shape since the occlusal margin should follow the height of contour.

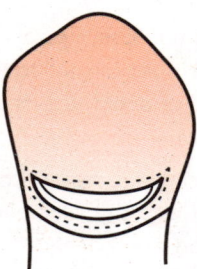

2. *Location of the Margins*

   – The *mesial, distal and gingival margins* follow the curvature of the gingivae and there is no demarcation between these margins.

   – The *occlusal or incisal margin* follows the curvature of the height of contour and with out including the height of contour.

3. *Internal Anatomy*

   – Internal angulation of the walls of this design is same as the Ferrier Design with the exception that there is no demarcation between the mesial-gingival and distal gingival walls.

Instrumentation

1. Use smaller instruments.

2. Spear bur is used to create reverse bevel dentinal form.

3. Angle former or the pointed end of a GMT can be used to sharpen the reverse bevel and starting points and to connect these retentive features with each other and with the rest of the preparation.

FINISHING AND POLISHING OF DIRECT GOLD RESTORATIONS

– The initial step in finishing procedure is to burnish the gold.

– A flat beaver-tail burnisher is used with heavy hand pressure to harden the surface gold.

– Then, a cleoid-discoid carver is used to continue the burnishing and or the gold knife is used to remove excess gold on cavosurface margin.

– If any excess gold is compacted, a green stone is necessary to remove the excess.

– Care should be taken to avoid abrading the surface enamel.

– Then a small round finishing bur is used to begin polishing.

– Polishing is performed with fine pumice followed by tin oxide or white rouge. These powdered abrasives are applied dry, with a soft webless rubber cup.

– Care should be taken to use light pressure.

– Gentle blows of air, should be used to cool the surface during polishing.

CHAPTER 12

CAST RESTORATIONS

INLAY

– *An indirect restoration involving proximal, occlusal surface (not morethan two surfaces), may cover one or more cusps but not all.*

CLASS - II INLAY

– *An indirect restoration involving proximal and occlusal surfaces and may cover one or more cusps but not all.*

INDICATIONS FOR INLAYS

1. A cavity whose width does not exceed one third the intercuspal distance.
2. Strong, self resistant cusps should be remained.
3. Indicated teeth have minimal or no occlusal facets.
4. The tooth is not to be an abutment for a fixed or removable prosthesis.

ONLAY

– *An indirect restoration, involving entire occlusal surface which covers all the cusps.*

CLASS-II ONLAY

– An indirect restoration which involves proximal surfaces of posterior tooth and caps all of the cusps.

INDICATIONS FOR ONLAYS

1. A cavity whose width is one-third to one half of the intercuspal distance.
2. In the tooth preparation, if the length: width ratio of the cusp is more than 1:1, but not exceeding 2:1, onlay can be considered.
3. In the tooth preparation, if length: width ratio of a cusp is more than 2:1 onlay is mandated.
4. Replacement of defective amalgam restorations.
5. When the restoration needs to splint the buccal and lingual cusps.
6. Restoration of posterior interproximal caries.
7. Restoration of posterior teeth with heavy occlusal wear.

CAST RESTORATIONS
INDICATIONS

1. Extensive tooth involvement.
2. Restoration of endodontically treated tooth.

3. Cracked teeth (vertically or diagonally).

4. Esthetics.

5. Repeated failures of amalgam restoration.

6. Worn teeth.

7. Fixed and removable denture retainers.

8. Low incidences of plaque accumulation and decay.

9. Patient preference.

CONTRAINDICATIONS

1. Developing and deciduous teeth.

2. High plaque / caries indices.

3. Occlusal disharmony.

4. Dissimilar metals

ADVANTAGES

1. High Strength.

2. Capable of reproduction of minute details also.

3. No significant tarnish and corrosion.

4. Very much biocompatible.

5. Long lasting.

DISADVANTAGES

1. Microleakage at the tooth cement casting junction.

2. Extensive tooth preparation.

3. Galvanism.

4. Needs multiple visits.

5. Some cast alloys have high abrasive resistance than that of enamel.

6. Not economical.

MATERIALS FOR CAST RESTORATIONS

Classification

1. *Class - I*
   - These are gold and platinum group based alloys.
   - These are sub divided into type I, II, III and IV gold alloys.

2. *Class - II*
   - These are low gold alloys with gold content less than 50%.

3. *Class - III*
   - These are non gold palladium based alloys.

4. *Class - IV*
   - These are nickel - chromium based alloys.

5. *Class - V*
   - These are castable, moldable ceramics.

PRINCIPLES OF TOOTH PREPARATION FOR CAST RESTORATIONS

- Tooth preparation is divided into,
  i. *Intra coronal tooth preparation.*
  ii. *Extra coronal tooth preparation.*

- *Intra Coronal Preparations* are mortise shaped having definite walls and floors joined at line and point angles.

- *Extra Coronal Preparations* are created by occlusal and axial surface reduction. In most of the cases, ends gingivally with no definite flat floor.

- There are 3 principles of tooth preparation,
  1. *Preparation path*
  2. *Apico occlusal taper of the preparation*
  3. *Circumferential tie*

1. PREPARATION PATH

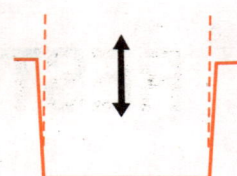

- The preparation should have a single insertion path, opposite to the direction of the occlusal load.

- *This path is usually parallel to the long axis of the tooth crown.*

- *This feature helps in the retention of restoration and decreases its micromovements during function.*

2. APICO - OCCLUSAL TAPER / INLAY TAPER

- *The concept is, intracoronally the cavity walls must diverge from the floor of the preparation to external surface and extracoronally walls must converge from the cervical to the occlusal surface.*

- *Taper permits an unobstructed removal of the wax pattern and seating of the subsequent casting.*

- Generally, the axis of taper for a Class - I or II preparation is parallel to the long axis of the tooth and for a Class - V, it is perpendicular to the long axis of the tooth.

- The taper should be on an average of 2 - 5° from the path of preparation.

- The amount of taper is influenced by certain factors, i.e. greater the wall length is the more taper will be but not to exceed 10° and greater the need for retention, the less taper will be.

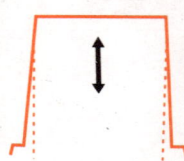

3. CIRCUMFERENTIAL TIE

– *The peripheral marginal anatomy of the preparation is called circumferential tie.*

– If the margin ends on enamel, enamel walls should fulfill all requirements.

  1. Enamel must be supported by sound dentin.
  2. Enamel rods forming the cavosurface margin should be continuous with sound dentin.
  3. Enamel rods forming the cavosurface margin should be covered with restorative material.
  4. Angular cavosurface angles should be trimmed.

– *For the occlusal and gingival walls in intracoronal cavity preparations the tooth circumferential tie will be in the form of a bevel. (which is a plane of a cavity wall or floor directed away from the cavity preparation).*

BEVELS

Definition

– Bevels are the flexible extensions of a cavity preparation allowing the inclusion of surface defects, supplementary grooves or other areas on the tooth surface.

Types

– According to their shape and type of tissue involvement they are divided into,

1. Partial Bevel

  – Involves the part of the enamel wall, not exceeding two-thirds of its dimension.
  – *Usually not used in cast restorations.*
  – *Used to trim weak enamel rods from margin peripheries.*

2. Short Bevel

  – Includes the entire enamel wall, but not dentin.
  – *Used mostly with Class - I alloys especially for type I and II.*

3. Long Bevel

  – Includes all of the enamel wall and upto one half of the dentinal wall.
  – It is the most frequently used bevel for the first three classes (Class - I, II and III) of cast materials.
  – *Advantage :* Preserves the internal 'boxed-up' resistance and retention features of the preparation.

4. Full Bevel

  – Includes all of the dentinal and enamel walls of the cavity wall or floor.

– It's use should be avoided except in cases where it is impossible to use any other form of bevel.
– *Disadvantage :* Deprives the preparations internal resistance and retention form.

5. Counter Bevel

  – Given opposite to an axial cavity wall, on the facial or lingual surface of the tooth with the gingival inclination facially or lingually.
  – It is used for the capping of cusps to protect and support them.

6. Hollow ground (concave) bevel

  – It is prepared in a concave form. This allows more space for cast material bulk; a design feature needed in special preparations to improve materials castability retention and better resistance to stresses.
  – It is ideal for Class - IV and V cast materials.

Functions

1. Produce obtuse angled marginal tooth structures which is the bulkiest and strongest configuration of any marginal tooth anatomy.
2. Producing an acute angled margin will be most amenable to burnishing for that alloy.
3. Reduce the error factors (space between cast and tooth substances).
4. Major retention forms for cast restoration.
5. Gingival bevels bring the gingival margins as cleansable or protected areas.

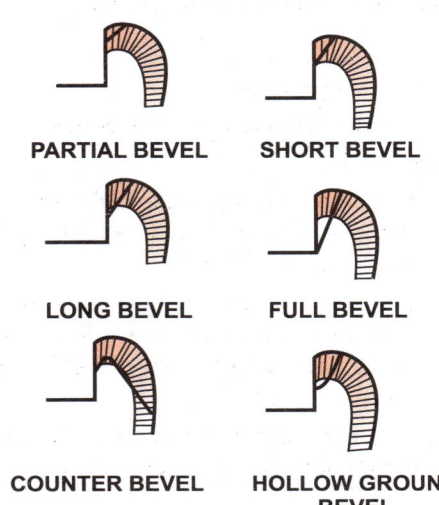

PARTIAL BEVEL   SHORT BEVEL   LONG BEVEL   FULL BEVEL   COUNTER BEVEL   HOLLOW GROUND BEVEL

FLARES

Flares are the flat or concave peripheral portions of the facial and lingual walls.

Types of flares

1. Primary Flare

- It is the conventional and basic part of the circumferential tie facially and lingually for an intra coronal preparation.
- It always has a specific angulation, i.e. 45° to the inner dentinal wall proper.
- It may be a hollow ground in the preparation for a non noble alloy or cast ceramics.

Functions and Indications

- Perform the same functions as bevels.
- They bring the facial and lingual margins of the cavity preparations to cleansable, finishable areas.
- Indicated for any facial or lingual proximal wall of an intra coronal cavity preparation.

2. Secondary Flare

- It is a flat plane superimposed peripherally to a primary flare.
- It can be prepared in a hollow ground form also
- Unlike primary flares, secondary flares may have different angulations, involvement and extent depending on their function.

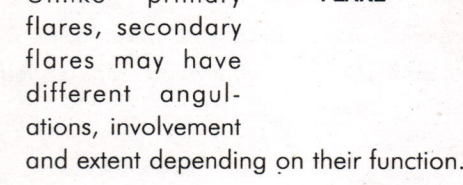

SECONDARY FLARE

PRIMARY FLARE

Functions and Indications

- Perform the same functions as bevels.
- In addition,
  - Provide obtuse angulation of the marginal tooth structure in a teeth with very widely extended lesions bucco lingually.
  - Bring the facial and lingual margins to finishable, cleansable areas in the teeth with very broad contact areas or malposed contact areas.
  - Avoid marginal failures due to peripheral marginal undercuts in ovoid teeth.

Circumferential Tie Constituents for Extracoronal Preparations : (Finishing Lines)

- *For extra coronal preparations, circumferential tie will be in one of the following forms.*

1. Chamfer finishing Line

- A concave extracoronal finish line that possesses greater angulation than a knife edge with less width than a shoulder.
- Is an obtuse angled gingival termination.
- Most universally used design for Class - I, II and III cast materials.
- Most practical type of finishing line for subgingival extra coronal preparations.
- *Contra indicated for Class - IV and V cast materials due to their poor castability.*

Advantages

1. Assures bulk
2. Definite marginal termination with little tooth involvement (0.5 mm maximal depth)

Disadvantage

- Limited burnishability of the marginal cast alloy.

2. Knife edge (feather edge) finishing line

- Circumferential tie consistent with the involvement of least tooth structure.
- If the margin is on enamel, it involves part of the enamel only.
- Used only for very castable burnishable type of alloy (preferably type II Gold alloys).
- It should be located on accessible areas of the tooth surface for proper finishing.
- Indicated when minimal axial depth is required for biologic or anatomic purposes.
- *Contra indicated for Class-III, IV and V cast materials.*

Advantages

1. Involvement of least tooth structure.
2. Blends easily and efficiently with bevelled constituents.

Disadvantage

- Possibility for indefinite termination for the casting.

3. Bevelled shoulder finishing line

- Most tooth structure is involved.
- It can be used for any class of cast materials.
- It is indicated when (i) a definite gingival floor, with all its components (wall proper and bevel) is needed for resistance, retention purposes, (ii) maximum bulk of the cast is needed marginally for materials that are limited in their castability and difficult to burnish.

Advantages

1. Blends easily with bevelled constituents.
2. Maximal reduction of marginal problems of internal spacing.

3. Ideal design for subgingivally located margins.

4. **Hollow ground (concave) bevel**
   - It is actually an exaggerated chamfer or a concave bevelled shoulder.
   - Tooth involvement is greater than a chamfer and less than a bevelled shoulder.
   - Ideal finishing line for Class - IV and V cast materials.

   Advantages
   1. Good transitional continuity with the beveled portion.
   2. Helps in stabilization of the casting.

TOOTH PREPARATION FOR CLASS - II CAST METAL INLAYS

A. INITIAL CAVITY PREPARATION

   - Carbide burs are used to develop the vertical internal walls of the preparation suggested burs are the No. 271 and the No.169L.
   - *Throughout the preparation, the cutting instruments are oriented to develop the vertical walls to attain a single 'draw' path (usually the long axis of the tooth crown) so that the completed preparation should have no undercuts (draft).*
   - The *gingival - to-occlusal divergence* of these preparation walls may range from *2 to 5 degrees* per wall from the line of draw.

1. **Occlusal Step**
   - With the No. 271 carbide bur holding parallel to the long axis of the tooth crown, enter the fossa / pit closest to the involved marginal ridge using a punch cut to a depth of 1.5 mm to establish the depth of the pulpal wall.
   - Maintain the long axis of the bur parallel to the long axis of the tooth crown at all times.
   - Maintaining the initial depth and the same bur orientation, extend the preparation outline along the central groove fissure to include the mesial fossa/pit.
   - Extend to include faulty facial and lingual fissures radiating from the mesial pit.
   - The facial and lingual extension in the mesial pit region should provide the desired dovetail retention or which resists distal displacement of the inlay.
   - Continuing at the initial depth extend the occlusal step distally into distal marginal ridge

sufficiently to expose the junction of the proximal enamel and the dentin.

   - While extending distally, progressively widen the preparation to the desired faciolingual width to facilitate the proximal box preparation.
   - The increased faciolingual width enables the facial and lingual walls of the box to project perpendicularly to the proximal surface at positions that will clear the adjacent tooth by 0.2 to 0.5 mm.

2. **Proximal Box**
   - Continuing with the No. 271 carbide bur isolate the distal enamel by cutting a proximal ditch.
   - The mesiodistal width of the ditch should be 0.8 mm and prepared approximately two-thirds (0.5 mm) at the expense of dentin and one third (0.3 mm) at the expense of enamel.
   - While penetrating gingivally extend the proximal ditch facially and lingually beyond the caries to the desired position of the facioaxial and linguoaxial line angles.
   - When preparing the proximal portion of the preparation, maintain the side of the bur at the specified axial wall depth regardless of whether it is in dentin, caries, old restorative material or air.
   - The axial wall should follow the contour of the tooth faciolingually.
   - Then with the No. 271 carbide bur, make two cuts one at the facial limit of the proximal ditch and the other at the lingual limit extending from the ditch perpendicularly toward the enamel surface.
   - Extend these cuts until the bur is nearly through the marginal ridge enamel. This weakens the enamel by which the remaining isolated portion is held. However, the remaining enamel wall often breaks away during cutting.
   - Plane the distofacial, distolingual and gingival walls by hand instruments to remove all undermined enamel.
   - The preparation should result in margins that clear the adjacent tooth by 0.2 to 0.5 mm.
   - Shallow (0.3 mm deep) retention groves may be cut in the facioaxial and linguoaxial line angles with the No: 169 L carbide bur. They are indicated especially when the prepared tooth is short.

B. FINAL CAVITY PREPARATION

1. Removal of infected carious dentin and pulp protection

- A slowly revolving round bur (No. 2 or No. 4) or spoon excavator may be used to remove the carious infected dentin.

- Light cured glass ionomer cement may be applied to the shallow (or moderately deep) excavated regions to the depth and form of the ideally prepared surface.

- In the deep carious lesions, calcium hydroxide liner is placed and then light cured GIC is given.

- For this situation, to increase the retention of base retention coves are placed with No. 1/4 carbide bur.

2. Preparation of Bevels and Flares

- A slender, flame shaped, fine grit diamond instrument is used to bevel the occlusal and gingival margins and to apply the secondary flare on the distolingual and distofacial walls.

- This should result in 30-40 degree marginal metal on the inlay. This cavosurface design helps to seal and protect the margins and results in a strong enamel margin with an angle of 140-150 degree.

- Using the flame shaped diamond instrument rotating at high speed, prepare the lingual secondary flare.

- During the secondary flare preparation, the long axis of the instrument should be held parallel to the line of draw, with a slight mesio lingual tilt for the assurance of draft.

- Bevel the gingival margin by moving the instrument facially along the gingival margin. The instrument should be tilted slight mesially to produce a gingival bevel with the correct steepness to result in 30 degree marginal metal if not the bevel will be too steep resulting in gingival bevel metal that is too thin (less than 30 degree metal) and thus too weak.

- *The width of the gingival bevel should be 0.5 to 1 mm.*

- Complete the gingival bevel and then prepare the facial secondary flare.

- The same flame shaped, fine grit diamond instrument is also used for occlusal bevels.

- The width of the cavosurface bevel on the occlusal margin should be approximately one-fourth the depth of the respective wall.

- The resulting occlusal marginal metal of the inlay should be 40 degree metal; thus the occlusal marginal enamel is 140 degree enamel.

- Failure to apply a bevel in these regions leaves the enamel margin weak and subject to injury by fracture and also results in metal alloy that is difficult to burnish.

- The diamond instrument is also used to bevel lightly the axiopulpal line angle.

- Thus, the desirable metal angle at the margins of inlays is 40 degree, except at the gingival margins, where the metal angle should be 30 degree.

PROXIMAL MARGIN DESIGNS

- The designs vary according to,
  1. The extent and location of tooth structure loss.
  2. Tooth form and its relationship with adjacent teeth.
  3. Need for retention convenience.

- The various designs are,
  1. Box
  2. Slice
  3. Auxiliary slice
  4. Modified flare

1. Box

- The box design is used with the proximo occlusal preparation for the direct method of wax pattern formation.

- A proximo occlusal cavity will have its buccal and lingual proximal walls finished so that the cavosurface angle formed 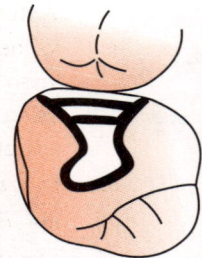 by the proximal flare and the tooth surface will be at right or slightly obtuse angles. A cervical bevel is given to provide a lap joint for finishing.

2. Slice

- It involves conservative preparation of the proximal surface to establish the buccal and lingual extent of the finish lines and to provide a lap joint for finishing.

- Slices are placed on the buccal and lingual proximal surfaces independently.

– The slice may extend to the cervical floor or terminate at a point occlusal to the cervical floor.

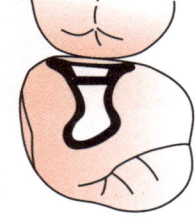

– Teeth with the square tooth form require a slice preparation that extends to the cervical floor.

– Teeth with tapering or ovoid forms require a slice preparation extending short of the cervical floor.

– Beveling of the proximal cavosurface with slice assures sound enamel margin and well adapted casting margin.

3. Auxiliary Slice

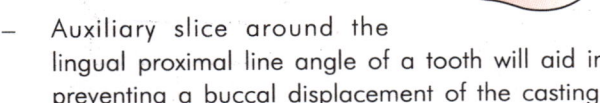

– It wraps partially around the proximal line angles and thus provides additional tooth support.

– It enhances resistance form with minimal tooth structure removal.

– Auxiliary slice around the lingual proximal line angle of a tooth will aid in preventing a buccal displacement of the casting.

– Auxiliary slice around the buccal line angle will aid in preventing the lingual displacement of the casting.

4. Modified Flare

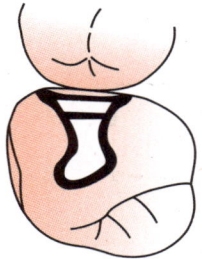

– It is a hybrid between the box and slice preparations.

– Buccal and lingual proximal walls are initially formed with minimal extension and then prepared in a plane that only slightly reduces the proximal wall dimension.

IMPRESSION PROCEDURE FOR CAST METAL RESTORATIONS

– The indirect technique is the most accurate and dependable one.

– The most common impression materials used for indirect casting technique are the Polyvinyl Siloxanes.

Polyvinyl Siloxane Impression

Advantages

1. Excellent reproduction of detail.

2. Excellent dimensional stability.

3. Easy to mix.

4. Have no unpleasant odor or taste.

Tray Selection

– The custom resin tray made over 2 to 3 mm wax spacer on the study cast is required.

Technique

– Two viscosities of impression material are used,

  1. Light bodied material - to inject around the preparation.

  2. Heavy bodied material to fill the tray.

– 2 dispensers are needed. These dispensers are loaded with the cartridges that contain the accelerator and base pastes.

– Using one dispenser to mix and fill the impression tray with the heavy bodied impression material.

– Then use the other dispenser to mix and inject the light bodied impression material on the prepared teeth and fill the opened gingival sulci and prepartions over and beyond the margins with material from the syringe.

– And also light bodied material is injected on the occlusal surfaces of the unprepared adjacent teeth.

– After filling and covering the teeth, now seat the loaded tray over the region.

– Once the material is set, remove it from the mouth by a quick, firm pull that is directed as much as possible in line with the draw of the preparation.

– Inspect the impression carefully.

FINISHING AND POLISHING OF CAST METAL RESTORATIONS

– The grooves, pits and inaccessible areas are smoothened by rubber abrasive points.

– Brush the occlusal surface with a soft bristle disc and tripoli polishing compound, running the disc parallel to the grooves.

– A small felt wheel with polishing compound is used on the proximal and other accesible areas to attain lustre.

– A felt or chamois wheel and rouge can be used for high sheen.

DIFFERENCES BETWEEN THE CLASS - II CAVITY PREPARATION FOR *SILVER AMALGAM AND CAST RESTORATIONS*

Preparation feature	Silver Amalgam	Cast Restoration
1. Outline form:	– narrow	– Wide
2. Cavity width:	– 1/4th of inter cuspal distance.	– 1/3rd of intercuspal distance.
3. Cavity depth:	– more	– less
4. Cavity walls:	– converge occlusally.	– parallel or diverge occlusally.
5. Cavosurface bevel:	– not given (Butt joint)	– given (Lap joint)
6. Line and Point angles:	– rounded and axio pulpal line angle is bevelled.	– well defined and axio pulpal line angle is slightly rounded.
7. Reverse bevel:	– not given	– given
8. Secondary retention:	– only locks are given	– only grooves are given.

CHAPTER 13

NON-CARIOUS LESIONS

– Non carious lesions may be classified into,
   1. Attrition
   2. Abrasion
   3. Erosion
   4. Localized Non-Hereditary enamel hypoplasia
   5. Localized Non-Hereditary Enamel Hypocalcification
   6. Localized Non-Hereditary Dentin hypoplasia
   7. Localized Non-Hereditary Dentin Hypocalcification
   8. Discolourations
   9. Malformation
   10. Amelogenesis imperfecta
   11. Dentinogenesis imperfecta
   12. Trauma

ATTRITION

– *Attrition is defined as the loss of surface tooth structure resulting from direct frictional forces between contacting teeth.*

– Attrition affecting occlusal surfaces results in flattening of their inclined planes, in facet formation and reverse cusp formation.

– Attrition affecting proximal surfaces results in flat, faceted proximal contours and sometimes concave proximal surfaces.

– Attrition increases in patients with parafunctional mandibular movements, i.e. bruxism.

– *Attrition is a physiologic process.*

EFFECTS OF ATTRITION

1. **Occluding surface attrition (Occlusal wear)**
   The effects are,
   – Loss of vertical dimension of the tooth
   – Cheek biting
   – Gingival irritation
   – Decay
   – Tooth sensitivity

2. **Proximal surface attrition (proximal surface faceting)**
   The effects are,
   – Increased susceptibility to caries
   – Hindering of cleansability
   – Drifting of teeth
   – Overall reduction of the length of dental arch
   – Decreased interproximal space

CAUSES OF ATTRITION

– They are of two types, i.e.

1. Physiological attrition
2. Pathological attrition

1. Physiological attrition

– Attrition is constant and is proportionate to the age of individual.

– Attrition also occurs in proximal surface in the contact point areas.

2. Pathological Attrition

i *Abnormal occlusion.* Ex: crowding of teeth and malposed teeth.

ii *Abnormal chewing habits.* Ex: Bruxism and chronic persistent chewing of coarse and abrasive foods or other substance.

iii *Structural defects* in teeth. Ex: Amelogenesis imperfecta, Dentinogenesis imperfecta.

TREATMENT

1. For pulpally involved teeth, endodontic therapy or extraction depending on its restorability and role in the stomatognathic system.

2. Treating of parafunctional activities.

3. Resolving of myofunctional, TMJ or any other symptoms in the stomatognathic system.

4. Occlusal Equilibration is performed after the reliving of all notable symptoms.

– Occlusal equilibration is defined as the selective grinding of tooth surfaces which include rounding and smoothening of the peripheries of the occlusal tables and also the creation of adequate overlap between the working inclines.

5. Protection of exposed sensitive dentinal areas and obliteration of actual carious lesions. Protection is by fluoride solution and obliteration is by proper temporary restoration.

6. *Restorative modalities* : metallic restorations are used to replace lost tooth structure due to attrition which is at high stress concentration areas.

ABRASION

– *Abrasion is defined as the mechanical wearing away of the teeth.*

– Occurs most frequently on incisal and occlusal surfaces.

– *Abrasion is a pathologic process* which is usually inseparable from attrition and / or erosion.

TYPES OF ABRASION (CAUSES)

– Based on the etiologic factor,

1. Tooth brush abrasion (most predominant).

2. Pipe smoking 'depression abrasion'.

3. Abrasion due to tobacco chewing.

4. Proximal abrasion due to the forcing of a tooth pick, inter dental stimulator, etc.

5. Abrasion due to professional habits such as cutting of sewing thread with incisors, holding and pulling of nails with anterior teeth.

6. Iatrogenic tooth abrasion, i.e. between porcelain teeth and opposing natural teeth; between cast alloy restoration of high abrasion resistance and opposing natural teeth.

1. Toothbrush Abrasion

– Occurs cervically, mostly on the facial surface of canines and bicuspids. It is usually on the left side for right handed persons and vice versa for left-handed people.

– The extent of abrasion is depend on the following,

– Horizontal direction of brushing is most detrimental.

– The larger and more irregular the abrasive particles the more the abrasion will be.

– The higher the percentage of abrasives in the dentifrice, the more the abrasion will be.

– Silica abrasives are much more abrading than phosphate and carbonate ones.

– The greater the diameter of brush bristles, the more the abrasion will be. Natural bristles are more abrasive than synthetic bristles.

– Type of tooth tissues being abraded : The most resistant tissues to abrasion are enamel especially occlusally and the least resistant is cementum. Dentin abrades very easily at cervical region.

SIGNS AND SYMPTOMS

1. Lesion is linear shape in outline.

2. Peripheries of the lesion are angularly demarcated from the surrounding tooth surface.

3. Surface of the lesion is extremely smooth and polished.

4. The surrounding walls of the lesion make a V - shape by meeting at an acute angle axially.

5. Stimulating (with hot, cold or sweets) or probing of the lesion can elicit the pain.

2. Pipe smoking 'depression abrasion'

   – An abrading depression on the occlusal surfaces of teeth at antero-lateral portion of the arch coinciding with the intraoral location of the pipe stem.

   Pica-syndrome

   – It is due to the habit of chewing clay (mud), has a specific occlusal abrasion pattern and other systemic disorders.

TREATMENT

1. Preventive

   – Correct or avoid ill-fitting metal clasps and dentures.

   Discontinuation of the habits of chewing tobacco, gum, toothpick, etc.

2. Restorative

   a. *Milder cases :* Limiting of the lateral extrusions of the mandible, excessive movements of the mandible by placing gold- foil restorations or inlays, building up of a cusp.

   b. *Moderate cases :* 'shoeing' method is employed, i.e. cutting cavities in the abraded surfaces and placing gold-foil restorations, inlays or onlays, making no attempt to restore original tooth forms.

   c. *Extensive cases :* operation of restoring vertical dimensions or `opening the bite' may be attempted, placing crowns or inlays on the posterior teeth, bridges or removable dentures in any existing spaces and building up and restoring to original form the anterior teeth with restorations or porcelain crowns.

EROSION

   – Erosion is the chemical or chemico-mechanical wearing away in such a manner that broad, shallow, smooth, highly polished excavations or depressions are made in the enamel and dentin on surfaces not subject to mastication.

   – Erosion is the pathologic process.

CAUSES

A. Mechanical Factors

   – The action of the muscles of the lips and cheeks and of the tooth brush against the affected surfaces.

B. Chemical factors

   1. Diseases of suboxidation or faulty metabolism resulting in excessive formation of acid sodium phosphate, acid calcium phosphate or both.

   2. Excess of lactic acid in the saliva.

   3. Excess of acid salts excreted from the blood by the salivary or mucous glands.

   4. Excess of alkaline salts or bases present in the saliva.

   5. Solution of the organic matrix by bacterial enzymes and later dissolution of the inorganic material.

   6. Excessive use of extraneous acids such as lemonjuice, vinegar, grapefruit and grapes.

   7. Acid vapours from nitric acid and sulfuric acids, acting in the mouths of workers in factories.

   8. Acidity from a local acidosis in the periodontal tissues as a result of traumatic occlusion.

SIGNS AND SYMPTOMS

1. No demarcation between the lesion and adjacent tooth surface.

2. Lesion's surface is glazed.

3. Erosion rate is same for enamel, dentin and cementum.

4. Adjacent gingiva and periodontium are almost always sound and healthy.

5. Presence of tooth sensitivity.

6. Carious lesions usually do not found on tooth surfaces attacked by erosion.

7. Erosion affects upper teeth more than lower teeth especially on the facial surface of cuspids and premolars; Facial surface of lower anterior teeth is a common location for erosion.

TREATMENT

A. Preventive

   i. *General*

   – Rx is directed against faulty metabolism including such features as regulation of the diet, exercise, fresh air, massage.

   – Plenty of pure water should be drunk or as a substitute some of the carbonated or `spring' waters.

   ii. *Local*

   – Prevention and cure of periodontal disturbances.

   – Stiff toothbrushes and gritty dentifrices should be abandoned.

B. Restorative

   – In the advanced cases, extend the cavity margins well beyond the eroded area and insert porcelain inlays, gold inlays, or gold foil restorations.

CHAPTER 14

DENTIN HYPERSENSITIVITY

DEFINITION

- `Sensitive or Hypersensitive dentin' implies an abnormal sensitiveness of an exposed area of dentin, exhibiting itself in the form of reflex or localized pains, sometimes in the absence of apparent external sources of irritation, or otherwise as a result of the contact of heat and cold, salt, sweet and acid substances or of foods and instruments.
- Pain is sharp, transient and well localized.

CAUSES

1. The action of caries, erosion, abrasion, cracks and fractures of the enamel.
2. The careless use of scalers.
3. Recessions of the gingivae.
4. Changes of temperature.
5. Action of salt, sweet and acid substances.

THEORIES OF DENTIN HYPERSENSITIVITY

1. **Dentin innervation theory**
   - This theory states that dentin hypersensitivity occurs due to direct stimulation of nerve fibers present in dentin.
2. **Odontoblast transmission theory**
   - It states that dentin hypersensitivity occurs due to direct stimulation of odontoblastic processes that are present in dentinal tubules.
3. **Hydrodynamic theory of dentin sensitivity**
   - Proposed by BRANTHROM.
   - Well accepted theory.
   - Dential tubules contain dentinal fluid, Odontoblastic processes, Nerve fibers.
   - Dentinal fluid composition is similar to tissue fluid and it fills the entire length of tubule.
   - The odontoblastic cell processes and nerve fibers extend only very little distance into the dentinal tubules from their origin in the pulp.
   - This theory states that the fluid in the dentinal tubules can be affected by mechanical, thermal and osmotic stimuli. Movement of the dentinal fluid within the tubules in either direction stimulates nerves in the dentin or pulp which result in a painful response.
   - Various stimuli that can alter the dentinal fluid flow in an exposed dentin are,
     1. Temperature changes, i.e. hot / cold food
     2. Sweets

3. Dental drill
4. Compressed air
5. Chiselling

MANAGEMENT

- It depends on cause,
  1. Restorative method.
  2. Nonrestorative method.

1. Restorative method

- When hypersensitivity is associated with significant loss of tooth structure, restorative methods are used.
- Cervical defects like abrasion erosion and abfraction can be treated by using Glass Ionomer or composites with proper pulp protection if required.
- Dental Caries can be treated with suitable metallic or non metallic restoration.
- Cracked tooth syndrome is treated with full crowns.
- Faulty restorations should be removed and then restored temporarily. Once the symptoms of sensitivity subsides tooth is permanently restored.

2. Nonrestorative Method

- If the loss of tooth structure is insignificant and generalized, then Nonrestorative methods are indicated.

Various treatment Modalities

1. Resin impregnation technique
2. Iontophoresis
3. Topical fluoride application
4. Application of calcium hydroxide
5. Chemical agents, i.e. potassium oxalate, silver nitrate
6. Medicated tooth paste
7. Dentin bonding agent
8. Lasers
9. Desiccation

1. Resin Impregnation Technique

- Exposed dentin surface is cleaned.
- Surface is etched with phosphoric acid for 5 sec.
- Rinsing and drying for 20 sec.
- Immediately an enamel bonding agent is applied on the surface which results in quick penetration of resin into the tubules and bonding resin is then cured.

2. Iontophoresis

- Iontophoresis is the transfer of ions under electrical pressure through electrodes having opposite charge.
- In this process, 1 - 2% sodium chloride or solution containing potassium, Zincions etc are applied.
- These ions are forced into the tubules by applying electrical force through electrodes.
- Fluoride ions react with calcium, get precipitated in tubules and there by blocks the tubules.
- They also reduce the excitability of a- delta nerve fibres and reduce dentin sensitivity.

3. Topical fluoride Application: (Fluoride Varnish)

- 30% Sodium fluoride Paste is used.
- Fluoride varnishes at regular intervals can reduce sensitivity by promoting remineralization and they also have antibacterial effects.

4. Application of Calcium hydroxide

- Used especially in Root cementum exposures.
- A paste of calcium hydroxide is placed over exposure area and covered and protected by periodontal paste dressing.

5. Chemical Agents

- Potassium oxalate when applied on the dentinal tubules, calcium oxalate is formed within the tubules and blocks dentinal tubules.
- Single application will be effective for 6 months.
- Potassium ions also have the ability to reduce the alpha delta nerve fibre excitation.
- Silver nitrate is rarely used.

6. Use of Medicated Tooth Paste

A. *Tooth Paste with strontium chloride*

- Strontium reacts with phosphate in the dentinal fluid to form strontium phosphate crystals and block the tubules.
- It also stimulates (1) the formation of secondary dentin, (2) can bind to the collagen matrix of the tubules and there by reduces the diameter of tubules.

B. *Tooth paste with 5% Potassium nitrate*

- Potassium reduces the excitability of peripheral a- delta nerve fibers.
- Promotes mineralization.

C. Tooth paste containing 0.7% sodium mono fluoro phosphate

 – Promotes crystallization and mineralization inside the dentinal tubules.

Formalin

 – Formalin combines with dentinal fluid which contains fluorine.

 – Precipitates inside the tubules to occlude the dentinal tubules.

7. Use of Dentin Bonding Agents

 – Various recently available Dentin bonding agents have been found to be useful in treating hypersensitivity.

 – These bonding agents contain resins like HEMA, META, etc.

8. LASERS

 – LASERS are used to melt and recrystallize the surface tooth structure and there by occlude the dentinal tubules.

 – This method provide the result which lasts quite long.

 – Commonly used LASER is Nd-YAG.

9. Desiccation

 – Dry heat is applied by the use of electrically heated blasts of compressed air.

 – The cavity may be moistened first with absolute alcohol or acetone, then the heat is applied, until the cavity is thoroughly desiccated.

CHAPTER 15

MISCELLANEOUS

CAD - CAM SYSTEMS

- *CAD - CAM* is expanded as *Computer Aided Design and Computer Aided Machining Systems*
- They provide an alternative method to produce metal, ceramic, or composite restorations without the need for processes that require two or more patient appointments for a given type of restoration or prothesis.
- This processing method was developed in the early 1980s.

Processing Method

- CAD-CAM system electronically or digitally records surface coordinates of the prepared tooth and stores these retrieved data in the memory of a computer.
- The image data can be retrieved immediately to mill or grind a metal, ceramic, or composite prosthesis by computer control from a solid block of the chosen material.
- Within minutes, the prosthesis can be fabricated and placed in a prepared tooth and bonded or cemented in patients mouth in a period ranging from 10 min to 1 hr.

Advantages

1. Homogeneous, high quality material
2. Negligible porosity
3. No need of making impression
4. Reduced chair side time
5. Single appointment
6. Good patient acceptance

Disadvantages

1. Costly equipment
2. Lack of computer controlled processing support for occlusal adjustment technique
3. Technique sensitive
4. Poor marginal fit

COPY MILLING PROCESS

Definition

- *The process of cutting or grinding a structure using a device that traces the surface of a master metal, ceramic or polymer pattern and transfers the traced special positions to a cutting station where a blank is cut or ground in a manner similar to a key cutting procedure.*

Processing Method

– It is based on the principle of tracing the surface of a pattern that is then replicated from a blank of ceramic, composite or metal that is ground, cut or milled by a rotating wheel whose motion is controlled by a link through the tracing device.

– It has been in use since 1991.

– The pattern to be traced is made from a blue colored resin based composite.

– Ex : Celay; Mikrona Technologies, Switzerland.

Disadvantages

1. Costly equipment
2. Poor marginal fit

LASERS

– *LASER* stands for *Light Amplification by Stimulated Emission of Radiation.*

– Lasers are devices that produce beams of coherent and very high intensity light.

– Various types of lasers are used in dentistry.

– Most commonly used are, Nd:YAG and Er:YAG.

Uses

1. *Soft tissue applications*

    i. Pulpotomy

   ii. Pulp extirpation

  iii. Apicoectomy

  iv. Gingivectomy

   v. Frenectomy

  vi. Curettage

  vii. Lesion excision

viii. Hemostasis

  ix. Incision and drainage of abscesses

2. *Hard tissue applications*

    i. Caries removal

   ii. Cavity preparation

  iii. Enamel etching

  iv. Enameloplasty

3. *Non-surgical procedures*

    i. Curing of materials

   ii. Instrument sterilization

4. *Root canal procedures*

    i. Access cavity preparation

   ii. Biomechanical preparation

  iii. Root canal debridement and cleaning

5. *Endodontic surgical procedures*

    i. Flap preparation

   ii. Cutting the bone to prepare a window access to the apex of the root.

  iii. Root end preparation for retrograde filling.

  iv. Removal of pathological tissues.

Advantages

1. Blood less
2. Painless

MICRO AND MACRO ABRASION

– It is an alternative for the reduction or elimination of superficial discolorations.

– They result in the physical removal of tooth structure and therefore, are indicated only for stains or enamel defects that do not extend beyond a few tenths of a millimeter in depth.

MICROABRASION

– *A technique involving the surface dissolution of the enamel by the acid along with the abrasiveness of the pumice to remove superficial stains or defects.*

Uses

– The following defects can be removed by microabrasion technique, i.e. incipient carious lesions, fluorosis discolorations extending with in the 0.2 to 0.3mm deep, small localized idiopathic white or light-brown areas and developmental discolored spots to some extent.

Advantages

1. Better control of the removal of tooth structure.
2. Superior patient acceptance.

MACROABRASION

– *A technique of removal of the defect using a 12-fluted composite finishing bur or a fine grit finishing diamond in a high-speed handpiece.*

Precautions

1. Use light
2. Apply intermittent pressure
3. Careful monitoring of removal of tooth structure.

4. Use Air-water spray to maintain the hydrated stage of tooth.

Uses

– Technique is used for the removal of localized, superficial white spots (not subject to conservative, remineralization therapy) and other surface stains or defects.

Advantages

1. Faster
2. No need of rubberdam application
3. Easy removal of defect

Disadvantages

1. Technique sensitive.
2. Should be extreme cautious.

AIR ABRASION

Definition

– A method of removal of tooth structure with the use of finely graded $27.5\,\mu$ alluminium oxide powder administered under compressed air through a fine tip.
– Air abrasion uses the kinetic energy principle, in which particles bounce off the tooth and blasts the decay away.

Uses

1. To remove any stains or decay from teeth.
2. To expose hidden cavities, which can then be removed and a filling added.

Advantages

1. Virtually painless procedure.
2. Produce no vibration and no heat from friction.
3. No harm to soft tissues.
4. Preservation of tooth structure.
5. Little or no discomfort.
6. Shorter chair side time.
7. Operate very quitely (hence preferred in treating young patients who would normally be afraid of the dentist's drill).

Limitations

1. Cannot be used to remove interproximal caries.
2. Cannot be used to prepare a tooth for larger restoration such as amalgam.

MICROLEAKAGE

Definition

– *Flow of oral fluid and bacteria into the microscopic gap between a prepared tooth surface and a restorative material.*

Consequences

– The biocompatibility of a restoration is altered by the leakage process, which may cause a number of undesirable events, i.e.
   1. It may allow bacteria or bacterial products to reach the pulp and cause infection.
   2. It may encourage the breakdown of the material.
   3. It may discolour the margins of the restoration.
   4. Post operative sensitivity.

Detecting methods of Microleakage

– Dyes
– Chemical tracers
– Radioactive isotopes
– Neutron activation analysis
– Scanning electron microscopy
– Bacterial studies
– Electrochemical studies
– Air pressure
– Artificial caries
– Pain perception
– Reverse diffusion method

Microleakage around the Restorations

Amalgam

– If the restoration is properly inserted, leakage decreases as the restoration ages in the mouth. This may be caused by corrosion products that form along the interface between the tooth and the restoration sealing the interface and thereby preventing leakage. Accumulation of corrosion products is slower for high-copper alloys.

NANOLEAKAGE

– If the resin penetrates the collagen network of the dentin but does not penetrate it completely, a much smaller gap (<0.1 mm) will exist between the mineralized matrix of the dentin and collagen-resin hybrid layer. This much smaller gap allows *Nanoleakage.*

- It reduces the longevity of the dentin-resin bond.
- This degradation process may gradually increase the gap size until microleakage begins to occur.
- Nanoleakage is not known to occur between restorations and enamel because enamel does not contain organic mass and therefore no collagenous matrix into which a resin may be embedded.

FINISHING AND POLISHING OF THE RESTORATIONS

- *Finishing is the process of removal of excess and contouring the restoration, and which is done immediately after the placement of restoration.*
- Smooth surface does not tarnish, corrode, gives shiny appearance, no surface deposition. Hence, the polishing of restoration is done to achieve the smooth surface.

Goals
- The goals of finishing and polishing procedures are to obtain the,
  1. Desired anatomy
  2. Proper occlusion
- Reduction of roughness, gouges and scratches which were produced by contouring and finishing instruments.

Polishing Materials
- They are supplied in paste and powder.

Polishing Agents
- Rubber cup, Brittle brush, Diamond points, Abrasive points, wheels and cylinders, etc.
- Polishing pastes are applied with soft felt points, muslin (Woven cotton fabric) wheels, prophylaxis rubber cups or buffing wheels.
- A nonabrasive material should be used as an applicator while using polishing pastes.
- For polishing, initially coarse abrasives and finally fine abrasives are used.
- Polishing should be done at slow speeds only.
- High speed results in heat generation which causes damage to the pulp.
- Dry polishing is not advocated because it releases vapours from the restoration and generates frictional heat.

BENEFITS
- Finishing and polishing provide three benefits of dental care.

1. *Oral health*
   - A well contoured and polished restoration promotes oral health by resisting the accumulation of food debris and pathologic bacteria.
2. *Function*
   - Oral function is enhanced with a well-polished restoration because food glides more freely over occlusal and embrasure surfaces during masticatons.
   - Smooth surfaces minimize wear rates on opposing and adjacent teeth.
   - Rough material surfaces lead to the development of high-contact stresses that can cause the loss of functional and stabilizing contacts between teeth.
3. *Esthetics*

REACTION OF THE PULP TO IRRITATING STIMULI

- The reaction will be in one of the following ways,
  1. ### Healthy Reparative Reaction
     - It is the most favourable response.
     - It consists of, formation of sclerotic dentin and/or calcific barrier. These are followed by normal secondary dentin.
     - It occurs without any disturbances in the pulp tissues.
  2. ### Unhealthy Reparative Reaction
     - It is fairly favourable.
     - It consists of, degeneration of the odontoblasts, followed by the formation of the dead tracts.
     - It is accompanied by mild pathological clinical changes of reversible nature in the pulp, which results in the formation of tertiary dentin.
  3. ### Destructive Reaction
     - Most unfavourable response.
     - It begins with the loss of odontoblasts and the outer protective layer of the pulp.
     - The resulting reaction will be inflammation, abscess formation, finally necrosis of the pulp.
     - In any event, pulp tissues can not recuperate from these pathologic changes.

Pulpal Response During Cavity Preparation
- It depends on many factors,
  1. Thermal injury
  2. Frictional heat

3. Vibration

4. Desiccation of dentin

5. Pulp exposure

6. Smear layer

7. Remaining dentin thickness

8. Agents for cleaning, drying and sterilization

9. Acid etching

— Sharp hand cutting instruments are the most biologically acceptable cutting instruments.

— Rotary cutting instruments (burs) are also biologically acceptable if used over effective depth of 2 mm and more with proper coolants.

— Rotary abrasive instruments (stones) are not recommended for cutting in vital dentin as their abrasive action elevates the temperature of surrounding dentin.

— The less the effective depth, the more destructive reaction will be.

— Heat generation not only creates destruction of pulp, but it can also coagulate protoplasm and even char dentin and enamel.

— Desiccation creates a disturbance in the osmotic pressure of dentinal tubules, increases the permeability of the dentin.

— Excessive Vibration can cause,

  — disruption of the odontoblasts in the opposite side of the pulp chamber.

  — edema

  — fibrosis of pulp tissues.

  — change in ground substance of the pulp.

  — reduction in the predentin formation.

  — microcracks in enamel and in non elastic dentin.

— Excessive Frictional heat : Coronal dentin develops a pinkish hue very soon after the dentin is cut. This pinkish hue represents vascular stasis in the sub odontoblastic capillary plexus blood flow. A dark colour indicates thrombosis.

Section II

Endodontics

CHAPTER 01

INTRODUCTION TO ENDODONTICS

Definition

– Endodontics is that branch of dental science which deals with the diagnosis, prevention and treatment of diseases and injuries of the pulp and associated periradicular conditions.

– It includes the study of basic sciences like biology of normal pulp, etiology for the various diseases and pathology of human dental pulp along with morphology and physiology.

Aims and Objectives

1. Diagnosis of the diseases of the pulp.
2. To identify and determine etiological factors responsible for pulpal and periapical disease.
3. Measures to prevent diseases of the pulp and periapical tissues.
4. Selection of cases for treatment.
5. To provide care which is proper and consistent with the knowledge and experience.
6. To determine reasonable prognosis for the cases selected for the treatment.
7. To evaluate or assess the completed endodontic procedures.

Scope of Endodontics

– Formerly, endodontic treatment confined itself to root canal filling techniques by conventional methods, even endodontic surgery was considered to be in the field of oral surgery.

– Modern endodontics has a much wider field and includes the following,
    1. diagnosis of oral pain.
    2. protection of healthy pulp from disease or injury.
    3. pulp capping
    4. pulpotomy
    5. root canal treatment of infected root canals.
    6. Surgical endodontics, which includes apicoectomy, hemi-section, root amputation and replantation.

"Father of Modern Endodontics"

– Dr. Louis Grossman

CHAPTER 02

DENTAL PULP AND PERIRADICULAR TISSUES

- The dental pulp consists of vascular connective tissue contained within the rigid dentinal walls.
- *Primary Function* of the pulp is the elaboration of dentin to form the tooth and to protect against and to repair the effects of noxious stimuli.

ZONES OF PULP
- Pulp is divided into,
  1. odontoblastic zone
  2. cell-free zone
  3. cell-rich zone
  4. central zone

I. ODONTOBLASTIC ZONE
- The odontoblastic cell bodies form the odontoblastic zone.
- In this odontoblastic zone capillaries and unmyelinated sensory nerves are around the odontoblastic cell bodies.

1. *Predentin layer*
- It is the first formed dentin, located adjacent to the pulp tissue.
- It is 2 to 6 μm wide.
- It is uncalcified dentin.
- Dentinogenesis includes the production, deposition and calcification of a matrix. This matrix is the predentin layer deposited around the odontoblastic process and is found between the calcified dentin and the odontoblastic zone.
- This is a protein carbohydrate complex consisting of proteoglycans, phosphoproteins, plasma proteins, glycoproteins and collagen fibrils.

Primary Dentin
- Primary dentin is formed before the teeth erupts and is divided into Mantle and Circum pulpal dentin.
- a. *Mantle Dentin*, the first calcified layer of the dentin deposited against the enamel; forms the dentinal side of the dentino enamel junction.
- b. *Circum pulpal dentin* is the dentin formed after the layer of mantle dentin.
- It forms initial shape.

2. *Secondary Dentin*
- It is a narrow band of dentin bordering the pulp and representing that dentin formed after root completion.

- Secondary dentin is elaborated after eruption of the teeth.

- It can be differentiated from primary dentin by the sharp bending of the tubules producing a line of demarcation.

- It is deposited unevenly on primary dentin and has incremental patterns and tubular structures less regular than those of primary dentin.

- For ex : secondary dentin is deposited in greater quantities in the floor and roof of the pulp chamber than on the walls.

- This deposition of secondary dentin protects the pulp.

- It is also formed in response to Calcium hydroxide cement due to its high pH.

3. **Peritubular Dentin**

- The dentin that immediately surrounds the dentinal tubules is termed peritubular dentin.

- It forms the walls of the tubules in all but the dentin near the pulp.

- It is hyper mineralised (about 40%) than intertubular dentin.

- It is twice as thick in outer dentin than in inner dentin.

- It differs from intertubular dentin,

   - in lacking collagenous fibrous matrix.

   - a zone of increased radiographic and electron density.

- When dentin is routinely demineralised, the peritubular dentin will be lost as it lacks the stabilizing feature of collagen.

- By its growth, it constricts the dentinal tubules to a diameter of $1\,\mu m$ near the DEJ.

- It is the *most highly mineralised part of dentin*.

- It is not found in interglobular areas.

4. **Intertubular Dentin**

- The main body of dentin is composed of intertubular dentin.

- It is located between the zones of peritubular dentin.

- Organic matrix is the main content.

5. **Interglobular Dentin**

- Sometimes mineralization of dentin begins in small globular areas that fail to coalesce into

a homogenous mass, which results in zones of hypo-mineralization between the globules. These zones are known as Interglobular dentin or interglobular spaces.

6. **Reparative Dentin**

- *Also known as irregular or reactionary or tertiary dentin.*

- It is laid down by the pulp as a protective response to noxious stimuli.

- These stimuli can result from caries, operative procedures, restorative materials, abrasion, erosion or trauma.

- The reparative dentin is deposited in the affected area at an average rate of $1.5\,\mu m$ per day.

- Deposition depends on the severity and duration of the injury to the odontoblasts.

- When there is mild stimulus for a prolonged period of time, produces slightly irregular tubules.

- Aggressive carious lesion or abrupt stimulus stimulates the production of reparative dentin with fewer and more irregular tubules.

7. **Dead tracts**

- Dentin areas characterized by degenerated odontoblast process give rise to dead tracts.

- They appear black in transmitted and white in reflected light.

- Those areas show decreased sensitivity and more seen in older teeth.

- They are probably the initial step in the formation of sclerotic dentin.

8. **Sclerotic or Transparent Dentin**

- Dentin that has more mineral content than normal dentin is called Sclerotic dentin.

- It occurs ahead of demineralization.

- It is seen in slowly advancing carious lesion or under old restoration and in the roots of elderly people.

- It is shiny and more dark in colour.

- It reduces the permeability of the dentin and thus prolong the pulp vitality (decreases the tubular lumen diameter).

- Therefore, it is difficult to bond a restorative material to sclerotic dentin.

II. CELL FREE ZONE (Zone of Weil)

— It is a acellular zone of the pulp located centrally to the odontoblastic zone.

— This zone contains some fibroblasts, mesenchymal cells and macrophages although called `cell free'.

— Main constituents of this zone are plexus of capillaries, the nerve plexus of Raschkow and the ground substance.

— This zone is more prominent in the coronal pulp.

III. CELL RICH ZONE

— This zone is located central to the cell free zone.

— Its main components are ground substance, fibroblasts with their product the collagen fibers, undifferentiated mesenchymal cells and macrophages.

IV. CENTRAL ZONE

— The central zone or pulp proper contains blood vessels and nerves that are embedded in the pulp matrix together with fibroblasts.

— From their central location blood vessels and nerves send branches to the periphery of the pulp.

ANATOMY OF THE PULP CAVITY

PULP CAVITY

— *It is the central cavity within a tooth and is entirely enclosed by dentin expect at the apical foramen.*

— Pulp cavity may be divided into *coronal portion, pulp chamber, radicular portion and root canal.*

— In anterior teeth the pulp chamber gradually merges into the root canal and this division becomes indistinct.

— In multirooted teeth the pulp cavity consists of a single pulp chamber and usually three root canals although the number of canals can very from one to five.

— *Roof of the pulp chamber* consists of dentin covering the pulp chamber occlusally or incisally.

— A *Pulp horn* is an accentuation of the root of the pulp chamber directly under a cusp or developmental lobe.

— The *floor of the pulp chamber* runs parallel to the roof and consists of dentin bounding the pulp chamber near the cervix of the tooth particularly dentin forming the furcation area.

— The *canal orifices* are openings in the floor of the pulp chamber leading into the root canals. These are continuous with both the pulp chamber and root canals.

— The *walls of a pulp chamber* derive their names from the corresponding walls of the tooth surface, such as the buccal wall of a pulp chamber.

— The *angles of a pulp chamber* derive their names from the walls forming the angle such as the mesio buccal angle of a pulp chamber.

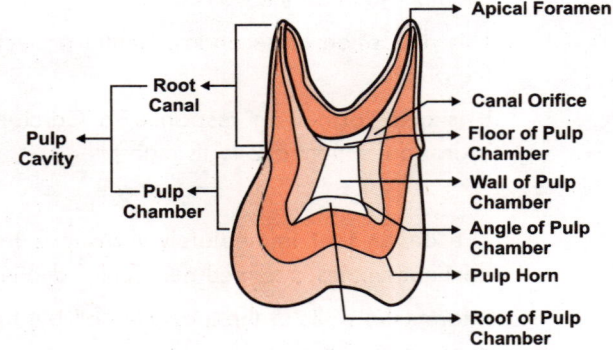

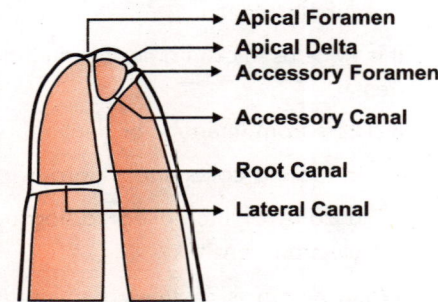

ROOT CANAL

— *It is that portion of the pulp cavity from the canal orifice to the apical foramen.*

— It is divided into three sections, i.e. coronal, middle and apical thirds.

Accessory Canals or Lateral Canals

— These are lateral branchings of the main root canal generally occuring in the apical third or furcation area of a root.

— Sometimes a distinction can be made between an accessory canal and a lateral canal.

— Lateral canal is an accessory canal that branches to the lateral surface of the root and may be visible on a radiograph.

Apical Foramen

– *An aperture at or near apex of a root through which the blood vessels and the nerves of the pulp enter or leave the pulp cavity.*

Accessory Foramina

– *An orifice on the surface of the root communicating with a lateral or accessory canal.*

– The periodontal vessels curve around the root apex of a developing tooth and become entrapped in Hertwig's epithelial root sheath which resulting in formation of the lateral and accessory foramina during calcification.

Apical Stop

– A barrier at the preparation end is an apical stop.

Apical Seat

– Lack of a complete barrier but the presence of a constriction represents an apical seat.

Open Apex

– The apical preparation resembles an open cylinder, i.e. neither barrier nor constriction.

– No apical seat will be created.

Apical Constriction
(minor apical diameter or apical stop)

– It is the apical portion of the root canal having the narrowest diameter.

– This position may vary but is usually 0.5 to 1.0 mm short of the center of the apical foramen.

– The minor diameter widens apically to the foramen (major diameter) and assumes a funnel shape.

TYPES OF ROOT CANAL CONFIGURATIONS

1. Weine's Classification

1. Type I : Single canal from the pulp chamber to the apex.

2. Type II : Two separate canals leaving the chamber but merging short of the apex to form only one canal.

3. Type III : Two separate canals leaving the chamber and exiting the root in separate apical foramina.

4. Type IV : One canal leaving the pulp chamber but dividing short of the apex into two separate and distinct canals with separate apical foramina.

2. Vertussi's Classification

– They are of 8 types,

1. Type I : Single root canal which exits as one single canal.

2. Type II : There will be two canals which exit as single canal.

3. Type III : Single canal which divides into two at the coronal 1/3 and rejoin at apical 1/3 and exit as one.

4. Type IV : Two canals which are exiting as two canals.

5. Type V : Single canal splitting into two.

6. Type VI : Two canals joining together at cervical 1/3 as one and again dividing into two in the apical 1/3.

7. Type VII : Single canal splitting and joining and again splitting into two.

8. Type VIII : Single canal splitting into three.

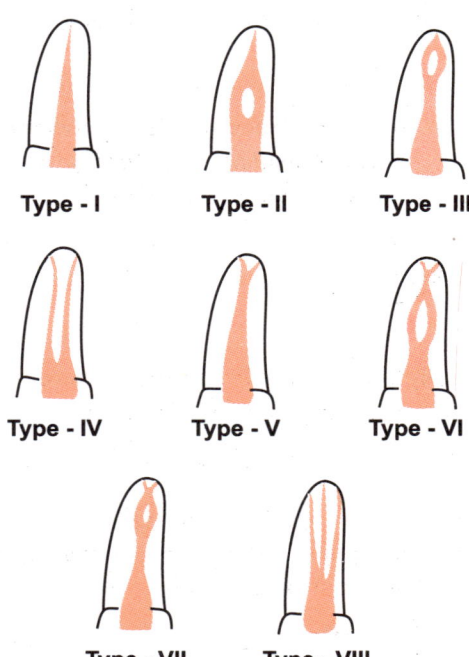

– The pulp horns that are most likely to be exposed during cavity preparation are,

1. *mesiobuccal horn of upper molars.*

2. *mesiolingual horn of lower molars.*

NORMAL PERIRADICULAR TISSUES

– The periradicular tissues consists of, the cementum which covers the teeth. Alveolar process which forms the bony troughs containing the roots of the teeth.

– Periodontal ligament whose collagen fibers embedded in the cementum of the roots to the surrounding tissues.

MORPHOLOGY OF THE PULP

PULPS OF MAXILLARY TEETH

Central Incisor

– *It is shovel shaped coronally with three short horns on the coronal roof.*

– Tapering down to a triangle root in cross section with the point of the triangle pointing lingually.

Lateral Incisor

– It is small and spoon shaped coronally changing to a round evenly tapering root to the apex.

Cuspid

– It is *the longest pulp* with an elliptical cross section buccolingually and distally inclined apex.

First Premolar

– It has a large occlusocervical pulp chamber with a mesial concavity extending from the root surface onto the cervical third of the pulp chamber.

– The coronal chamber divides into two smooth funnel shaped roots.

Second Premolar

– Coronally it is similar to first premolar except it has only one root which begins to taper at about its midpoint.

Molars

– Molars have a roughly rectangular cervical cross section with greatest dimension buccolingually and demonstrating a mesiobuccal prominence.

– There are 3 roots
    – The lingual is longest.
    – The distobuccal is shortest and straight.
    – The mesiobuccal is curved and flattened buccolingually with its convex meisal surface.
    – From the first to third molar the coronal pulp chambers get smaller and roots get closer together.

PULPS OF MANDIBULAR TEETH

Central Incisor

– *It is the smallest pulp in the dentition.*

– It is long and narrow with a flattened elliptical shape in cross section buccolingually.

Lateral Incisor

– It is similar to central incisor but smaller in all dimensions.

Cuspid

– It is similar to, but shorter than the maxillary canine.

– Its root begins tapering at about its midpoint ending in a distally inclined apex.

First Premolar

– It looks like a small mandibular canine with an insignificant or missing lingual pulp horn.

Second Premolar

– The lingual horn is smaller than the buccal horn and is about the dimension of the mandibular canine.

– In cross section it is often roundly triangular or sometimes rectangular.

Molars

– The coronal cross section is rectangular with the mesiodistal dimension greatest.

– Displays a mesiobuccal prominence.

– The horn heights from highest to lowest are mesiobuccal, mesiolingual, distobuccal, distolingual.

– There are two roots,
    – Distal is shorter and straighter and singular.
    – Mesial is longer, curved and often double.
    – From first to third the roots get smaller and closer together.

APICAL CLOSURE

– While calcification and cementum deposition at the apex continue throughout life, apices can be considered as fully formed several years after eruption, and approximate ages are given below:

Tooth	Apical Closure (Years)
I – PRIMARY TEETH	
Upper CI	1 ½
LI	2
C	3 ¼
M₁	2 ½
M₂	3
Lower CI	1 ½
LI	1 ½
C	3 ¼
M₁	2 ¼
M₂	3
II – PERMANENT TEETH	
Upper	10
CI	11
LI	13 – 15
C	12 – 13
I$_{PM}$	12 – 14
II$_{PM}$	9 – 10
I$_M$	14 – 16
II$_M$	18 – 25
III$_M$	
Lower	9
CI	10
LI	12 – 14
C	12 – 13
I$_{PM}$	13 – 14
II$_{PM}$	9 – 10
I$_M$	14 – 15
II$_M$	18 – 25
III$_M$	

CHAPTER 03

DISEASES OF THE DENTAL PULP

CAUSES OF PULP DISEASE
- According to Grossman,

I. PHYSICAL
A. Mechanical
1. Trauma
    a. Accidental
    b. Iatrogenic dental procedures
2. Pathologic wear
3. Crack through the body of tooth
4. Barometric changes

B. Thermal
1. Heat during cavity preparation.
2. Exothermic heat during setting of cement.
3. Conduction of heat and cold through deep restorations with out a protective base.
4. Frictional heat during the polishing of restorations.

C. Electrical
- Galvanic Shock.

II. CHEMICAL
A. Phosphoric aid, acrylic monomer etc.
B. Erosion (acids)

III. BACTERIAL
A. Toxins associated with caries.
B. Direct invasion of pulp from caries or trauma.
C. Anachoresis

- According to Ingle,

I. BACTERIAL
A. Coronal Ingress
1. Caries
2. Fracture
    i. Complete
    ii. Incomplete
3. Non fracture trauma
4. Anamolous tract,
    i. dens invaginatus
    ii. dens evaginatus
    iii. radicular lingual groove

B. Radicular ingress
1. Caries

2. Retrogenic infection
   i. periodontal pocket
   ii. periodontal abscess
3. Hematogenic

II. TRAUMATIC

A. Acute
1. Coronal fracture
2. Radicular fracture
3. Vascular stasis
4. Luxation
5. Avulsion

B. Chronic
1. Adolescent female bruxism
2. Traumatism
3. Attrition or abrasion
4. Erosion

III. IATRAL

A. Cavity preparation
1. Heat of preparation
2. Depth of preparation
3. Dehydration
4. Pulp horn extensions
5. Pulp hemorrhage
6. Pulp exposure
7. Pulp incertion
8. Impression taking

B. Restoration
1. Insertion
2. Fracture
   i. complete
   ii. incomplete
3. Force of cementing
4. Heat of polishing

C. Intentional extirpation and root canal filling

D. Orthodontic movement

E. Periodontal curettage

F. Electro surgery

G. Laser burn

H. Periradicular curettage

I. Rhinoplasty

J. Osteotomy

K. Intubation for general anesthesia

IV. CHEMICAL

A. Restorative materials
1. Cements
2. Plastics
3. Etching Agents
4. Cavity Liners
5. Dentin Bonding Agents
6. Tubule Blockage Agents

B. Disinfectants
1. Silver Nitrate
2. Phenol
3. Sodium Fluoride

C. Desiccants
1. Alcohol
2. Ether
3. Others

V. IDIOPATHIC

A. Aging

B. Internal Resorption

C. External Resorption

D. Hereditary Hypophosphatemia

E. Sickle cell anemia

F. Herpes zoster infection

G. HIV and Aids

CLASSIFICATION OF PULP DISEASES

- According to Grossman,
- Based on clinical features,

I. Pulpitides (Inflammation)

A. *Reversible*
1. Symptomatic (acute)
2. Asymptomatic (Chronic)

B. *Irreversible*
1. Acute
   a. Abnormally responsive to cold
   b. Abnormally responsive to heat
2. Chronic
   a. Asymptomatic with pulp exposure
   b. Hyperplastic pulpitis
   c. Internal resorption

II. Pulp Degeneration

    A.   Calcific (Radiographic Diagnosis)

    B.   Others (Histopathologic diagnosis)

III. Necrosis

BARODONTALGIA (AERODONTALGIA)

– Toothache occurring at low atmospheric pressure experienced either during flight or during a test run in a decompression chamber.

– Barodontalgia has generally been observed in altitudes over 5,000 feet but it is more likely to occur at 10,000 feet or above.

– A tooth with chronic pulpitis can be symptomless at ground level, but it may cause pain at high altitude because of reduced pressure.

Treatment

– Lining the cavity with a varnish or a base of zinc phosphate cement, with a subbase of ZOE cement in deep cavities helps to prevent barodontalgia.

PATHWAYS OF BACTERIAL INVASION OF THE PULP

BACTERIA

– The most common cause of pulp injury is bacterial.

– Once bacteria have invaded the pulp, the damage is almost always irreparable.

– The bacteria most often recovered from infected vital pulps are streptococci, but many other microorganisms from diphtheroids to an aerobes have also been isolated.

– Microorganisms reach the dental pulp in various ways

    1.   *Through the open cavity*, i.e. by dental caries, traumatic injuries or operative procedures.

    2.   *Through the dental tubules* following carious invasions, restorative procedures.

    3.   *Through the lymphatic or haematogenous route (Anachoresis)*.

    4.   *Through the gingival sulcus or periodontal ligament*, i.e. microorganisms and other irritants from the periodontal tissue through exposed dental tubules reach the lateral and accessory canals or apical and lateral foramina.

    5.   *Through a broken occlusal seal* or faulty restoration of a tooth previously treated by endodontic therapy.

    6.   *Through extension of a periapical infection* from adjacent infected teeth.

ANACHORESIS

– It is the transportation of microbes through the blood or lymph to an area of inflammation such as a tooth with pulpitis.

1. REVERSIBLE PULPITIS

Definition

– *A mild to moderate inflammatory condition of the pulp caused by noxious stimuli in which the pulp is capable of returning to the uninflamed state following removal of the stimuli.*

Etiology

– Trauma

– Thermal shock

– Excessive dehydration of the cavity with alcohol or chloroform.

– Galvanism

– Chemical stimulus

– Bacteria from caries

Clinical Features

– Sharp pain lasting for few seconds to minutes.

– Pain on taking cold food, cold beverages and cold air.

– Does not occur spontaneously and does not continue when the stimulus is removed.

Diagnosis

1.   Based on symptoms

2.   Clinical tests: cold test

Differential Diagnosis

– Irreversible pulpitis

Treatment

– Best treatment is prevention.

– Prevention of dental caries.

– Early insertion of filling if a cavity develops.

– Desensitization of neck of teeth where gingival recession occurs.

– Cavity varnish or base application before insertion of filling.

– Care in cavity preparation and polishing.

– Removal of noxious stimuli.

2. IRREVERSIBLE PULPITIS

Definition

- *A persistent inflammatory condition of the pulp symptomatic or asymptomatic caused by a noxious stimuli.*

Etiology

- Bacterial invasion through dental caries is most common.
- Chemical, thermal or mechanical causes.
- Reversible pulpitis may deteriorate into irreversible pulpits.

Clinical Features

Early stage

- *Pain:* Sharp, piercing or shooting and generally severe, intermittent or continuous type.
- May occur by sudden temperature changes particularly to cold, sweet and pressure from the packing food into the cavity.
- Exacerbation of pain on changing position, lying down or bending over (pain during nights while sleeping is observed).
- Referred pain from upper posterior tooth to temple or sinuses.
- From lower posterior tooth to ear.

Later Stage

- Pain is more severe, boring, gnawing or throbbing.
- Slight exposure of the pulp.
- Patient often kept awake at night by the pain.
- Pain is increased by heat and may be relieved by cold.

Diagnosis

1. Inspection

- Discloses a deep cavity
- Pulp exposure
- Greyish skum like layer over the exposed pulp and surrounding dentin
- Eroded pulp surface

2. Radiography

- Exposure of the pulp
- Caries under a filling

3. Thermal test

Differential Diagnosis

- Reversible pulpitis.

Treatment

- Pulpectomy
- Pulpotomy for posterior tooth as an emergency procedure.
- Extraction of the tooth if it is unrestorable.

3. CHRONIC HYPERPLASTIC PULPITIS (PULP POLYP)

Definition

- *A productive pulpal inflammation due to an extensive carious procedure of a young pulp.*
- It is characterized by the development of granulation tissue, covered at times with epithelium and resulting from long standing low grade irritation.

Etiology

- Slow progressive carious exposure of the pulp.
- For the development of hyperplastic pulpitis, a large open cavity, a young resistant pulp and a chronic low grade stimulus are necessary.

Clinical Features

- Symptomless except during mastication, food bolus may cause discomfort.

Diagnosis

Clinical Examination

- Seen in children and young adults.
- Appearance of polypoid tissue. A fleshy, reddish pulpal mass fills most of the pulp chamber or cavity or even extends beyond the confines of the tooth.

Radiography

- Large open cavity with direct access to the pulp chamber.

Differential Diagnosis

- Proliferating gingival tissue.

Treatment

- Pulpectomy

4. INTERNAL RESORPTION

Definition

- *An idiopathic slow or fast progressive resorptive process occurring in the dentin of the pulp chamber or root canal of teeth.*

Etiology

- Unknown
- May be history of trauma

Clinical Features

- Asymptomatic

- *Pink Spot:* Internal resorption is manifested in the crown as a reddish area.
- It represents the granulation tissue showing through the resorbed area of the crown.

Diagnosis

- Common in maxillary anterior teeth.
- During routine radiographic examination.
- On radiograph: round or ovoid radiolucent area in the root canal or pulp chamber.

Differential Diagnosis

- External root resorption.
- In internal resorption, resorptive defect is more extensive in the pulpal wall than on the root surface.

Treatment

- Pulp extripation.
- RCT with plasticized gutta-percha.
- If root perforation occurs seal it with calcium hydroxide.

5. PULP DEGENERATION

- The early stage of pulp degeneration does not usually cause definitive clinical symptoms.
- The tooth is not discolored and the pulp may react normally to electric and thermal tests.
- As degeneration of the pulp progresses the tooth may become discolored and the pulp will not respond to stimulation.

Types

1. *Calcific Degeneration*

- In this, part of the pulp tissue is replaced by calcific material, i.e. pulp stones or denticles are formed.
- It may occur either with in the pulp chamber or root canal, but it is generally present in the pulp chamber.
- In another type of calcification, the calcified material is attached to the wall of the pulp cavity and is an integral part of it.
- They are considered to be harmless concretions although referred pain in a few patients has been described to the presence of these calcifications in the pulp.

2. *Atrophic Degeneration*

- No clinical diagnosis exists.
- Pulp tissue is less sensitive than normal.

- Fewer stellate cells are present and intercellular fluid is increased.
- Observed histopathologically in pulps of older people.

3. *Fibrous Degeneration*

- Characterised by replacement of the cellular elements by fibrous connective tissue.
- On removal from the root canal such a pulp has the characteristic appearance of a leathery fibre.
- This disorder causes no distinguishing symptoms to aid in the clinical diagnosis.

4. *Pulp Artifacts*

- Fatty degeneration of the pulp along with reticular atrophy and vacualization of the odontoblasts are probably artifacts caused by poor fixation of the tissue specimen.

5. *Tumor Metastasis*

- Metastasis of tumor cells to the dental pulp is rare except possibly in terminal stages.

6. NECROSIS OF PULP

Definition

- *Necrosis is death of the pulp. It may be partial or total, depending on whether part of or the entire pulp is involved.*

Types

1. Coagulation necrosis
2. Liquefaction necrosis.

Etiology

- Caused by any noxious stimulus injurious to the pulp such as bacteria, trauma and chemical irritation.

Symptoms

- An otherwise normal tooth with a necrotic pulp causes no painful symptoms.
- Discolouration of the tooth is first indication that pulp is dead.
- Discolouration is either greyish or brownish and may lack its usual brilliance and luster.
- Tooth is a symptomatic and the radiograph is non diagnostic.

Diagnosis

History of pain

- Severe pain lasting from a few min. to a few hours followed by complete and sudden cessation of pain.

Radiographic Examination

- Shows a large cavity or filling. An open approach to the root canal and thickening of periodontal ligament.
- *Cold Test, Electric pulp and test cavity:* Negative response.

Treatment

- Root canal therapy.

CRACKED TOOTH SYNDROME

Definition

- *Incomplete fractures through the body of the tooth may cause pain of apparently idiopathic origin - is referred to as cracked tooth syndrome.*
- A patient may complain of poorly localized pain from an unidentified posterior tooth on biting or the application of cold drinks.
- Clinically and radiographically, there is often no evidence of caries, and the offending tooth may not be heavily restored.
- Affected tooth responds to electrical stimulation.

- Careful examination of the teeth, particularly with an intra oral light may reveal one with vertical hairline cracks.
- Mandibular molars are most frequently affected.
- The pain may be reproduced if the patient is asked to close with an object such as a cotton roll placed between that and the opposing teeth.
- When this fails to produce a response, cold in the form of ice may be applied on the tooth and a hypersensitive response will indicate the offending tooth.
- *Mechanism of pain on biting :* The crack contains bacteria whose toxins pass down the dentinal tubules to cause pulpal inflammation. As the cusp is wedged by chewing there is fluid movement in the crack and the communicating tubular which elicits pain in an already sensitive tooth.

Treatment

- The treatment depends on whether there have been symptoms of reversible or irreversible pulpitis.
- *In case of Reversible pulpitis :* If there is a loose cusp, any restoration should be removed together with the loose cusp and is restored to the shape and size of the cavity. If there is no loose cusp, tooth may be temporarily crowned to relieve from pain.
- *In case of Irreversible pulpitis :* Pulp extirpation and RCT.

CHAPTER 04

DISEASES OF THE PERIRADICULAR TISSUES

- Pulpal disease is only one of several possible causes of diseases of the Periradicular tissues.
- Neoplastic disorders periodontal conditions developments factors and trauma can Periradicular diseases.

CLASSIFICATION

1. **Acute Periradicular diseases**
   - Acute alveolar abscess.
   - Acute apical periodontitis,
     - i. Vital
     - ii. Non Vital
   - Acute exacerbation of a chronic lesion (Phoenix abscess).

2. **Chronic Periradicular diseases with areas of rarefaction**
   - Chronic alveolar abscess
   - Granuloma
   - Cyst

3. **Chronic Periradicular disease with area of condensation**
   - Condensing osteitis

4. **Other Periradicular lesions**
   - External root resorption.
   - Diseases of the Periradicular tissues of non odontogenic origin.

1. ACUTE ALVEOLAR ABSCESS

Synonyms
- Acute abscess
- Acute apical abscess
- Acute dentoalveolar abscess
- Acute periapical abscess
- Acute radicular abscess

Definition
- *A localized collection of pus in the alveolar bone at the root apex of a tooth following death of the pulp with extension of the infection through the apical foramen into the Periradicular tissues.*

Etiology
- Result of trauma, chemical or mechanical irritation
- Bacterial invasion of the dead pulp tissue.

Symptoms

Local
- Severe throbbing pain with swelling of overlying soft tissue.

- — Swelling progresses and tooth becomes mobile.
- — Formation of sinus tract in the labial or buccal mucosa.
- — Distorted patient appearance.

General

- — Pale, irritable, week, loss of sleep, headache, malaise.
- — Temperature : 99 - 103° F.
- — Fever with chills.
- — Intestinal statis manifested with coated tongue and foul breath.

Diagnosis

1. *Clinical*
   - — Subjective symptoms.
   - — Tender on percussion.
   - — Tender on palpation of apical muscosa.
   - — Mobile and extruded tooth.

2. *Radiographic*
   - — A cavity, a defective restoration, thickened periodontal ligament space, evidence of breakdown of bone in the region of the root apex.

Differential Diagnosis

- — Periodontal abscess
- — Irreversible pulpitis.

Treatment

- — Establishment of drainage
- — Debridement
- — After the subsidation of symptom perform RCT.

2. ACUTE APICAL PERIODONTITIS

Definition

- — *A painful inflammation of the periodontium as a result of trauma, irritation and infection through the root canal regardless of whether the pulp is vital or non vital.*

Etiology

- — *Vital tooth - occlusal trauma.*
   - — Recently inserted restoration extending beyond the occlusal plane.
   - — Wedging of a foreign object between teeth.
   - — By a blow to the teeth.
- — *Non Vital tooth -* Sequela of the pulpal disease iatrogenic.

Clinical Features

- — Pain and tenderness
- — Tooth may slightly sore
- — Tooth may be extruded

Diagnosis

1. Known history of a tooth under treatment.
2. *Clinical examination* : tender to percussion.
3. *Radiographic* : thickened periodontal ligament.

Differential Diagnosis

- — Acute alveolar abscess.

Treatment

- — Treat the cause
- — RCT

3. ACUTE EXACERBATION OF A CHRONIC LESION (PHOENIX ABSCESS)

Definition

- — *An acute inflammatory reaction superimposed on an existing chronic lesion such as a cyst or granuloma.*

Etiology

- — Periradicular disease.
- — Bacteria released from root canal during instrumentation may trigger acute response.

Symptoms

- — At onset, tooth may be tender to touch.
- — As inflammation progresses tooth may be elevated in its socket and may become sensitive.
- — Mucosa over the radicular area appears red and swollen.

Diagnosis

- — Most commonly associated with the initiation of RCT.
- — History of trauma.

Differential Diagnosis

- — Acute irreversible pulpitis.

Treatment

- — An emergency condition
- — Drainage and debridement
- — RCT

4. CHRONIC ALVEOLAR ABSCESS

(Chronic Suppurative Apical Periodontitis)

Definition

- — *A long standing low grade infection of the periradicular alveolar bone.*

Etiology

- Sequela of the death of the pulp.
- May result from a pre-existing acute abscess.

Clinical Features

- Generally asymptomatic.
- At times detected only during routine radiography or because of the presence of sinus tract.
- When open cavity present drainage occurs through root canal.

Diagnosis

Clinical examination

- Shows a cavity, a composite, acrylic or metalic restoration or a gold or jacket crown under which pulp may be dead without causing symptoms.

Differential diagnosis

- Periradicular diseases.
- Periapical osteo fibrosis/ cementoma / ossifying fibroma.

Treatment

- Elimination of infection
- Root Canal Therapy

5. GRANULOMA

Definition

- *A growth of granulomatous tissue continuous with the periodontal ligament resulting from death of the pulp and the diffusion of bacterial toxins from the root canal into the surrounding periradicular tissues through the apical and lateral foramina.*

Etiology

- Death of the pulp.
- Irritation of the periapical tissue that stimulates a productive cellular reaction.
- In some cases a granuloma is preceded by a chronic alveolar abscess.

Symptoms

- Usually asymptomatic.
- A granuloma may not produce any subjective reaction, except in rare cases when it breaks down and undergoes suppuration.

Diagnosis

1. Routine radiographic examination.
2. It is not tender on percussion and is not loose.
3. Palpation.
4. Electric pulp test and thermal test.

5. Patient may give a history of pulpalgia that subsided.

Differential Diagnosis

- Cementoma / periapical osteofibrosis.

Treatment

1. Removal of cause of inflammation.
2. RCT.

6. RADICULAR CYST

Definition

- *A slowly growing epithelial sac at the apex of a tooth that lines a pathologic cavity in the alveolar bone.*
- The lumen of the cyst is filled with a low concentration of protenaceous fluid.

Etiology

- Death of the pulp followed by stimulation of the epithelial cells of Malassez.

Clinical Feature

- Symptomless swelling
- Tooth become mobile
- Distortion of the face
- Maxilla is more commonly affected that mandible

Diagnosis

Radiograph

- Break in the continuity of lamina dura.
- Oval shaped radiolucency more than 2 cm.

Differential Diagnosis

- Granuloma
- Normal bony cavity such as incisive foramen
- Globulomaxillary cyst
- Traumatic bone cyst

Treatment

- Marsupilization
- Root canal therapy

7. CONDENSING OSTEITIS

Definition

- *The response to a low grade chronic inflammation of the periradicular area as a result of a mild irritation through the root canal.*

Etiology

- Mild irritation from pulpal disease that stimulates osteoblastic activity in the alveolar bone.

Symptoms

– Asymptomatic

– Discovered during routine radiographic examination

Diagnosis

Radiographic Examination

– Appears as a localized area of radiopacity surrounding the affected root. It is an area of dense bone with reduced trabecular pattern.

Treatment

– RCT

8. EXTERNAL ROOT RESORPTION

Definition

– A lytic process occuring in the cementum or cementum and dentin of the roots of teeth.

Etiology

– Unknown.

– The suspected cause is periradicular inflammation due to trauma, excessive forces, granuloma, cyst, central jaw tumours, replantation of teeth, bleaching of teeth, impaction of teeth.

– If no cause is evident the disorder is called Idiopathic resorption.

Symptoms

– Asymptomatic.

– When the root is completely resorbed the tooth becomes mobile.

– If the external root resorption extends into the crown it will give the appearance of pink tooth seen in internal resorption.

– Root resorption of the type called replacement resorption or ankylosis, in which the root is gradually replaced by bone, renders the tooth immobile.

Diagnosis

– Radiographic examination.

Differential Diagnosis

– Internal root resorption.

Treatment

– Treatment varies with the etiologic factor.

– If the external resorption is caused by extension of pulpal discase into the supporting tissues, Root canal therapy will usually stop the resorptive process.

– External resorption produced by excessive forces from orthodontic appliances can be stopped by reducing those forces.

– In patient with external resorption due to replantation of teeth, preparation of the root canal and obturation with calcium hydroxide paste may stop the resorptive process.

CHAPTER 05

ENDODONTIC MICROBIOLOGY

ROOT CANAL FLORA

Streptococcus viridans	-	63%
Staphylococcus albus	-	17%
Diphtheroid bacilli	-	6.5%
Staphylococcus aureus		
Bacillus proteus		
Streptococcus haemolyticans		

Gram Positive

- Streptococci
- Staphylococci
- Corynebacteria
- Yeast

Gram Negative

- Spirochetes
- Neisseria
- Bacteriods
- Fusobacterium
- Pseudomonas
- Coliform bacteria

BACTERIOLOGIC EXAMINATION

1. Culture media

- Not all microorganisms in root canal grow in readily available culture media especially the obligate anaerobes which destroy due to exposure to air, chemical agents such as sodium hypochlorite. Several media are satisfactory for culturing material from root canals.

- They are:

  1. Brain heart infusion broth with 0.1% agar.
  2. Trypticase Soy broth with 0.1% agar (TSA).
  3. Thioglycollate broth or Brewer's Thioglycollate broth.
  4. Glucose ascites broth.
  5. TSA + 0.1% agar facilitates growth of anaerobes.
  6. TSA + 5% ascitic fluid or 10% horse serum enables fastidious organisms to grow.
  7. Viability medium for growth (VMG).
     - Streptococci
     - Non Sporing anaerobes
  8. Stuarts transporting medium
  9. Moiler's base culture medium : contains veal, veal heart, peptone products in an agar gel and certain supplements.

2. Taking the culture

- The dressing from the previous visit is removed from the root canal and is discarded.

- A sterile absorbent point is inserted into the canal with a wiping motion, to cleanse the canal surface of any trace of medicament.

- The point is removed and discarded.

- The purpose of wiping the root canal is to prevent the transfer to the culture medium of any intracanal medicament which could inhibit bacterial growth and could result in a false negative culture.

- A fresh, sterile absorbent point is now inserted into the apical foramen and is allowed to remain there for atleast 1 min to absorb as much periapical exudate and microorganisms from the root canal as possible.

- The absorbent point is removed with sterilized cotton pliers held with the thumb, index and middle fingers while the plug or cap of the test tube is removed with the little finger and palm of the same hand.

- The test tube is held in the other hand and is tilted slightly to prevent air contamination.

- The absorbent point is drapped into the medium, the tip of the tube is flamed and the plug or cap is replaced and the culture tube is incubated properly.

3. Anaerobic Culturing

- Culturing obligate anaecrobes is a fastidious process that requires special equipment and media used in a temperature controlled oxygen free environment.

A. *Periradicular sample*

- Using an aseptic technique, insert the sterile needle of a leur lock syringe into the periradicular space (i.e. swelling), aspirate fluid eject any air inside the syringe barrel immediately, insert the needle through the rubber septum stopper by an anaport vial and eject the fluid.

- The Anaport vial, a 10 ml vial with a rubber septum stopper from which the gas been removed, should be transported to any anaerobic culturing depot usually located in a hospital or health care institute with in 4 hours after taking the sample.

B. *Root canal sample*

- Aseptically prepare an access cavity into the pulp chamber.

- Inject a few drops of prereduced, anaerobically sterilized medium into the chamber, pump the medium into the root canal with a sterile endodontic file aspirate the fluid with a leurlock syringe, eject any air from the syringe barrel immediately insert the needle through the rubber stopper of an anaport vial and eject the fluid.

- Transport the sample to an anaerobic culturing depot within 4 hours.

4. Culture Reversal

- A negative culture that becomes a positive culture by the time of obturation.

- It may be due to,
  - Improper care in taking the culture.
  - Possible leakage between treatments.
  - Capability of the culture medium to sustain growth of the microorganisms.

- It is advisable to allow more than 48 hours between taking the culture and filling the root canal, preferably 96 hours or more and it is recommended that the culture tube be re-examined immediately before obturating a canal to make certain that no evidence of growth is present.

5. Interpretation

- Culture tube is held against a white background.
- Turbidity indicates growth of organisms.
- If culture medium remains clear, it indicates sterility.

1. *False Positive Culture*

- May be there if there is inadequate sterilization of operating field, leakage from rubber dam, unstcrile paper points, break on loss of real from previous dressings.

2. *False Negative culture*

May be seen when there is inadequate absorption of exudation by paper points presence of antimicrobial agents of root canal and absence of inactivation of culture medium or when there is insufficient incubation.

CHAPTER 06

CLINICAL DIAGNOSTIC METHODS

HISTORY AND RECORD

– To avoid irrelevant information and to prevent errors of omission in clinical tests, the clinician must establish a routine for examination.

– Questions concerning the patients chief complaint, past medical history and past dental history are reviewed.

I. SUBJECTIVE SYMPTOMS

– The symptoms which are felt by patient like pain, swelling, lack of function or esthetics.

– Whatever may be the reason but patients chief complaint is best starting point for a correct diagnosis.

Pain

– One should ask the patient about:

– The kind of pain

– Its location

– Its duration

– What causes it

– What alleviates it

– Whether it is referred to any site or not.

– It is important to know whether the pain is localized to particular teeth (or) diffuse type of pain surrounding areas.

– Generally, pulpal pain is described by a patient in one of 2 ways.

1. *Sharp, Piercing and Lancinating Pain*

– Consistent with those usually associated with excitation of the `A Delta' nerve fibers in the pulp.

– Usually localized.

– Response promptly to cold.

2. *Dull, boring, gnawing and excruciating pain*

– Consistent with those resulting from exitation and slower rate of transmission of the `C' nerve fibers in the pulp.

– Usually diffused

– Responds abnormally to heat more than to cold and with symptoms that can be referred to other sites.

Duration of Pain

– The duration of pain is also diagnostic.

– At times pulpal pain lasts only as long as irritant is present.

– At other times, it lasts for minutes to hours.

– The pain may be either intermittent or constant.

– A tooth with fleeting pulpal pain that disappears on removal of the irritant has an excellent chance of recovery without the need for endodontic treatment.

– *Acute Reversible Pulpitis (Hyperemia)* is characterized by pain of short duration, caused by a specific irritant that disappears as soon as the irritant is removed. The pain is usually localized and is more responsive to cold than to heat.

– If the pain persists or if it occurs without any apparent cause the pulpitis usually be irreversible and the patient will require endodontic therapy.

– Abnormal dental pain caused by heat usually requires endodontic treatment.

– Pain that occurs on changing the position of the head, awakens the patient from sleep or occurs during mastication of food in a cariously exposed tooth usually indicates a need for endodontic treatment.

– Spontaneous pain and pain of long duration are symptoms of irreversible pulpitis.

II. OBJECTIVE SYMPTOMS

– Are determined by tests and observations performed by the clinicians.

– These tests are as follows,

1. Visual and tactile inspection
2. Percussion
3. Palpation
4. Mobility and depressibility
5. Radiographs
6. Electric pulp test
7. Thermal tests (hot and cold)
8. Anesthetic test
9. Test cavity preparation
10. Occlusal Pressure Test

1. VISUAL AND TACTILE INSPECTION

– Simplest clinical test.

– A thorough visual, tactile examination of the hard and soft tissue relies on checking the three `C's, i.e.

– Colour

– Consistency

– Contour

– In soft tissue such as gingiva, deviation from the healthy pink colour is readily recognized when inflammation is present.

– A change in contour occurs with swelling and the consistency of soft, fluctuant or spongy tissue differs from that of normal, healthy, firm tissue and is indicative of a pathologic condition.

– Similarly teeth should be visually examined using the three 'C's.

– A normal appearing crown has a life like translucency and sparkle that is missing in pulpless teeth.

– Staining may be caused by old amalgam restorations, root canal filling materials and medicaments or systemic medications such as Tetracycline Staining.

– Many discolourations are the result of diseases commonly associated with necrotic, gangrenous pulps, internal or external resorption and carious exposure.

– Crown fractures should be examined because fractures, wear facets and restoration change the crowns contour.

Technique

– One uses ones eyes, fingers, an explorer and the periodontal probe.

– The patient's teeth and periodontium should be examined in good light under dry conditions.

2. PERCUSSION

– This test enables one to evaluate the status of the periodontium surrounding a tooth.

– The tooth is struck a quick, moderate blow initially with low intensity by using the handle of an instrument to determine whether the tooth is tender.

– A sensitive response differing from that of the adjacent teeth, usually indicates the presence of periodontitis.

– Although percussion is a simple method, it may be misleading if used alone.

– To eliminate bias on the part of the patient one must change the sequence of the teeth percussed on successive tests.

– And also one should change the direction of the blow from the vertical occlusal to the buccal or lingual surface of the crown and strike separate cusps in a differing order.

– One must not percuss a sensitive tooth beyond the patient tolerance.

3. PALPATION

- Act of determining by tactile sense which will dictate the consistency of tissues.

- Done with the fingertip, using light pressure to examine tissue consistency and pain response.

- Its value lies in locating the swelling over an involved tooth and determining the following,

    - Whether the tissue is fluctuant and enlarged sufficiently for incision and drainage.

    - The presence, intensity and location of pain.

    - The presence and location of adenopathy.

    - The presence of bone crepitus.

- Diagnostically when the posterior teeth are infected the submaxillary lymphnodes become involved.

- Infection of the lower anterior teeth may cause swelling of the submental lymphnodes.

- Percussion, palpation, mobility depressibility are tests of the periodontium rather than of the pulp.

4. MOBILITY TEST

- Used to evaluate the integrity of the attachment apparatus surrounding the tooth.

- *Objective:* To determine whether the tooth is firmly or loosely attached to its alveolus.

- The test consists of moving a tooth laterally in its socket by using the fingers or preferably the handles of two instruments.

- The amount of movement is indicative of the condition of the periodontium, the greater the movement the poorer the periodontal condition.

5. DEPRESSABILITY TEST

- It consists of moving a tooth vertically in its socket.

- The test is done with the fingers or with an instrument.

- When depressability exists, the chance for retaining the tooth ranges from poor to hopeless.

- *First Degree Mobility*: A noticeable movement of the tooth.

- *Second Degree Mobility*: Movement of a tooth with in a range of 1mm.

- *Third Degree Mobility*: Movement greater than 1 mm or when the tooth can be depressed.

- Endodontic treatment should not be carried out on teeth with third degree mobility unless mobility is reduced when pressure in the peridontium has been relieved. For ex: this situation could occur in the case of an acute apical abscess if sufficient drainage was established and pus escaped after the root canal was opened sufficiently enlarged and left patent.

6. RADIOGRAPHY

Uses

- Shows the presence of caries that may involve or may threaten to involve the pulp.

- Number, course, shape, length and width of root conals.

- The presence of calcified material in the pulp chamber or root canal.

- The presence of internal and external root resorption.

- The calcification or obliteration of the pulp cavity.

- The thickening of the periodontal ligament.

- The resorption of cementum.

- The nature and extent of periapical and alveolar bone destruction.

- Thus, radiographs provide pertinent information concerning diagnosis, prognosis, case selection, instrumentation, obturation and repair of bone and cementum.

Limitations

1. Pulpal status (ex: Necrosis) cannot be determined in the radiograph.

2. Radiographic differentiation of different periapical lesions is difficult like periapical granuloma, chronic periapical abscess or cyst; to be accurate, histologic examination is necessary.

3. Lesion in the cancellous structure of bone cannot be detected radiographically until it is penetrated or reached the cortical bone.

4. Periapical radiolucency does not indicate diseased tooth all the time.

5. It cannot give a true picture of bacteriologic or pathologic conditions.

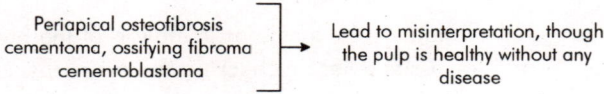

Periapical osteofibrosis cementoma, ossifying fibroma cementoblastoma → Lead to misinterpretation, though the pulp is healthy without any disease

7. OCCLUSAL PRESSURE TEST

- Most frequent complaint from the patients is pain on biting or chewing.

- The test which stimulates the pain on biting or chewing is the occlusal pressure test.

– The pain may be due to apical periodontitis, apical abscess and incomplete tooth fractures.

Method

– It can be tested by biting on an orange wood stick, a Burlew rubber disc or a wet cotton roll.

8. PULP VITALITY TESTS

1. Electric pulp testing
2. Thermal testing
   i. Heat Testing
   ii. Cold Testing
3. Anesthetic testing
4. Test cavity preparation
5. Thermography
6. Transillumination

1. ELECTRIC PULP TESTING

– It is one of the most useful tool in endodontics.
– Pulp testers are designed to elicit response by electrical excitation of neural elements in the pulp.
– They only suggest whether a tooth is *vital / non vital*.

Technique

– Describe the test to the patient in such a way, that will reduce anxiety and will eliminate a biased response.
– Isolate the area of teeth to be tested with cotton rolls and saliva ejector and air dry all the teeth.
– Check the electric pulp tester for function and determine that current is passing through the electrode.
– Apply an electrolyte (tooth paste) on the tooth electrode and place it against the dried enamel of the crowns on the occlusobuccal or incisolabial surface.
– It is important to avoid contacting any restoration in the tooth or the adjacent gingival tissue with the electrolyte or the electrode or else this would cause a false and misleading response.
– Retract the patients cheek away from the tooth electrode with the free hand. When this hand contacts with the patients cheek, it completes the electrical circuit.
– Turn the rheostat slowly to introduce minimal current into the tooth and increase the current slowly. Ask the patient to indicate when sensation occurs by using such words as tingling or warmth. Record the result according to the numeric scale on the pulp tester.

– Repeat the foregoing for each tooth to be tested.
– *Accuracy depends on,*
   1. Accuracy of apparatus.
   2. State of mind of the patient whether the patient is apprehensive or relaxed.
   3. Individual threshold response.
   4. Patient under sedative medication.
   5. Recently erupted teeth with incomplete root formation.
   6. Recently traumatized teeth.
   7. Teeth with extensive restoration and a pulp protecting base.

False Positive Response

1. Conductor / Electrode contact with a large metal restoration (Bridge, Class - II restoration) or the gingiva.
2. Patient anxiety.
3. Liquefaction necrosis.
4. Inadequate isolation.
5. Multirooted tooth.

False Negative Response

1. Patient premedicated with analgesics, narcotics, alcohol tranquilizers.
2. Inadequate contact of electrode with the enamel.
3. Recently traumatized tooth.
4. Excessive calcification in the canal.
5. Dead batteries or forgetting to turn the pulp tester.
6. Recently erupted tooth with an immature apex.
7. Partial necrosis.
8. Clinician wearing surgical gloves.
9. Presence of pulp protecting materials under restoration.
10. Patient's high pain threshold.

Disadvantages

1. No indication is given of the state of the vascular supply, which would give a more reliable measure of the vitality of the pulp.
2. Readings taken from posterior teeth may be misleading since the chances of presence of some combination of vital and non vital root canal pulps.
3. Cannot be used on crowned tooth. In such a case we have to prepare a cavity and use the pulp tester.

4. False positive readings may be due to stimulation of nerve fibres in the periodontium.

5. Anxiety can cause false positive response.

6. It may elicit response from the periodontium.

7. False positive response may be seen in liquefaction necrosis of the pulp due to transmission of current from the liquid.

Examples of Electric Pulp testers

1. Digilog pulp tester (battery operated).

2. Pelton - Crane Compact (Transistorized battery operated electric pulp tester).

3. Battery operated Parkell pulp tester.

4. Analytic Technology pulp tester.

5. Neotest Automatic digital pulp tester (ADP).

Precaution

– *Electric pulp testers should not be used on patients who have a pacemaker because of the possible electrical interference.*

2. THERMAL TESTING

– *It involves the application of cold and heat to a tooth to determine sensitivity to thermal changes.*

– *A response to cold indicates a vital pulp regardless of whether that pulp is normal or abnormal.*

– *An abnormal response to heat usually indicates the presence of a pulpal or periapical disorder requiring endodontic treatment.*

A. Heat Testing

– Usually done by using a hot gutta-percha / hot burnisher / hot air / hot water.

Procedure

– 3.0 mm of the end of a stick of pink gutta-percha is heated in a flame for 2 seconds and is applied to the suspected tooth.

Precautions

– Tooth surface is lightly coated with vaseline to prevent the sticking of guttapercha.

– First a normal contralateral tooth should be tested and then the affected tooth is tested.

Observation

1. *No response* - necrosis, gangrene, chronic abscess.

2. *Mild to moderate response* - normal pulp.

3. *Painful response which subsides after the removal of stimulus* - reversible pulpitis.

4. *Painful response which continues even after the removal of stimulus*—Irreversible pulpitis, acute alveolar abscess, acute pulpitis.

B. Cold Testing

– It is done by using an air blast, cold drink, ethylene chloride, fluori-methane, sticks of ice, carbon dioxide snow (dry ice).

– Excess cold may cause pulpal damage or crazing lines in the enamel.

– The CO_2 dry ice stick is preferred for testing as it does not affect adjacent teeth.

– When testing with a cold stimulus, one must begin with the most posterior tooth and proceeds towards the anterior teeth because such sequence will prevent melting of ice water from dripping in a posterior direction and possible excitation of non tested tooth by giving false response.

Observations

1. *No response* - Non vital or false negative.

   Examples of negative response

   – Calcification of immature opening.

   – Recent trauma to the tooth.

   – Patient is premedicated.

2. *Moderate response* - normal pulp.

3. *Painful response which subsides immediately after the stimulus is removed* - Reversible pulpitis / hyperemia.

4. *Painful response which may remain even after removal of stimulus* - irreversible pulpitis.

   – In case of hyperemia, there may be a quick response and in chronic pulpitis, may be a delayed response.

– However thermal tests are not as accurate as an electric pulp test.

3. ANESTHETIC TESTING

– This test is restricted to patients who are in pain at the time of the test, when the usual tests have failed to enable one to identify the tooth.

Objective

– To anesthetize a single tooth at a time until the pain disappears and is localized to a specific tooth.

Technique

– Using either infiltration or intraligamentary injection, inject the most posterior tooth in the area suspected of being the cause of pain.

- If pain persists when the tooth has been fully anesthetized, anesthetize the next tooth mesial to it and continue to do so until the pain disappears.

- If the source of pain cannot be determined, whether in maxillary or mandibular teeth, an inferior alveolar injection should be given.

- Cessation of pain naturally indicates involvement of a mandibular tooth and localization of the specific tooth is done by the intraligamentary injection when the anesthetic has spent itself.

- This test is a last resort and has an advantage over the *test cavity preparation* during which iatrogenic damage is possible.

4. TEST CAVITY PREPARATION

- It is performed when the other methods of diagnosis are failed.

- The test cavity is made by drilling through the enamel dentin junction of an unanesthetized tooth.

- The drilling should be done at slow speed and without a water coolant.

- Sensitivity or pain felt by the patient is an indication of pulp vitality. If so, no endodontic treatment is indicated. A sedative cement is then placed in the cavity and the search for the source of pain continues.

- If no pain is felt, cavity preparation may be continued until the pulp chamber is reached.

- If the pulp is completely necrotic endodontic treatment can be continued painlessly in many cases without anesthesia.

5. THERMOGRAPHY

- Not widely used.

- It uses crystal to determine the vitality.

- It determines vitality by measuring the temperature of the tooth.

- A non vital tooth has no blood supply so there is lower surface temperature than a vital tooth.

- But this test is impractical and so not used.

6. TRANSILLUMINATION

- Strong fibre optic light helps to distinguish both vital and necrotic pulp in young patients.

- It will also help in diagnosing vertically fracture crowns when a beam of strong fibre optic light is passed.

- The light does not pass across the fracture line so that the part of the tooth nearest to the light is bright and beyond fracture remains dark.

- Necrosed tooth appear opaque and dark because of breakdown by blood in the pulp chamber.

CHAPTER 07

ENDODONTIC ARMAMENTARIUM

CLASSIFICATION OF ENDODONTIC INSTRUMENTS

I. GROSSMAN'S CLASSIFICATION

- Root canal instruments are divided into 4 types according to their function.

1. Endodontic Explorers (Exploring Instruments)

- To locate the canal orifice.
- To determine or assist in obtaining patency of the root canal.
  Ex: 1. *Smooth broaches*
  2. *Endodontic explorers*

2. Debridement Instruments (Extirpating Instruments)

- To extirpate the pulp.
- To remove debris and other foreign material.
  Ex: *Barbed broach.*

3. Root canal shaping Instruments

- To shape the root canal laterally and apically.
  Ex: 1. *Reamers*
  2. *Gates - Glidden drill*
  3. *Files*

4. Obturating Instruments

- To cement and pack guttapercha into the root canal.
  Examples
  1. *Pluggers (flat end-for vertical condensation)*
  2. *Spreaders (pointed end-lateral condensation)*
  3. *Lentulospirals (to deliver sealer or paste to the root canal)*

II. I.S.O. AND FDI CLASSIFICATION

1. Group - I : Hand use only

- Hand operated instruments such as *barbed and smooth broaches, reamers, K,H, and R files, plugger, spreaders, etc.*

2. Group - II : Engine driven Instruments

- Same instruments as described above. But the handles of these instruments have been replaced by latch type adapter for insertion into low speed handpieces.
- These instruments consist of two parts.
  1. An operative cutting head
  2. Latch type of attachment

3. Group - III : Engine driven latch type - drills

- Similar to Group - II these instruments have latch attachment but are fabricated from a single piece of metal. So latch, shaft and cutting head are made of a single piece. Ex: Gates glidden drill, Peeso reamer.

4. Group - IV : Root canal points
- They are usually the materials used. Ex: Guttapercha points, Absorbable points.

STANDARDIZATION OF ENDODONTIC INSTRUMENTS

- Earlier, root canal instruments were manufactured according to the manufacturer's wish with no definite specifications regarding length, diameter, shape and length of the cutting instrument.
- *Ingle and Levine* using a electrode microcomparator found variations in diameter and taper for the same sizes of instruments and later suggested some recommendations to maintain uniformity.

Ingle and Levine Recommendations

1. *Instruments shall be numbered from 10 to 100 - 150. The numbers advance by 5 units, to size 60 and then by 10 units to size 100.*

2. *Each number shall be representative of the diameter of the instrument in hundredths of a millimeter at the tip.*

   Ex: No: 10 is 10/100 or 0.1 mm at the tip

   No: 25 is 25/100 or 0.25 mm at the tip

   No: 90 is 90/100 or 0.9 mm at the tip

3. *The working blade (flutes) shall begin at the tip, designated site D_1 and shall extend exactly 16 mm up the shaft, terminating at designated site D_2. The diameter of D_2 shall be 32/100 or 0.32 mm greater than of D_1.*

   Ex: A No: 20 reamer shall have a diameter of 0.20 mm at D_1 and a diameter of 0.20 plus 0.32 or 0.52 at D_2.

   This sizing ensures a constant increase in taper of 0.02 mm per mm for every instrument regardless of size.

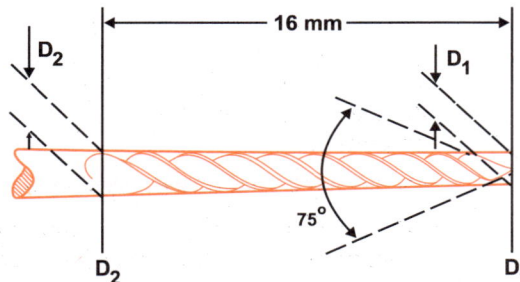

D_1 - diameter at the tip,

D_2 - diameter at the tip end of the cutting blade,

The tip angle of the instrument should be $75 \pm 15°$.

Other Specifications (were added later)

1. *The tip angle of an instrument should be $75 \pm 15°$.*

2. *Instrument sizes should increase by 0.05 mm at D_1 between Numbers: 10 and 60. Ex: Numbers: 10,15 and 20. They should increase by 0.1 mm from Numbers: 60 to 150. Ex: Numbers 60, 70 and 80.*

3. *06 and 08 have been added for increased instrument selection.*

4. *In addition, instrument handles have been colour coded for easier recognition.*

- Stainless steel root canal instruments are used more often today than carbon steel instruments because of their more flexibility, less likely to fracture, less susceptible to corrosion.

- The finer sizes of reamers and files have low resistance to torque (pressure used to rotate instrument for cutting and shaping) and break using less force than larger instruments when they bind in a root canal.

- As a result small instruments are manufactured from square blanks, which are more resistant to torque, fractures, and large instruments are manufactured from triangular blanks, to improve their cutting efficiency.

- Instruments are available in lengths of 21, 25, 28 and 30 mm.

- Ordinarily, instruments of 25 mm long are used, but occasionally 21mm instruments are needed for molars especially when the patient cannot open the mouth wide and 28 and 30 mm instruments are necessary for cuspids and other teeth in which a 25 mm instrument cannot reach the apical foramen.

- Reamers are also available in 40 mm lengths for use in preparing root canals for endodontic treatment.

Colour Coding of Handles of Instruments

6	–	Pink	30	–	Blue
8	–	Grey	35	–	Green
10	–	Purple	40	–	Black
15	–	White	45	–	White
20	–	Yellow	50	–	Yellow
25	–	Red			
			150		

EXPLORING INSTRUMENTS

1. ENDODONTIC EXPLORER

- A double ended instrument with long tapered tines at either a right or an obtuse angle. This design facilitates the location of canal orifice.

– These instruments are very stiff and should not be inserted into canals or used for condensing guttapercha.

– Explorers should never be heated.

EXTIRPATING INSTRUMENTS

1. BARBED BROACH
Uses
– To extripate the pulp.
– To remove debris and other foreign material, absorbent points, cotton pellets, etc.

Manufacture
– It is manufactured from a tapered, round, soft iron wire in which angle cuts are made into the surface to produce barbs.

Available as
– A variety of sizes from *triple extra fine to extra coarse*.
– Barbs are used to engage the pulp as the broach is carefully rotated within the canal until it begins to meet resistance against the walls of the canal.
– Barbed broaches break easily especially if they bind in the root canal hence root canal should be enlarged before insertion of the broach.

Selection
– By comparing the size of the broach with the size of the last instrument used in the root canal or an estimated size of the image in a radiograph. One should select a barbed broaches that fits loosely into the apical third of the root canal.
– A barbed broach that is too wide does not permit removal of all the pulp tissue or it may force the pulp apically as the broach is inserted in the canal.

Technique
– The root canal is irrigated with a 5.2% solution of sodium hypochlorite and the barbed broach is introduced until one notes unforced contact with root canal walls.
– The broach is withdrawn about 1 mm and is rotated 360° to engage the pulp tissue and it is withdrawn again to remove this tissue.
– When the root canal is unusually wide as in young teeth even a coarse barbed broach may not be able to engage and remove the massive pulp tissue.

– In such cases, two fine barded broaches are inserted into the canal and are rotated at the same time until the pulp tissue is engaged and removed.

Sterilization
– A barbed broach can be cleaned by scrubbing with a bur brush.
– To clean a broach which has tissue tags or necrotic debris, place it in a 5.2% sodium hypochlorite solution for half an hour and then broach is rinsed in running water, air dried and is sterilized in dry heat.

2. RASPS or R - Type Files
– This is similar in design to barbed broach, but have shallower and more rounded barbs.
– Used to enlarge the root canal but usually produce rough wall of the root canal. So it is not preferred often.

INSTRUMENTS FOR CLEANING AND SHAPING OF ROOT CANALS

I. REAMERS
1. Physical Characteristics
– Manufactured from stainless steel triangular blank.
– Has less number of flutes.
– Do not break easily unless they have an undetected steel shaft or until the instrument is strained or deformed.
– Flutes are loosely twisted.

2. Functional Characteristics
– Used with a rotating - pushing motion limited to a quarter - to a half turn to engage their blades into the dentin and withdrawn - penetration, rotation and retraction.
– The cut is made during retraction.

II. FILES
1. K - file (Kerr manufacturing company)
– Has got the name from its manufacturing company.
– Manufactured from stainless steel square blank.
– Does not break easily unless they have an undetected steel shaft or until the instrument is strained or deformed.
– Flutes are tightly twisted.
– K - files can be used as `PATHFINDER' (to locate the root canal orifices).

2. K - Flex Files
    — Manufactured from rhomboidal or diamond shaped blanks.
    — Designed for more flexibility and cutting efficiency.
    — Has alternating high and low flutes for more efficiency.

3. Hedstroem Files (H-Files)
    — Manufactured from a round stainless steel wire machined to produce spiral flutes resembling cones or as crew or christmas tree appearance.
    — When placed in contact with the root canal wall the cutting edges contact the wall at angles approaching 90 degrees and when the instrument is withdrawn exert an effective honoring action. Cut in one direction only - retraction.
    — Used in wide opened canals (Blunder bluss canals).
    — Used to flare the canal from the apical region to the occusal or incisal orifice.
    — Fragile and fractures easily.
    — Higher cutting efficiency than K - Instruments.
    — Also used to engage and remove retained instruments, gutta-percha and silver points.

4. Uni Files (Modification of H-File)
    — Manufactured from round stainless steel wire by cutting two superficial grooves to produce flutes in a double helix design.
    — Resemble H-file in appearance.
    — Less subject to fracture.
    — Less efficient.

5. S - File (Modification of H - File)
    — Manufactured from a solid piece of stainless steel wire that produces a sharp cutting edge.
    — Has a double cutting edge.
    — Similar to unifile except that the angles of the flutes remain uniform where as pitch and depth of the flutes increases from the tip to the handle.
    — Stiffer than H-files.
    — Has 90° cutting tip.
    — Can be used for straight or curved canals.
    — Used either as a reamer or file.

6. Flexofile
    — Manufactured by Dentsply maillefer.
    — Manufactured in the same way as the K - file but using a more flexible stainless steel alloy.
    — It has more flutes than K - file.
    — It has a non-cutting (Batt) tip and a triangular cross-section so the cutting flutes are sharper ond there is more scope for debris removal.

    Advantages
    1. More cutting efficiency
    2. Resistance to fracture

7. Niti Files (Nitinol Files)
    — The name Nitinol was derived from the elements that make up the alloy, i.e. Nickel and Titanium and `nol' for the Naval ordinance Laboratory (who manufactured it for the first time).
    — Nitinol instruments should be used with a rotational or reaming motion and are effective in the shaping of root canals.

    Advantages
    1. More flexible
    2. Better conformation to canal curvature
    3. Resistance to fracture
    4. Less wear
    5. Super elasticity
    6. Enhanced canal negotiation
    7. Faster instrumentation
    8. No need to pre curve

8. Greater Taper (GT) hand files
    — Were designed by Buchanan.
    — Are made from Ni-Ti.
    — The set of four hand files of varying tapers, 0.12 - 0.16, all have a tip size of ISO 20.
    — They have pear-shaped handles and each file is designed for different areas and types of canals. For ex: 0.12 GT file is suited to canal orifices of relatively straight canals of large apical diameter, 0.06 GT file is suited to the apical third in a thin or curved canal.
    — Used in a sequence of counter clockwise and clockwise rotations.
    — They are intended to allow the creation of a predetermined funnel-shaped canal with fewer instruments than using the ISO series.

9. Series 29 Files
    — In accordance with ISO specifications for traditional hand instruments sizes, the

percentage difference between tip diameters of sizes 10 -15 is 50%, whilst between sizes 55 and 60 is 9%. This variable percentage changes are leading for procedural errors such as ledging, difficulty in negotiating narrow and curved canals.

- These instruments are based on a constant percentage change of diameter at *D*, instead of the variable linear dimensional changes.
- These are made with a constant 29% increase in tip diameter between successive sizes.

Functional Characteristics of Files

- Inserted into the root canal to the apex laterally pressed against one side of the canal wall and withdrawn with a pulling motion or respiring motion.
- The cutting action of the file can be effected in either a filing (rasping) or reaming (drilling).

COMPARISON BETWEEN REAMERS AND FILES

Reamers	Files
1. Made of stainless steel.	1. Made of stainless steel.
2. Used with push motion and rotation quarter to half turn.	2. Used with pull or rasping motion.
3. Has less number of flutes.	3. Has more number of flutes.
4. Flutes are loosely twisted.	4. Flutes are tightly twisted.
5. Manufactured from triangular blanks.	5. Manufactured from square blanks.

OBTURATING INSTRUMENTS

1. PLUGGERS (Condenser)

- Have smooth and flat apical tips.
- These are used for condensation of gutta-percha during obturation.
- Used primarily for vertical condensation.

Selection of pluggers

- 3 or 4 pluggers to be used in the coronal, middle and apical thirds of the canal must be persecuted to ensure their lose fit.

2. SPREADERS

- Spreaders are long tapered pointed instruments.
- Available in wide variety of lengths and taper.
- Used to condense the filling material laterally against the canal walls creating space for insertion of additional auxiliary cones.
- Spreaders should always be fit into the an empty canal to ensure that the force is absorbed by the gutta-percha and not the canal walls selection of spreaders.
- Spreaders are available that have been numbered to match the instrument size. Spreader of the same apical instrument size or one size larger is chosen so that it reaches to within 1.0 to 2.0 mm but will not penetrate the apical orifice.

3. LENTULO SPIRALS

- Used for coating sealer on root canal walls.
- Used in clockwise rotary motion.

MOTIONS OF INSTRUMENTATION

- These are also referred to as *envelops of motion*.
- They are useful for generating or controlling the cutting activity of an endodontic file.
- The motions are,
1. Filing
2. Reaming
3. Turn and Pull
4. Watch - Winding
5. Watch - Winding and Pull
6. Balanced force instrumentation

1. Filing

- *It indicates a push - pull action with the instrument.*
- Filing is an effective technique with hedstroem type instruments since they do not engage during the insertion and cut efficiently during the withdrawal motion. The *disadvantage* is that it can cause stripping of the canals.

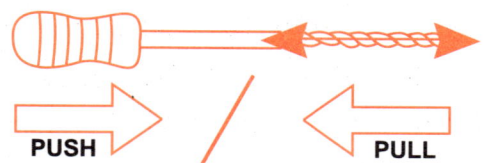

PUSH / **PULL**

2. Reaming

- *It indicates clockwise or right-hand rotation of an instrument.*
- The instrument must be restrained from insertion to generate a cutting effect.
- *Disadvantage* of this motion is increased instrument fracture.

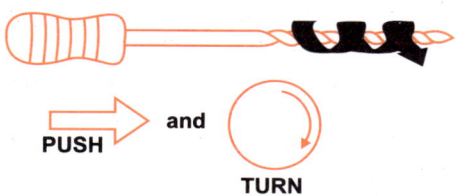

PUSH and **TURN**

3. Turn and Pull

- *It is a combination of reaming and filing.*
- The file is inserted with a quarter turn clockwise and inwardly directed hand presure (i.e., reaming) positioned into the canal. By this action the file is subsequently withdrawn (i.e. filing).
- It is an effective motion where the instrument is not forcefully pushed towards the apex and the preparation depths are allowed to diminish with each subsequent instrument.
- *Disadvantages* are, the process is tedious and time consuming.

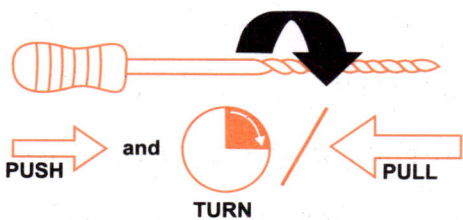

PUSH and **TURN** / **PULL**
BACK AND FORTH

4. Watch - Winding

- It is the back and forth oscillation of a file (30 to 60) right and (30 to 60) left as the instrument is pushed forward into the canal.
- The back and forth movement of k-type files and reamers causes them to plane dentinal walls efficiently.
- This motion is very useful during shaping.

Advantages

1. Less aggressive than turn and pull motion.
2. Reduced apical ledge formation.
3. It is effective with all k- type files.

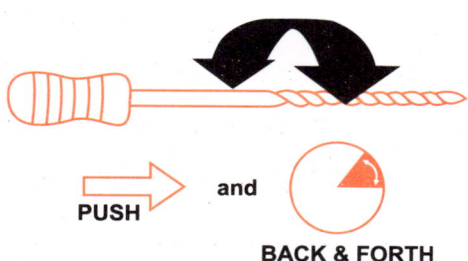

PUSH and **BACK & FORTH**

5. Watch - Winding and Pull

- It is used primarily with Hedstroem files.
- An inward pressure is mentioned while the file is gently rocked right and left , when that insertion stops, all rotation is ceased and the instrument is withdrawn from the canal.

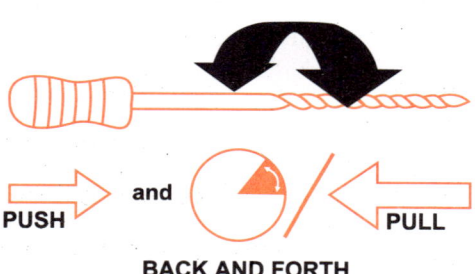

PUSH and **PULL**
BACK AND FORTH

6. Balanced force instrumentation

- It is the most efficient way to cut dentin.
- It is specifically designed to operate k - type endodontic instruments and should not be used with Broach type or Hedstroem type instruments, since either possesses left hand cutting capacity.
- It is introduced by *Roane et.al* in 1985.
- *He described the technique as "positioning and pre-loading an instrument through a clockwise rotation and then shaping the canal with a counter clockwise rotation".*
- The technique is, the file is pushed inwardly and rotated one quarter - turn clockwise. It is then rotated more that one half - turn counter clockwise. These alternate motions are repeated until the file reaches working length.

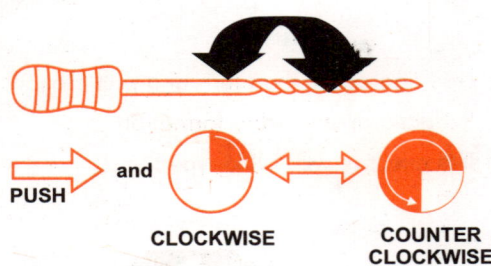

PUSH   and   CLOCKWISE   COUNTER CLOCKWISE

MECHANICAL INSTRUMENTATION

1. Engine Driven Instruments
2. Power Driven Instruments
3. Ultrasonic and sonic Instruments

1. ENGINE DRIVEN INSTRUMENTS

- Can be used for opening root canals.
- They should not be used for canal preparation except as a last resort.
- The rapid revolution of an engine driven reamer, file or broach can create a ledge, a perforation or an obstruction especially when the instrument breaks after it binds particularly in the apical region where the root canal is narrow.

Available as

- Two engine driven contra angle hand pieces namely,
  1. Giromatic
  2. Racer

1. Giromatic

- Activates a stainless steel barbed broach or reamer in the root canal through a 900 reciprocating arc at a speed upto 1000 cycles / min.

Disadvantages

- It may pack the dentinal shavings in the canal.
- Less effective for preparing root canals.
- Longer time is needed for preparation.
- Had a tendency to create ledges and to produce flaring at the apex.

2. Racer

- Uses a standard file and oscillates the file in the root canal.
- The instruments length can be adjusted to the working length using this contra angle.

Disadvantages

- Debris may be forced ahead of the instrument with resulting clogging of the canal or pushing of debris into periapical tissue.

Precaution

- When engine driven instruments are used, access to the apical foramen must be made first with hand instruments.

2. POWER DRIVEN INSTRUMENTS

Available as

1. Gates Glidden drills
2. Peeso Reamers

1. Gates Glidden Drill

- *Has a long thin shaft ending in a flame shaped head with a safe tip to guard against perforations.*
- The flame head cuts laterally and is used with gentle, apically directed pressure.
- The long shaft is designed to break at the neck, i.e. narrowest diameter that lies adjacent to the hand piece.
- If the drill binds during use, it will fracture at the neck of the shaft and extrude from the tooth.
- The fractured segment is easily removed by grasping the broken shaft with pliers and pulling it out of tooth.

Uses

- Used to remove the lingual shoulder during access preparation for anterior teeth.
- To enlarge root canal orifices.
- To clean and shape the cervical third of root canals in the step back preparation.

2. Peeso Reamer

- Has long, sharp flutes connected to a thick shaft.
- It cuts laterally and is primarily used for the preparation of post space when gutta percha has been removed from the obturated root canal.

Precaution

- Both gates glidden and peeso reamers are made of hardened carbon steel that corrodes easily.
- These aggressive cutting instruments are inflexible and should be used with slow speed

and with extreme caution to prevent overinstrumentation and perforations.

3. ULTRASONIC AND SONIC INSTRUMENTS

- Have been developed for cleaning and shaping root canals.

- Ultrasonic instrument consists of a piezoelectric ceramic unit that generates ultrasonic waves which activate a magneto strictive stack hand piece.

- The hand piece holds a k-file or a specially designed diamond file that when activated produces movements of the shaft of the file between 0.01 and 0.004 at a frequency of 20000 to 25000/ sec.

- The oscillating movements produces cutting action of the file and creates a ultrasonic wave of sodium hypochlorite irrigant solution, which is delivered along the side of the file into the root canal.

- Before ultrasonic instrumentation the apical third of the root canal should be hand instrumented to at least the size of a No: 15 file.

- In curved root canals, a precurved No:15, endosonic file is introduced into the canal to working length (1mm short of the apical foramen) and is activated.

- After activation, the file is moved in a circumferential manner with a smooth push pull stroke along the walls of the canal for a period of 1 min.

- The procedure is repeated with No:20 and 25 files.

- The ultrasonic file should be inserted into the root canal to the working length before activation to prevent ledge formation.

- The apical third of the canal should be filed cautiously to prevent transportation of the apical root canal and foramen.

Sonic Hand Pieces

- Sonic hand pieces operate at 1500 to 6500 cycles / min when filing inside root canals.

- They are similar in shape and weight to dental hand pieces and are attached to existing air and water lines.

- These instruments are used in a manner similar to the ultrasonic system in instrumentation of the root canals.

- The only difference is that the sonic system uses water as an irrigant and does not usually require diamond files for the flare of the preparation.

SOTOKAWA'S CLASSIFICATION OF INSTRUMENT DAMAGE

- Sotokawa classified the types of damage to instruments as,

  - He found that No. 10 file is the most frequently damaged instrument.

  - He described the progression of breakage as "first a starting point crack develops on the file's edge and then metal fatigue fans out from that point, spreading towards the file's axial center".

1.	Type I	:	Bent instrument.
2.	Type II	:	Stretching or straightening of twist contour.
3.	Type III	:	Peeling-off metal at blade edges.
4.	Type IV	:	Partial clockwise twist.
5.	Type V	:	Cracking along axis.
6.	Type VI	:	Full fracture.

CHAPTER 08

PRINCIPLES OF ENDODONTIC TREATMENT

PRINCIPLES OF ENDODONTICS

- Grossman has proposed principles which have to be followed systematically during endodontic treatment,

   1. Strict asepsis.

   2. Instruments should be confined to the root canal only.

   3. Root canal should always be entered with fine instruments initially to minimise the possibility of forcing debris beyond the apex.

   4. Root canal should be enlarged even though it may be fairly wide already.

   5. Root canal should be flooded with antiseptic solution during instrumentation.

   6. The irrigant that is used for disinfection should be nonirritating to the periapical tissues.

   7. Fistula or sinus requires no special treatment.

   8. Successive negative culture should be obtained before filling the root canal.

   9. There should be hermetic seal between the filling and the canal wall both laterally and apically.

   10. Root canal filling material should be acceptable by the periapical tissues.

   11. Whenever there is an acute abscess, drainage should be established. Incision and drainage should be followed when the swelling is soft and fluctuant.

   12. Injection into the infected area should not be made.

   13. Not all the pulpless teeth are amenable to treatment and not all patients are candidates for endodontic treatment.

Endodontic Treatment includes the following,

1. Isolation : Rubber dam application.
2. Aseptic technique
   - Infection control
   - Sterilization
3. Debridement
4. Drainage
5. Chemprophylaxis
6. Immobilization
7. Avoidance of trauma

1. Rubber Dam

   - Refer under the Chapter "THE OPERATING FIELD".

2. Aseptic Technique

   - Infection control
   - Sterilization
   - Refer under the Chapter "STERILIZATION".

3. Debridement
   - It is a principle of surgery that an infected wound must first be cleansed mechanically.
   - In this removal of necrotic pulp is done with Sodium hypochlorite, Saline, Hydrogen peroxide.
   - This promotes the faster healing.

4. Drainage
   - When there is infection and swelling the drainage is done by incision.
   - When there is acute alveolar abscess with much edema is present drainage is done through the root canal or incision or by both.
   - Drainage through the root canal is preferable because it allows the pent up pus and gas to escape.

5. Chemoprophylaxis
   - Patient with a history of Rh fever or heart ailment involving the heart valves.
   - 2g Phenoxy methyl penicillin should be given 1hr before the operation and then 1g 6 hr postoperatively.

     OR
   - 1g Erythromycin 1 hr before treatment and 500mg 6 hour after treatment.

6. Immobilization
   - Immobilization is employed by the surgeon to rest an organ to allay pain or promote healing. Immobilization reduces the potential for spreading of microorganisms.
   - Immobilizing the affected tooth, i.e. relieving tooth from occlusal stress when it is in occlusion.
   - It also reduces the possibility of traumatising the periodontal ligament.

7. Avoidance of Trauma
   - Soft tissues should be handled gently.
   - We should not cause trauma to the soft tissues.
   - Instrument should not pass beyond the apical foramen.
   - The following measures are followed to prevent the instrument going beyond apical foramen,
     - Using Rubber stops or mechanical stops.
   - Careful study about radiographs.
   - Should visualize length, shape and outline of the canal before passing the instrument.

A. TREPHINATION

   - A means of relieving pain has been used from time to time. It is done by creation of surgical passage in the region of the root apex with bur or special drill.
   - We do not use this procedure normally.

Purpose

   - To provide a channel for the escape of blood and pus to relative the pressure of accumulated fluid or gas in the Jaw bone.

Prophylactic Trephination

   - Done to prevent post operative pain during single sitting endodontics.

Indications

1. Acute alveolar abscess where drainage through the root canal is inadequate and much pain or swelling is present.
2. Teeth with large areas of rarefaction.
3. When the root canal has been overfilled and pain or discomfort is present.
4. For post operative pain following obturation of the canal by conventional means.

B. CHEMICAL IRRITATION

   - Can do as much damage as mechanical trauma.
   - Irritating drugs should be confined to the root canal itself and should not be forced through the apical foramen where they may come into contact with the periradicular tissues.

     Ex: Careless irrigation of the root canal to an extent that either hydrogen peroxide or sodium hypochlorite solution is forced through the apical foramen causes considerable pain and edema.
   - Preference should always be given to non irritating root canal medicaments.

CHAPTER 09

STERILIZATION

CLASSIFICATION OF INSTRUMENT STERILIZATION (By SPAULDING)

- Based on the contact with different tissue types to determine whether sterilization or disinfection is required.

1. Critical Items

- Instruments that touch sterile areas of body or enter the vascular system and that penetrate the oral mucosa. Ex: scalpels, currettes, burs and files.

2. Semi-critical Items

- Instruments that touch mucous membrane but do not penetrate tissue. Ex : amalgam condenser, saliva ejectors.

3. Non-critical Items

- Items do not come in contact with oral mucosa but are touched by saliva or blood contaminated hands. Ex : Switches, counter tops, drawer pulls on cabinets.

STERILIZATION OF ENDODONTIC INSTRUMENTS

- Prior to any method of sterilization used, the instrument should first be cleansed of debris.
- The instruments should be wiped clean by squeezing the instrument blade with a gauze or cotton roll moistened with hydrogen peroxide or alcohol.

I. Chemical sterilization

- 2% Benzalkonium chloride in 50% isopropylalcohol.
- Swabbing with hydrogen peroxide followed by tincture of iodine.
- Ethyl alcohol (2 parts) + formalin (1 part) to destroy spore formers.

II. Cold sterilization

- Sterilization by cold chemical solutions.
- *Quaternary ammonium compounds:* Kills vegetative organisms.
- *Ethyl alcohol and isopropyl alcohol :* Kills Vegetative bacteria, TB bacilli.
- *Alcohol-formalin solution :* Kills Vegetative bacteria, T.B. bacilli, spores.
- *Ortho phenyl phenol and Benzyl para chlorophenol:* Kills Vegetative bacteria, TB bacilli, certain fungi and viruses but not spores.

III. Autoclaving

- Common method.
- **Method (According to Ingle) :** At 121°C at 15 psi for 15 - 40 minutes.

– The time depends on the items to be autoclaved, the size of the load and type of container used.

IV. Chemiclave / Chemical vapour sterilization / Harvey chemiclave

– Similar to autoclave.

– Solutions used are alcohol, acetone, formaldehyde, water.

Method

1. **According to Ingle** at 132°C at 20 psi for 20 min.

2. **According to Grossman**, at 135°C at 15 lbs for 10 - 15 min.

V. Dry heat sterilization

1. *Prolonged Dry heat*

– It sterilizes at 160°C for 2 hours.

2. *Rapid Dry heat sterilization*

– Small chamber, high speed dry heat sterilizer.

– Operated at 190°C, sterilize unpackaged instruments in 6 minutes and packaged instruments in 12 minutes.

3. *Intense Dry heat*

A. Hot salt sterilizer

– Apparatus consists of a metal cup in which table salt is kept at a temperature between 425°F - 475°F.

– A thermometer is used always to measure the temperature.

– *Root canal instruments such as broaches, files, reamers are sterilized for 5 sec.*

– *Absorbent points and cotton pellets for 10 sec.*

Advantages

– Use of ordinary salt instead of metal or beads.

– Eliminates the risk of clogging the root canal.

B. Glass Bead sterilizer

– Glass beads are effectively substituted for the hot salt sterilizer provided glass beads less than 1mm diameter.

– Larger beads are not effective in transferring the heat to the endodontic treatment.

Method

Temperature : 425 - 475° F (218 - 246° C)

Time : 5 sec

Disadvantage

– Only small instruments can be sterilized.

VI. Sterilization of some other endodontic instruments

1. Dappendish

– Swabbing thoroughly with tincture of thimerosal followed by alcohol.

– Swabbing is done under pressure with the intent of physically removing the debris and microorganisms.

2. Long handle instruments, tip of cotton pliers, blades of scissors and other instruments

– Dipping the working point in alcohol and flaming twice.

3. Bulky instruments such as cotton pliers, and cement spatulas

– Sterilized quickly by passing the working blades through a flame several times.

4. Mixing slab (glass slab)

– By swabbing the surface with tincture of thimerosal followed by a double swabbing with alcohol.

5. Gutta-percha cones

– May be kept sterile in screw-capped vials containing alcohol.

– Sterilized by immersing in 5.2% sodium hypochlorite for 1 min then rinse the cone with hydrogen peroxide and dry it between two layers of sterile gauze.

– **Alternative method** - immersion in polyvinyl pyrolidone iodine for 6 min.

6. Silver cones

– Sterilized by slowly passing them back and forth through a Bunsen flame for 2 or 4 times or by immersion in the hot salt sterilizer for 5 sec.

7. Burs

– Autoclave

– Dry heat sterilization

– Dipping in alcohol

8. Handpiece sterilization

– FDA and ADA recommend that reusable dental handpieces and related instruments should be heat sterilized between each patient use.

– Handpieces can be sterilized by steam, chemical vapor and ethylene oxide gas (ETO).

CAUSES OF STERILIZATION FAILURE

1. Improper instrument preparation.

2. Improper packaging of instruments.

3. Improper loading of the sterilizer chamber.

4. Improper temperature in the sterilization chamber.

5. Improper timing of the sterilization cycle.

6. Equipment malfunction.

MONITORING STERILIZATION

– Two methods are commonly used to monitor sterilization in office, i.e.

    1.   Process indicators

    2.   Biologic indicators

1. Process indicators

– Process indicators are usually strips, tape, or paper products marked with special ink that changes colour on exposure to heat, steam, chemical vapor or ETO.

– The ink changes colour when the items being processed have been subjected to sterilizing conditions.

– But a process indicator usually does not monitor how long such conditions were present.

2. Biologic indicators

– Biologic indicators are usually preparations of non pathogenic bacterial spores that serve as a challenge to a specific method of sterilization.

– If a sterilization method destroys spore forms that are highly to that method, it is logical to assume that all other life forms have also been destroyed.

– The bacterial spores are usually attached to a paper strip within a biologically protected packet.

– The spore packet is placed between instrument packages or within an instrument packages itself.

– After the sterilizer has cycled, the spore strip is cultured for a specific time Lack of culture growth indicates sterility.

CHAPTER 10

RATIONALE OF ENDODONTIC TREATMENT

According to Grossman

- Any injury to the pulp (due to caries trauma chemicals) can produce many changes.

- Micro-organisms in the root canal multiply sufficiently to grow out of root canal or the toxins produced by root canal flora may diffuse into periradicular area.

- As the micro-organisms are virulent, the host defence decreases and they destroy PMN leukocytes and leads to chronic abscess.

- The proteolytic enzymes released by the dead PMN leukocytes produce pus.

- Following changes occur due to noxious stimuli from the diseased dental pulp,

  - Periapical infection causing lesion peripical radiolucency at the apex.

  - Cellular changes like infiltration of lymphocytes, macrophages, PMN Lymphocytes, phagocytes, osteoclasts, fibroblasts which causes so many changes.

  - These changes in periradicular area due to the diffusion of toxins from root canal flora are experimentally demonstrated by FISH.

- Hence, it is necessary to go for endodontic treatment to remove the toxins in the root canal and which leads to healing, repair and establishment of tooth function and saving the tooth.

FISH ZONES

- Fish established experimental foci of infection in the jaws of guinea pigs by drilling openings in the bone and packing in wool fibres saturated with a broth culture of micro organisms.

- He found 4 well defined zones of reaction.

- They are,
  1. Zone of infection
  2. Zone of contamination
  3. Zone of irritation
  4. Zone of stimulation

1. Zone of Infection

- *Characterized by PMN Leukocytes.*
- Infection is present in the centre of the lesion.

2. Zone of Contamination

- *Characterized by Round Cell Infiltration.*
- Around the central zone, Fish observed cellular destruction not from bacteria themselves but also from toxins discharged from the central zone.

- Empty lacunae are appeared as the bone cells had died and had undergone autolysis.
- Lymphocytes were prevalent.

3. Zone of Irritation

- *Characterized by macrophages and osteoclasts.*
- Fish found evidence of irritation further from the central lesion as the toxins became more diluted.
- The collagen framework is digested by phagocytic cells and the macrophages while the osteoclasts destroy the bone tissue.
- Some amount of repair has seen histopathologically.

4. Zone of stimulation

- *Characterized by Fibroblasts and Osteoblasts.*
- At the periphery the toxin was mild enough to be a stimulant.
- In response to this stimulation collagen fibres were laid down by the fibroblasts, which acted both as a wall of defense around the zone of irritation and as a scaffolding on which the osteoblasts built new bone.
- The new bone is built in a irregular fashion.

According to Cohen

- The rationale of endodontic treatment is based on simple biologic principles.
- Because the pulp is surrounded by dentin it can not benefit fully from the body's natural inflammatory response.
- First, the microcirculatory system of the pulp lacks a significant collateral circulation, second the pulp consists of a relatively large volume of tissue for a relatively small blood supply. And finally, the pulp of the root canal system is locked into the unyielding walls of surrounding dentin.
- Because of caries, restorative producers or trauma, a vascular pulp may degenerate into a vascular necrosis.
- The necrotic material then seeps out of the portals of exit (POE) of the root canal and into the supporting vascular attachment apparatus, generating lesions of endodontic origin (LEO).
- If the root canal system is sealed permanently in three dimensions, then the resolution can be expected.
- Longevity of a tooth is not based on the pulp, but on the healthy attachment apparatus.
- Therefore, treatment must be based on the effectiveness of cleaning shaping and packing the root canal with a permanent, biologically inert root canal filling.

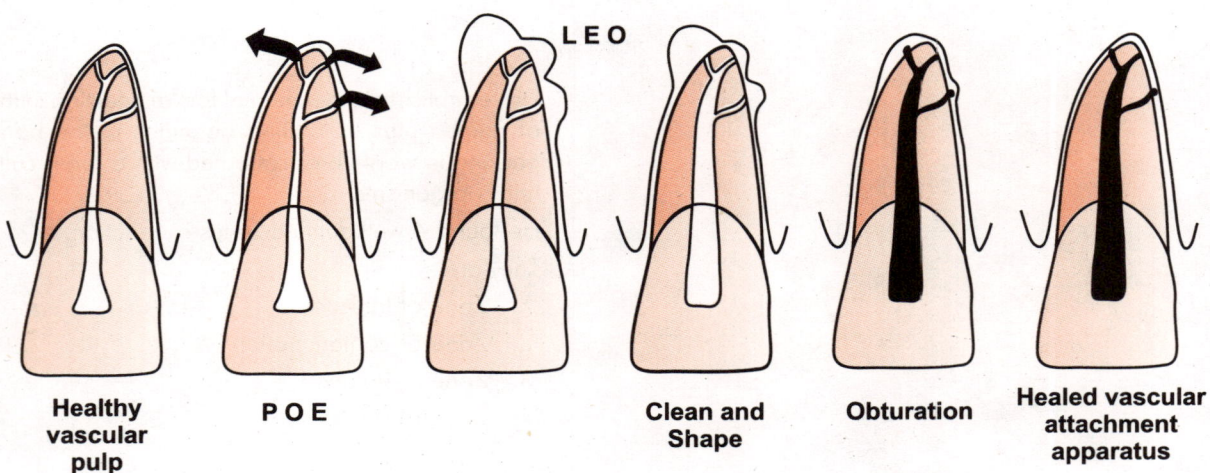

| Healthy vascular pulp | POE | LEO | Clean and Shape | Obturation | Healed vascular attachment apparatus |

CHAPTER 11

RCT:
AN OVERVIEW

– Once upon a time, if you had a tooth with a diseased nerve, you'd probably lose that tooth. Today with a special dental procedure called Root Canal Therapy you may save that tooth. Inside each tooth is the pulp which provides nutrients and nerves to the tooth, it runs like a thread down through the root. When the pulp is diseased or injured, the pulp tissue dies. If you don't remove it, your tooth gets infected and you could lose it. After the dentist removes the pulp the root canal is cleaned and sealed off to protect it. Then your dentist places a crown over the tooth to help make it stronger.

– Most of the time a root canal treatment is a relatively simple procedure with little or no discomfort, involving one to three visits.

– Best of all, it can save your tooth and your smile !

– The procedure for RCT is described below in brief.

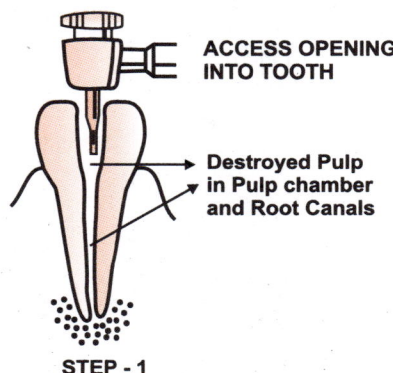

ACCESS OPENING INTO TOOTH

Destroyed Pulp in Pulp chamber and Root Canals

STEP - 1

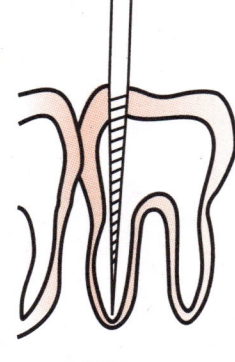

File used to remove dead pulp, debris and bacteria

STEP - 2

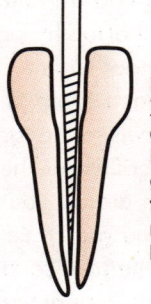

Examine by X - Rays to ensure the instruments go exactly to the end of the root and not beyond root

STEP - 3

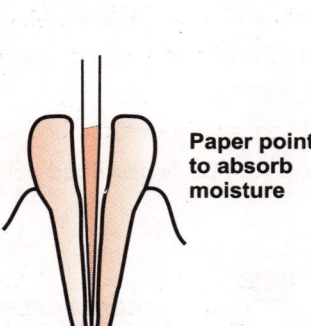

Paper point to absorb moisture

STEP - 4

Medicament

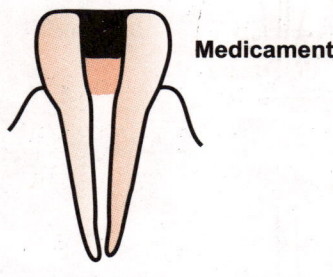

STEP - 5

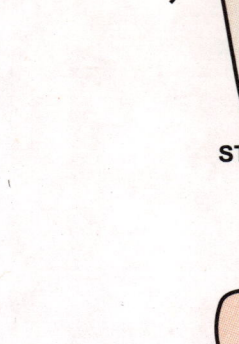

Fill with Gutta Percha points

STEP - 6

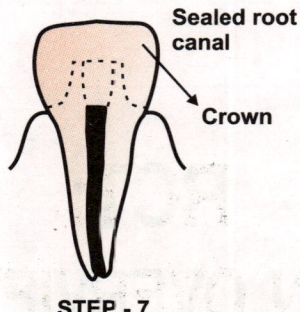

Sealed root canal

Crown

STEP - 7

CHAPTER 12

SELECTION OF CASES FOR ENDODONTIC TREATMENT

– Proper selection of cases is a must to ensure a successful endodontic treatment.

– The following factors are considered before the selection of cases for endodontic treatment,

1. Accessibility of the apical foramen through the root canal.

2. Restorability of the involved tooth.

3. General resistance of the patient.

– Endodontic treatment may be done when it is not contra indicated by the patient's health, provided the entire extent of the root canal can be instrumented, disinfected and obturated satisfactorily.

– *It is simpler to enumerate the contraindications as they are few in number than the indications.*

LOCAL CONTRAINDICATIONS

1. *Root Fractures :* Vertical fractures have a poor prognosis.

2. *Destruction* of the periapical tissues involving more than $1/3^{rd}$ of the length of the root.

3. *Obstructed root canal* of a pulpless tooth with a radiolucent area, i.e. curved root a tortuous canal, secondary dentin, a pulpstone that cannot be removed or by passed, a calcified or partially calcified canal a malformed tooth or a broken instrument.

4. *Bizarre anatomy*, i.e. incomplete development of root apex and death of the pulp.

5. *Accidental or pathologic perforations* of the root surface.

6. *Insufficient periodontal support.*

7. Massive internal or external *resorption*.

8. When there is persistent excessive *periapical exudate* that cannot be controlled prior to filling the root canal or when negative cultures cannot be obtained.

9. In cases of treatment, when a *foreign body* such as a fragment of guttapercha or of root canal filling material, lies in the periapical tissues of radiolucent teeth.

10. When an *acute infection* in a previously treated and filled pulpless tooth has occurred, treatment is indicated after the acute symptoms are controlled.

GENERAL CONTRAINDICATIONS

1. Systemic Conditions

– Patient's physical or mental condition, due to a chronic debilitating disease or old age would not enable them to tolerate endodontic treatment.

– In patient's with severe systemic disease such as active diabetes, syphilis, tuberculosis, a severe anaemia may not respond as readily to treatment; repair of periapical tissue may be delayed or may not occur as the potential for repair is reduced.

2. Small Mouth

– Access must be sufficient to allow placement of a rubberdam and a clamp.

3. Poor oral hygiene.

4. Patient's attitude

– Unless the patient is sufficiently well motivated a simpler form of treatment would be preferable.

CHEMOPROPHYLAXIS

– For the patients with a history of Rheumatic fever, with valvular heart damage, cardiovascular, renal diseases, hypertension, arteriosclerosis, patient with open heart operation or valve defect replaced by plastic substitutes.

– Antibiotic Pre-medication is as follows,

– 2 g Penicillin V 1 hour before the operation and 1 g Pencillin 6 hr after the operation.

OR

– 1 g Erythromycin 1 hour before the operation and 500mg Erythromycin 6 hr after the operation.

– Recommended by American Heart Association.

CHAPTER 13

PRINCIPLES OF ENDODONTIC CAVITY PREPARATION

– Here also Black's basic principles of cavity preparation are applied.

I. Endodontic coronal cavity preparation

1. Outline form
2. Convenience form
3. Removal of the remaining carious dentin
4. Toilet of the cavity

II. Endodontic radicular cavity preparation

1. Outline form
2. Convenience form
3. Toilet of the cavity
4. Retention from
5. Resistance form

A. CORONAL CAVITY PREPARATION

1. Outline form

– The outline form of the endodontic cavity must be correctly shaped and positioned to establish complete access for instrumentation from cavity margin to apical foramen.
– Access is obtained by drilling into the space and working the bur from within inside to the outside maintaining the circumferential contact all over.
– Dentinal wall overlying the pulp chamber should be removed.

Factors affecting outline form

i. Size of pulp chamber

– In young patients more extensive preparation is required than older patients where the pulp chamber has receded and it is small in all the three dimensions.
– A small orifice in the crown will not allow proper sized instruments and filling materials to pass through them.
– The access cavity preparation should be wider than the root canal.

ii. Shape of the pulp chamber

– It varies from tooth to tooth.

Anterior teeth

– The access preparation should diverge from the orifice towards the external surface of the tooth.

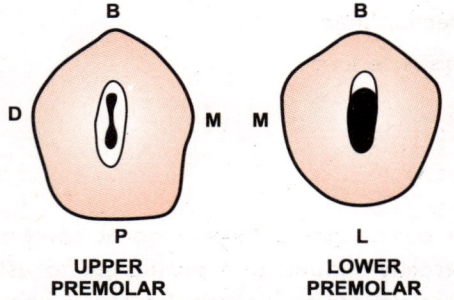

CENTRAL INCISOR   **LATERAL INCISOR**   **CANINE**

M = mesial ; D = distal

Upper premolars

– The access preparation should be oval shaped.

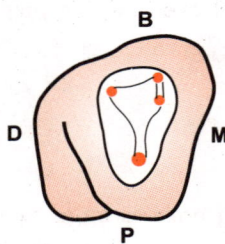

UPPER PREMOLAR   **LOWER PREMOLAR**

M = mesial; D = distal; P = palatal; B = buccal

Maxillary molars

– Normally triangular in shape.

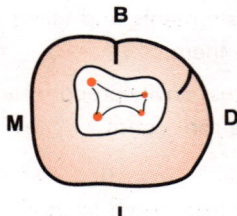

Mandibular molars

– Normally square shaped.

iii. Number and curvature of root canals

– In order to instrument each canal efficiently without interference cavity walls have to be extended to

allow the instruments to approach the apical foramen.

– When cavity walls are extended to improve instrumentation, the outline form is materially affected.

2. Convenience form

– Refers to convenient preparation and obturation of root canal.

– *Benefits of proper convenience form are*

1. Unobstructed access to canal orifices.

2. Direct access to the apical foramen.

3. Cavity expansion to accommodate the filling material.

4. Complete authority over enlarging instruments.

– Luebke has made the important point that an entire wall need not be extended in the event that instrument impingement occurs owing to a severely curved root or an extracanal.

– In extending only that portion of the wall needed to free this instrument, a cloverleaf appearance may evolve as the outline form. Hence Luebke has termed this a *'Shamrock Preparation'*.

3. Removal of remaining carious dentin and defective restorations

– Caries and defective restorations remaining in an endodontic cavity preparation must be removed for three reasons:

– To eliminate mechanically as many bacteria as possible from the interior of the tooth.

– To eliminate the discolored tooth structure, that may ultimately lead to staining of the crown.

– To eliminate the possibility of any bacteria laden saliva leaking into the prepared cavity.

4. Toilet of the Cavity

– After the removal of most of the debris any remaining necrotic debris should be flushed out during the toilet of the cavity.

– If the debris is carried out the root canal it may increase the bacterial population of the canal.

– Irrigation is done with sodium hypochlorite solution or hydrogen peroxide.

– The pulp chamber is dried with cotton rolls and use of air to dry the canal should be avoided.

- Even if air is used it should not be directed against the apex.
- If blasts of air escape from the apex, it may cause 'emphysema'.

Objectives / Advantages of Ideal Access Cavity Preparation

1. Permits complete debridement of the pulp chamber.
2. Permits visualisation of its floor.
3. Permits unimpeded placement of instruments into the root canals (straight line access).
4. Permits conservation of tooth structure.
- An axiom of canal preparation is the instruments should physically contact and plane the walls in order to loosen the tissue and debris for removal.

B. RADICULAR PREPARATION

1. Retention form
- Obtained in the apical third where 3-5 mm of walls are parallel to ensure firm seating of the primary cone or one should get a 'tugback' or resistance when the primary cone is inserted and with drawn. This is known as preparation of APICAL COLLAR.

2. Resistance form
- Obtained by maintaining natural apical constriction which is that key to successful therapy. It prevents the over extension of the filling material following condensation.

Objectives
- Debridement of the root canal.
- Shaping of the root canal to receive a filling.

CHAPTER 14

ROOT CANAL IRRIGANTS

- Irrigant is a liquid used to lubricate the canal walls and flushout the debris and microorganisms from the root canals.

Advantages

1. Rinses out the debris.
2. Lubricant facilitates instrumentation.
3. Dissolution of organic matter.
4. Smear layer removal.
5. Penetrates into inaccessible areas to instruments - extending the cleaning process.
6. Antibacterial properties.

IDEAL PROPERTIES

- It should,
    1. Be a tissue or debris solvent.
    2. Be able to dissolve or disrupt soft tissue, hard tissue remnants.
    3. Be non reactive to periapical tissues.
    4. Be a good lubricant.
    5. Act as disinfectant.
    6. Remove smear layer.
    7. Have low surface tension, i.e. promotes its flow into inaccessible areas.

IRRIGATING SOLUTIONS

1. Stream of hot water (140 -170° F).
2. Physiologic Saline
3. 30% Solution of urea
4. Urea peroxide solution in glycerin
5. Sodium hypochlorite - 5.2 %
6. Hydrogen peroxide
7. Anesthetic Solution
8. Solution of chloramines
9. Chlorhexidine gluconate (0.2%)

- Among these most commonly used are,
    - Sodium hypochlorite 5.2%
    - Hydrogen peroxide

In case of Acute Abscess

- Hydrogen peroxide is contraindicated.
- Distilled water or physiologic saline is used.
- The most popular and most advocated irrigant is sodium hypochlorite in various concentrations.

- *Alternate irrigation of sodium hypochlorite and H_2O_2 (3%) helps in producing `Effervescence'.*
- Interaction produces transient but energetic effervescence that mechanically forces the debris and micro-organisms out of the canal.

SODIUM HYPOCHLORITE (5.2%)

- Most widely used root canal irrigant.
- It is a reducing agent.
- *It contains 5% available chlorine.*
- It is less effective in narrow root canals than in wide root canals.

Mechanism of action

- The effervescent reaction of sodium hypochlorite pushes debris out of the root canal through the least resistant orifice.
- It has both antimicrobial and tissue solvent properties.
- It destroys the bacteria by two phases,
  1. Penetration into the bacterial cell.
  2. Chemical combination with the protoplasm of the bacterial cell that destroys it.

Disadvantage

- Potential toxicity causes tissue damage so all round isolation of tissues with a rubber dam is necessary.

Prevention of procedural errors with NaOCl

1. Avoid the forceful injection.
2. Using of specially designed side - venting needles.
3. Careful use in the presence of resorbed or open apices and perforation areas.

COMBINATION SOLUTIONS

1. EDTA (Ethylene Diamine Tetraacetic Acid)

- EDTA is used in conjunction with sodium hypochlorite.
- It is a chelating agent.
- EDTA removes the smear layer of dentin.
- In some instances reactions of the pulp to inflammation causes calcification and blockage of the root canal orifice. The blockage orifice can be opened by sharp endodontic explorer or by using slow speed small burs.
- If these procedures are not effective a chelating agent, i.e. EDTA is sealed in the pulp chamber for 24 hours.
- EDTA softens the dentin, calcified tissue and it can be removed and orifice opened by packing with an endodontic explorer.
- EDTA has distant antimicrobial properties.
- It is capable of causing mild irritation.
- EDTA is inserted by depositing a few drops in the pulp chamber with a syringe or pipette and then carefully pumping the solution into the canal.

2. RC - PREP

- It is a gel like commercial preparation developed by Stewart and collegues.

Composition

- EDTA - 15%
- Urea Peroxide - 10%
- Propylene glycol
- It is an effective lubricating and cleaning agent.
- It allows deeper penetration of medicament into the dentin.

CHAPTER 15

WORKING LENGTH DETERMINATION

Definition

– The distance from a coronal reference point to the point at which canal preparation and obturation should terminate (Glossary of Endondontics).

I. Objectives

1. To establish the length at which canal preparation and obturation has to be done.
2. Optimum length has been established at 1-2 mm short of the apex.
– *Over instrumentation* causes apical perforation, overfilling and pain.
– *Failure* to determine correct working length leads to,
   1. Incomplete instrumentation
   2. Ledge formation
   3. Underfilling with apical percolation
   4. Persistent pain and discomfort from retained pulp tissue

II. Methods

1. *Radiographic Methods*
   1. Grossman's method
   2. Ingle's Method
   3. Xeroradiography
   4. Radiovisiography (RVG)

2. *Non Radiographic Methods*
   1. Electrical resistance Method
   2. Audiometric Method
   3. Paper Point Method

Anatomic apex
– It is the tip or the end of the root determined morphologically.

Radiographic (major apical diameter) apex
– It is the tip or the end of the root determined radiographically.

RADIOGRAPHIC METHODS

1. GROSSMAN'S METHOD

Technique
– An instrument extending to the apical constriction is placed in the root canal which can be determined by digital tactile sense and a radiograph is taken.

– Stopper is placed at the level of incisal or occlusal reference point.

– Measure the length of the X - ray images of both the tooth and measuring instrument as well as actual length of the instrument in the canal.

Formula

$$\frac{A}{D} = \frac{C}{D} \Rightarrow \frac{\text{actual length of the tooth (A)}}{\text{actual length of instrument (B)}} = \frac{\text{Radiographic length of tooth (C)}}{\text{Radiographic length of instrument in the tooth (D)}}$$

$$\text{Actual length the tooth (A)} = \frac{\text{Radiographic length of tooth (C)}}{\text{Radiographic length of instrument in the tooth (D)}} \times \text{Actual length the instrument (B)}$$

$$A = \frac{C}{D} \times B$$

2. INGLE'S METHOD

– Preoperative radiographs are taken.

– From these the approximate length of the root canal is found by adjusting a occlusal rubber stop on the shaft of a file.

– From this, a length of atleast 1mm is reduced by moving the rubber stopper on the shaft.

– This is a safety measure.

– According to Ingle, it is to be observed for possible image distortion on the X-ray.

– After adjusting this, a radiograph is taken with the instrument in position.

– On the X - ray the difference between the tip of the instrument and the tip of the root is added to safety measure if it is short of the apex.

– If the instrument has gone beyond the apex, the measurement that is obtained is subtracted from the original measurement.

– Finally 1mm is reduced from final measurement so that the tip of the instrument will correspond to the apical foramen.

– In this method it is assumed that apical foramen is 0.5mm away from the radiographic root tip.

Example

Initial Measurement	-	23 mm
Safety Measure	-	(-) 01 mm
Tentative Working Length	-	22 mm
After taking radiograph, if it is short of 1.5 mm	-	(+) 1.5 mm
		23.5 mm
Adjustment for apical termination	-	(-) 1.0 mm
Final working length	-	22.5 mm

– Wein's modifications for Ingle's method,

1. If radiographically, there is no resorption of the root end or bone, shorten the length by the standard 1 mm.

2. If periapical bone resorption is apparent, shorten by 1.5 mm.

3. If both root and bone resorption are apparent shorten by 2 mm.

– This is because if there is root resorption, the apical constriction is probably destroyed hence the shorter move back up the canal. Also when bone resorption is apparent, probably there is also root resorption, even though it may not be apparent radiographically.

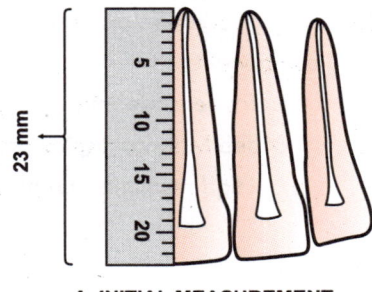

A. INITIAL MEASUREMENT

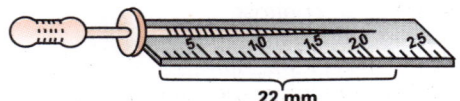

B. TENTATIVE WORKING LENGTH

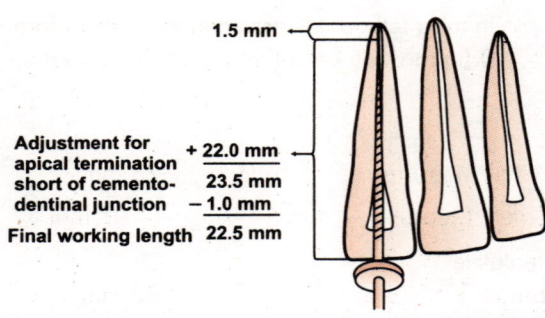

1.5 mm

Adjustment for apical termination short of cemento-dentinal junction

+ 22.0 mm
23.5 mm
− 1.0 mm

Final working length   22.5 mm

C. FINAL WORKING LENGTH

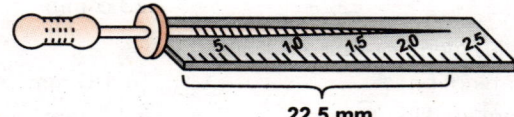

22.5 mm

D. SETTING THE INSTRUMENTS AT FINAL WORKING LENGTH

3. XERORADIOGRAPHY

- Not widely used in endodontics.
- They record images produced by an X-ray but differ from conventional radiography is that it does not require a wet chemical processing or dark rooms.
- Xeroradiographs are superior to conventional radiographs in that.
- Soft tissue and bone abnormalities are visible.
- Periapex is seen with greater sharpness.
- Better edge contrast.

4. RADIOVISIOGRAPHY (RVG)

- It produces diagnostically useful images at low radiation.
- It provides an instantaneous image on a monitor, while reducing radiation exposure by 80%.
- *It has 3 components*
  1. *Radio* : Has sensitive intra oral sensor.
  2. *Visio* : Video Monitor display processing Unit.
  3. *Graphy* : High resolution printers.

Advantages

- Reduction of radiation exposure.
- Instantaneous image and display.
- Control of contrast.
- Elimination of X - ray film.
- Ability to enlarge special areas.
- Potential for computer storage.

NON-RADIOGRAPHIC METHODS

- The main disadvantages of Radiographic methods are,
  - Radiation Exposure
  - No definitive interpretation
  - Time consuming
  - Due to morphologic variability of the root canal, apical foramen does not correspond to root tip.
  - Possible distortion
- To overcome these disadvantages some electrical devices which can determine the working length have been invented.

1. ELECTRICAL RESISTANCE METHOD

- Working length is determined by comparing the electrical resistance of apical periodontal membrane with the gingiva surrounding the tooth and both should be similar.

Technique

- A probe such as a file is attached to the electronic instrument with a cord and is inserted into the root canal till it contacts the periodontal ligament.
- The second probe is attached to the gingival.
- When the file touches the soft tissues, the electrical resistance gauges of both periodontal ligament and gingiva should have the same reading.
- By measuring the depth of probe, one can determine the working length.

2. AUDIOMETRIC METHOD

- Has slight variation from the electronic method.
- In this method a variation in the principle of electrical resistance of comparative tissue uses frequency oscillation sound to indicate when a similarity to electrical resistance has occurred by a similar sound response.

Technique

- Introduce an instrument into the gingival sulcus and induce an electric current until a sound is produced.
- The same procedure is repeated by introducing the instrument into the root canal and length is determined when the same sound is produced.
- These gadgets are commonly called 'APEX LOCATORS'.

APEX LOCATORS

- In many of these instruments, the event is signalled by a beep, flashing lights and digital reading.
- One electrode is attached to the chip and the other to the file and the patient forms the circuit.

Trade Names

Endo meter

Sonoexplorer

Neosone

Classification

1. First Generation

- Also known as 'resistance apex locators'.
- Measure opposition to the flow of direct current or resistance.

2. Second Generation

- Also known as `Impedance apex Locators'.
- Measure opposition to the flow of alternating current or impedance.

- *Disadvantage* : Root canal should be free from electroconductive materials to use this.

APEX FINDER

- This is a new instrument used to locate the apex, as well as the working length.
- Insert a fine plastic tapered shaft through a bevelled tube into the root canal.
- Resistance to withdrawal indicates that some barbs have engaged the apical region and the shaft is marked at this level of cusp tip.
- The distance between the barb and marker is determined.
- The barbs that are engaged with resistance will show apical inclination which will be in the opposite inclination of the other barbs.

MASTER APICAL FILE DETERMINATION

- Master Apical File (MAF) is defined as *the largest file that binds slightly at correct working length after straight line access.*
- It is determined of passively placing successively larger files until a size is reached that slightly binds at the tip.

CHAPTER 16

CLEANING AND SHAPING (BIOMECHANICAL PREPARATION) OF THE ROOT CANAL

CLEANING AND SHAPING

- Schilder defined the general objective of canal preparation as follows :
- Root canal system must be *cleaned and shaped, cleaned of their organic remnants and shaped to receive a three dimensional hermetic filling of the entire root canal space.*

AIMS OF ROOT CANAL PREPARATION

1. To reduce the bacterial load of the root canal.
2. To dissolute and debride the inflament and infected tissue.
3. To create a shape, which is suitable for obturation.

SCHILDER'S MECHANICAL OBJECTIVES OF ROOT CANAL PREPARATION

1. Develop a continuously tapering conical form in the root canal preparation.
2. Make the canal narrower apically, with the narrowest cross-sectional diameter at its terminus.
3. Make the preparation in multiple steps.
4. Never transport the foramen.
5. Keep the apical foramen as small as in practical.

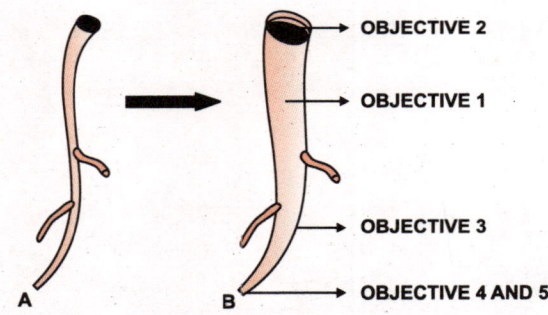

SCHILDER MECHANICAL OBJECTIVES

The `LOOK'

- Schilder refers to `the look' as the radiographic appearance of three - dimensional obturation, when all five mechanical objectives have been achieved.

MOTIONS OF CLEANING AND SHAPING

- There are six distinctive motion of files and reamers.

1. Follow

- Usually performs with files.
- They can be used during cleaning and shaping or any time an obstruction blocks the foramen.

2. Follow - Withdraw

- It is an in-and-out, passive motion that makes no attempt to shape the canal.
- File is the most useful instrument for this purpose.
- This motion is used when the foramen is reached, and the next step is to create the path from access cavity to foramen.

3. Cart

- Refers to the extension of a reamer to or near the radiographic terminus.
- Reamer should gently and randomly touch the dentinal walls and `cart' away debris.

4. Carve

- Carving is for shaping.
- Reamers are best for carving.
- Instrument should not be pressed apically but simply touches the dentin and shape on withdraw.

5. Smooth / Circumferential

- Usually accomplished by files.
- If the above procedures are followed, smoothing is not required.

6. Patency

- Achieved with files or reamers.
- It is used to clear any debris at the portal of exit.

PURPOSE OF CLEANING AND SHAPING

- Cleaning and shaping is the basis for endodontic therapy.
- Cleaning is a combined chemical and mechanical process.
- Shaping is purely mechanical.
- Cleaning removes affected, infected antigenic, and substrate material from the canal system.
- Shaping enlarges the canals diameter and smoothens the walls as it removes crevices, fissures and irregularities from the canal, and facilitates obturation.

RULES MUST BE FOLLOWED DURING CLEANING AND SHAPING

1. Straight line access.
2. The Length of the tooth should be correctly determined.

3. Instruments should be used in a sequence of sizes with periodic recapitulation, returning to smaller sizes to avoid blockage and ledging.
4. The instruments must be used as quarter to half turn in pull strokes.
5. Barbed broach should be used cautiously and only when the root canal is wide enough to permit their insertion and rotation without binding.
6. Should not force the instrument if it binds.
7. Clean, sterile instruments should be used.
8. Debris should not be forced through apical foramen.
9. Instrument should confine to root canal.
10. The apical portion of root canal 3-4 mm should be enlarged atleast 3 sizes greater than the first instrument that binds and until the walls are tapered without irregularities.

TECHNIQUES OF RADICULAR CAVITY PREPARATION

- There are two techniques present,
  1. Step - back preparation
  2. Step - down preparation

1. STEP - BACK PREPARATION

- Also called as *serial technique or telescopic preparation.*
- *Preparation starts at the apex with fine instruments and working one's way back up (or down) the canal with progressively larger instruments.*
- Designed to overcome instrument transportation in the apical third canal.

Technique

- *Mullaney* divided the preparation into two phases,
  1. *Phase - I* : apical preparation starting at the apical constriction.
  2. *Phase - II* : Preparation of the remainder of the canal, gradually stepping back while increasing in size.

1. *Phase - I: Apical Preparation*

- Apical portion of the canal is enlarged to atleast 25 to 30 sized instruments or the apical portion is enlarged using 1-2 sizes larger that the first file that binds.

2. Phase -II

- To complete the instrumentation of remaining portion of root canal by successively using larger instruments and each larger instrument should be kept 1 mm shorter than previous instrument.
- The remainder of the root canal is prepared in a step back manner.
- Thus the preparation steps back up the canal 1 mm and one larger instrument at a time.

Advantages

1. Less likely to cause periapical trauma.
2. Facilitates removal of more debris.
3. Greater flare that results from instrumentation facilitates packing of guttapercha by either lateral or vertical condensation.
4. One can obtain development of apical matrix or step which prevent overfilling of root canal.
5. Greater condensation pressure can be exerted which often fills lateral canals.

Objectives

- To keep the apical portion of preparation as small as possible, with an increasing taper throughout the remainder of the canal.
- In addition, the final apical preparation should be at or close to the original canal preparation.
- It creates a smooth flow and more tapered preparation from apical portion to coronal portion.

2. STEP DOWN TECHNIQUE (Crown Down Pressure less Technique)

- This involves cleaning and shaping of the canal from coronal third down to the apical third.
- Apical third is approached only after the coronal two third preparations.

Technique

1. Coronal and Midroot Preparation

- Working length is determined.
- Coronal (16 mm) is prepared with H-files or Gates Glidden of sizes 15 - 40.
- Each larger file is inserted shorter than its predecessor.

2. Apical Preparation

- It involves enlargement of the apex by 2-3 sizes from the first file that binds apically.

3. To do stepback to connect apical and coronal taper.

Advantages

1. Elimination of debris and microorganisms from the more coronal parts of the root canal system there by preventing inoculation of apical tissues with contaminated debris.
2. Elimination of coronally placed interferences that might adversely influence instrumentation.
3. Early movement of large volumes of irrigant and lubricant to the apical part of the canal.
4. Facilitation of accurate working length determination as coronal curvature is eliminated early in the preparation.

Clinical Benefits

1. Easy removal of pulp stones.
2. Enhanced tactile feedback with instruments by removal of coronal interferences.
3. Enhanced apical movement of instruments into the canal.
4. Enhanced working length determination due to minimal tooth contact in the coronal third.
5. Increased space for irrigant penetration and debridement.
6. Rapid removal of pulp tissue located in the coronal third.
7. Straight line access to the root curves and canal junctions.
8. Enhanced coronal movement of debris.
9. Decreased deviation of instruments in canal curvatures.
10. Decreased canal blockages.
11. Minimization of instrument separation.
12. Predictable quality of canal cleaning and shaping.
13. Faster preparation.

Biological Benefits

1. Rapid removal of contaminated, infected tissue from the root canal.
2. Removal of tissue debris coronally thereby minimizing pushing of debris apically.
3. Reduction of post operative pain.
4. Better dissolution of tissue with increased irrigant penetration.
5. Easy removal of smearlayer.

6. Enhanced disinfection of canal irregularities due to irrigant penetration.

RECAPITULATION

– Refers to repeated reintroduction and reapplication of instruments previously used through out the cleaning and shaping process inorder to create a well designed unclogged, smooth, evenly tapered unstepped root canals.

– The entire procedure is called **serial reaming** and filing and constant recapitulation.

EVALUATION CRITERIA FOR APICAL PREPARATION

– Three criteria are described.

1. Debridement

– Following preparation, the MAF tip is pressed against each wall on the outstroke. All walls should feel smooth.

2. Adequate taper

– The selected spreader or plugger passes easily to or within 1 mm of the working length with space left alongside for gutta percha.

3. Apical preparation

– A seat or a stop or neither is identified by using a file smaller than the MAF at the working length.

CHAPTER 17

DISINFECTION OF THE ROOT CANAL

DISINFECTION

- *It is the destruction of pathogenic microorganisms, presupposes adequate removal of pulp tissue and debris clearing and enlarging of the canal by biomechanical means and clearing of its contents by irrigation.*

- The four factors either predispose the teeth to infection or counteract disinfection whether it may be of a wound or the root canal of a pulpless tooth, i.e. trauma, devitalized tissue, dead spaces and accumulation of exudate.

- Disinfection of the root canal is accomplished by intra canal medication.

- Microorganisms present in the canal can invade the periapical tissue and may not only give rise to pain but also destroy the periodontium including bone.

- The intracanal medication reduces or eliminates the microbial flora present in the root canal.

INTRACANAL MEDICAMENTS

Functions of Intracanal Medicaments

A. *Primary functions*

1. Antimicrobial activity
2. Antisepsis
3. Disinfection

B. *Secondary functions*

1. Hard tissue formation
2. Pain control
3. Exudation control
4. Resorption control

Requirements

- It should,

    1. Be an effective germicide and fungicide.
    2. Be non irritating to the periapical tissue.
    3. Remain stable in solution.
    4. Have a prolonged antimicrobial effect.
    5. Be active in the presence of blood, serum and protein derivatives of tissue.
    6. Not interfere with repair of periapical tissues.
    7. Not stain tooth structure.
    8. Be capable of inactivation in a culture medium.
    9. Have low surface tension.
    10. Not induce a cell mediated immune response.

Classification

– May be classified arbitrarily as,

  A. Essential oils

  B. Phenolic compounds

  C. Halogens

  D. Other material

  E. Antibiotics ·

A. ESSENTIAL OILS

– These are weak disinfectants.

Eugenol

– Chemical essence of oil of clove and is related to phenol.

– Antiseptic and anodyne.

– Slightly more irritating than oil of clove.

B. PHENOLIC COMPOUNDS

1. Phenol

– A white crystalline substance which has a characteristic odour derived from coal tar.

– Liquefied phenol (carbolic acid) consists of 9 parts of phenol and 1 part water.

– Phenol is a protoplasm poison and produces necrosis of soft tissue.

2. Para - chlorophenol

– A substitution product of phenol in which chlorine replaces one of the hydrogen atoms ($C_6 H_4 OCl$).

– On trituration with gum camphor these substances combine to form an oily liquid.

– Harrison and Madonia have recommended 1% aqueous solution of parachlorophenol.

– Penetrates deeper into the dentinal tubules than camphorated chlorophenol.

3. Formocresol

– This substance is a combination of formalin and cresol in the proportions of 1:2 or 1: 1.

– It is a non specific bactericidal medicament most effective against aerobic and anaerobic Organisms found in a root canal.

4. Glutaraldehyde

– S'Gravenmade and Dankert have recommended it in low concentration (2%).

– It is a strong disinfectant and fixative.

– This colorless oil is slightly soluble in water and thereby has a slightly acidic reaction.

5. Crestatin (Metacresylacetate)

– A clear, Stable, oily liquid of low volatility.

– It has antiseptic and obtundant properties.

C. HALOGENS

1. Sodium Hypochlorite

– Sometimes used as an intracanal medicament.

– Sodium hypochlorite vapours were bactericidal, whereas those of formocresol, aqueous para-chlorophenol and camphorated chlorophenol were bacteriostatic.

– As the activity of sodium hypochlorite is intense but of short duration, the compound should preferably be applied to the root canal every other day.

2. Iodides

– Engstrom and Spangberg have recommended a 2% solution of Iodine of Potassium iodide as a root canal disinfectant.

– This compound consists of,

  – Iodine crystals - 2 parts

  – Potassium iodide - 4 parts

  – Distilled water - 94 parts

– Antibacterial effect is of short duration.

D. OTHER MATERIALS

1. Quaternary Ammonium

– The quats are compounds that lower the surface tension of solutions.

– 9-aminoacridine, an antiseptic but it may stain tooth structure.

2. Calcium Hydroxide

– It is best used as an intracanal medicament when one anticipates an excessive delay between appointments because it is efficacious as long as it remains within the root canal.

3. N2 (Sargentis Paste)

– A compound containing para formaldehyde as its primary ingredient, contains eugenol and phenyl mercuric borate and at times additional ingredients including lead, corticosteriods, antibiotics and perfume.

– An intracanal medicament and sealer.

– Available as 'RC-2B'.

4. Antibiotics
 – They should not be used routinely as an intra canal medicament as they cause allergy, development of resistance to microorganisms, drug toxicity.
 – **PBSC (Polyantibiotic pastes)** was used as an intracanal medicament.
 – It is seldom used nowadays.
 – PBSC Consists of,
   – Penicillin - effective against gram positive.
   – Bacitracin - effective against penicillin resistant microorganisms.
   – Streptomycin - effective against Gram negative.
   – Caprolate sodium - effective against fungi.

FREQUENCY OF MEDICATION

 – In accordance with general principles of root canal management disinfectant dressings should preferably be renewed in a week and not longer than 2 weeks.
 – Because dressing become diluted by periapical exudate and are decomposed by interaction with the micro-organisms.
 – Length of time for which the medicament remains effective depends on,
   1. Size of apical foramen
      – Wide apical foramen: washing of medicaments is quick. So they will not remain effective for long.
   2. Size of the dentinal tubules
      – Young teeth with little secondary dentin will allow greater diffusion of medicament.
      – So it will not remain effective longer in the canal for as long as older teeth.

3. Presence of Smear layer
 – Smear layer initially delays the release of components and can have the effect of not allowing the medicaments to reach the regions of infection or inflammation in suitable therapeutic concentrations.

4. Presence of remnants of pulp tissue
 – If pulp tissue is left in the canal, it will dissolve the medicaments and it will be rapidly cleared from the canal system.

5. Temporary sealing of the access cavity
 – If the access cavity is not effectively sealed, then medicaments will not last long due to dissolution

6. Medicament that is used
 – The material should be preferably in the past form and have low solubility.

ELECTROSTERILIZATION

 – It is a combined and simultaneous use of medicaments and direct electric current.
 – The process of sterilization depends upon the passage of direct current through an electrolyte.
 – A suitable Iridoplatinum electrode is selected which reaches the apex and fits the canal loosely.
 – The canal is flooded with Zinc Iodide Iodine solution.
 – The electrode is then inserted and retracted in the root canal in order to eliminate air bubbles, and pump the solution to the apex.
 – After the tooth electrode is adjusted, a hand electrode to be held in the hand and current is turned on gradually.
 – The patient is instructed to signal the operator by raising the hand when there is tingling sensation.
 – Amount of current tolerated by the patient is registered and duration of treatment is then calculated.

CHAPTER 18

TEMPORARY FILLING MATERIALS

DEFINITION

- *These are the materials used to seal the root canals to prevent from the leakage.*

REQUIREMENTS

- The material should,
    1. Be impervious to fluids of the mouth and bacteria.
    2. Hermetically seal the access cavity peripherally.
    3. Not cause pressure on the dressing during insertion.
    4. Set within a few min after insertion.
    5. Withstand the force of mastication.
    6. Be easy to manipulate and to remove.
    7. Harmonize with the colour of the tooth structure.

MATERIALS

1. CAVIT

- It is a moisture initiated, auto polymerized, premixed calcium sulfate-polyvinyl chloride acetate.
- **Composition** : zincoxide, calcium sulfate, glycol acetate, polyvinyl acetate, polyvinyl chloride, triethanolamine and red colouring.
- Thickness of at least 3.5 mm is necessary to prevent leakage.

Advantages

1. Superior sealing
2. Ability to withstand thermal changes.
3. Easy to insertion
4. Can also be used as retrograde filling material.

Disadvantages

- It was found that long periods between appointments predisposed the tooth to leakage.

2. INTERMEDIATE RESTORATIVE MATERIAL (IRM)

- It is a ZOE (Type - III) based cement to which reinforcing particles are added to improve the strength and toughness of the set material.
- Its longevity can extend a year or longer.
- There is no evidence of leakage.

3. TERM

- It is a light activated particle filled composite resin for which there is no need of acid etching prior to placement.
- Main component is Urethane Dimethacrylate polymer.

CHAPTER 19

ROOT CANAL SEALERS / CEMENTS

DEFINITION

– *These are the cements which are used in adjunct to obturating material to seal the canal perfectly.*

FUNCTIONS

1. Cementing the core material into the canal.
2. Filling of the discrepancies between the canal walls and core material.
3. Acting as a lubricant.
4. Bactericidal agent.
5. Acting as a marker for accessory canals, resorptive defects, root fractures and other spaces into which the main core material may not penetrate.

IDEAL PROPERTIES

– It should,
    1. Provide an excellent seal when sets.
    2. Produce adequate adhesion among the canal walls and the filling material.
    3. Be radiopaque
    4. Be non staining
    5. Be dimensionally stable
    6. Be easily mixed and introduced into canals.
    7. Be easily removed if necessary.
    8. Be insoluble in tissue fluids.
    9. Be bactericidal or discourage bacterial growth.
    10. Be non irritating to periapical tissues.
    11. Be slow setting, to ensure sufficient working time.

CLASSIFICATION

– Based on the composition,
    A. Eugenol sealers
        1. Grossman's sealer
        2. Kerr root canal sealer
        3. Wach's cement
        4. Rickert's sealer
        5. Tubli seal
    B. Non Eugenol sealers
        1. Chloropercha
        2. Diaket
        3. AH 26
        4. Paraformaldehyde cement

C. Resorbable pastes with therapeutic values
  - Zinc oxide eugenol paste + Iodoform + thymoliodide + camphorated phenol + paraformaldehyde.

1. GROSSMAN'S SEALER
  - It is a non staining sealer which meets ideal requisites.

Composition
Powder

Zinc oxide	-	42%
Staybelite resin	-	27%
Bismuth subcarbonate	-	15%
Barium sulfate	-	15%
Sodium borate anhydrous	-	1%

Liquid
  - Eugenol or oil of pigmenta leaf.
  - Powder and liquid is mixed to creamy consistency.
  - Different tests, to test for proper consistency are drop test and string test.

Drop Test
  - The cement is gathered and the spatula is held edgewise.
  - The cement should not drop off the spatula's edge in less than 10 to 12 seconds.

String Test
  - The mixed cement should string out for at least 1 inch when the spatula is raised from the glass slab.

2. CHLOROPERCHA
Composition
Powder
  Zinc oxide
  Canada balsam
  Rosin
  Guttapercha
Liquid
  Chloroform

3. DIAKET
  - It is a polyvinyl resin (polyketone).
  - It consists of a fine, pure white powder and a viscous, honey colored liquid.

Composition
Powder
  Zinc oxide
  Bismuth phosphate
Liquid
  Polyvinyl resin

Advantages
  - Good adhesion to teeth.
  - Rapid set
  - High tensile strength
  - Resistance to permeability

4. AH - 26
  - An epoxy resin containing a non toxic hardener.
  - Radiopacity is imparted by Bismuth oxide.

Advantages
  - Strong adhesive properties.
  - Provides good seal.

Disadvantages
  - Staining of tooth structure.
  - Insoluble in solvents.

5. RICKERT'S SEALER
  - It is germicidal.

Composition
Powder
  Zinc oxide
  Precipitated silver
  White resin
  Thymol iodide
Liquid
  Oil of cloves
  Canada balsam

Advantages
  1. excellent lubricating property
  2. excellent adhesion
  3. adequate setting time

Disadvantage
  - Possibility of discoloration of tooth (due to silver).

6. TUBLISEAL

Composition

Zincoxide

Bismuth trioxide

Oleoresins

Thymol iodide

Oils

Modifiers

Advantages

1. Excellent lubricating property.
2. Does not stain the tooth.

Disadvantage

– Rapid setting

7. WACH'S SEALER

– It is germicidal.

Composition

Powder

Zinc Oxide	-	10 g
Calcium phosphate	-	2 g
Bismuth subnitrate	-	3.5 g
Heavy magnesium oxide	-	0.5 g

Liquid

Canada balsam	-	20 ml
Oil of Clove	-	6 ml

Advantages

– Low tissue irritation
– Adequate setting time
– Limited lubricating qualities

CHAPTER 20

OBTURATION OF THE ROOT CANAL

– *Obturation* It is the final phase of Root Canal Therapy, refers to filling the entire root canal completely and densely with a non-irritating, air - tight sealing agent.

OBJECTIVES

1. To prevent percolation and microleakage of periapical exudate into the root canal space.
2. To prevent reinfection.
3. To create a favourable biologic environment for the process of tissue healing to take place.

APPROPRIATE TIME FOR OBTURATION (OR WHEN TO OBTURATE)

– Root Canal should be obturated when,

1. Tooth is asymptomatic-no tenderness and pain.
2. The canal is dry
3. There is no sinus tract
4. There is no foul odor
5. Successive negative culture is obtained.
6. The temporary filling is intact.

OBTURATING MATERIALS OR ROOT CANAL FILING MATERIALS

REQUIREMENTS FOR AN IDEAL ROOT CANAL FILLING MATERIAL

– It should,

– Be easily introduced

– Be liquid or semi solid and should become solid

– Seal laterally and apically

– Be impervious to moisture

– Not shrink

– Be bacteriostatic

– Not stain tooth

– Not irritate periapical tissues

– Be easily removed

– Be sterile or sterilizable

– Be radiopaque

– They are the bulk that will fill the canal space

– They may or may not be used in conjunction with sealer.

CLASSIFICATION OF OBTURATING MATERIALS

1. Pastes

- Chloropercha
- Calcium Hydroxide
- N_2

2. Solids

a.	*Semirigid Flexible*	Silvercones
b.	*Rigid*	Vitallium implants
c.	*Plastic*	Gutta-percha
		Epoxy resin acrylate
d.	*Cements*	Zinc oxide eugenol

1. GUTTA-PERCHA (GP)

- Most widely used and accepted root canal filling material.
- GP is a hydrocarbon resembling a rubber in origin.
- Pure GP is not used.

Composition

Zinc Oxide	-	66 % (filled)
Gutta-percha	-	20% (Matrix)
Heavy metal surfaces	-	11% (radiopacifier)
Waxes or resins	-	3% (plasticizer)

- GP is manufactured in two different shapes,

1. Standardized

- The standardized sizes co-ordinate with the ISO sizes of the root canal file.
- They are used primarily as the main core material for obturation.

2. Non standardized

- They are more tapered from the tip or point to the top.
- These are usually designated as extra fine, fine - fine, medium-fine, fine-medium, medium, medium-large, large and extra large.
- These are used as secondary and auxillary cones.
- GP may come in either pellet form or in cannulas for the injectable thermoplastic obturation techniques.
- It is available in heatable syringes for thermo mechanical techniques.

- Gutta-percha cones have become available containing an iodoform component called medicated gutta-percha, an this enhances the anti microbial properties.

Advantages

1. As it is plastic, it adapts and seals better with irregularities and contour of canal.
2. It is least toxic or inert.
3. Tissue tolerant or non allergic.
4. Radiopaque
5. It will not discolour the tooth structure.
6. It does not shrink after insertion unless it is plasticised by a solvent / heat.
7. It does not encourage bacterial growth.
8. It can be easily sterilized and easily removed from root canal when necessary.

Disadvantages

1. It lacks rigidity so difficult to place in narrow canals and canals with extreme curvature.
2. Lacks adhesive quality hence used with a sealer.
3. Can become brittle with age.
4. It can be easily displaced by pressure.

Technique to rejuvenate the aged brittle cone

- By momentary immersion in hot tap water (55°C) followed by instant cooling in cold tap water.

2. SILVER CONES

- Are usually used in fine, tortuous canals as a solid core.
- May also as a retro-grade root canal filling.

Advantages

1. Made of pure silver.
2. When extreme curvatures are present, it can be conveniently used.

Disadvantages

1. Non adaptability
2. Corrosion
3. Difficulty in removal for re-treatment and for restorative reasons.
4. Post space preparation while trying to remove a portion of silver point it may disturb the apical seal or cause lateral perforation.

MASTER CONE SELECTION

- There are 4 methods to determine the proper fit of master cone,
    1. Visual Test
    2. Tactile Test
    3. Patient response
    4. Radiograph

1. Visual test

- Grasp the measured point at a position with in 1mm short of the prepared length of the canal with cotton pliers.
- Then the point is carried into the canal until the cotton pliers touch the external reference point of the tooth.
- If the working length of the tooth is correct and the point goes completely to position, the visual test has been passed unless the point can be pushed this position.
- This can be determined by grasping 1 mm further back on the point and attempting to push it apically.

2. Tactile test

- It determines whether the point tightly fits the canal or not.
- In the event the apical 3-4 mm of the canal have been prepared with near parallel walls (in contrast to a continous taper), some degree of force should be required to seat the point and once it is in position, a pulling force should be there to dislodge it. This is known as 'TUG BACK'.
- If tugback is present tactile test is passed.

3. Patient response

- Patient's who are not anesthesitized during a treatment of non-vital pulp or at the second appointment of vital pulp may feel the GP penetrating the foramen.
- Adjustments can be made until it is completely comfortable.
- This is a good test when the position of the foramen cannot be determined accurately by radiograph or by tactile sensation.

4. Radiograph Test

- After visual and tactile test its position must be checked by the radiograph.
- The film must show the point extending to within 1 mm from the tip of the preparation.

OBTURATION TECHNIQUES FOR GUTTA-PERCHA

1. Single cone technique
2. Lateral condensation technique
3. Vertical condensation technique or warm gutta-percha technique.
4. Combination of lateral and vertical condensation techniques.
5. Inverted cone method
6. Rolled cone technique
7. Sectional method
8. Chemically plasticized gutta-percha technique.
9. Compaction (McSpadden technique)
10. Thermoplasticized injection moulded method.

1. SINGLE CONE TECHNIQUE

Indications

1. Can be used where the primary cone fits snugly in the apical third of root canal.
2. When the root canal is round with minimum taper.

Technique

- Rubberdam is placed and the contents of the canal are removed.
- Selection of cone should be done using the No. of the last instrument used to enlarge the canal.
- Cone is placed to the predetermined length.
- Radiograph is taken to check for lateral and vertical fit.
- Root canal cement should be mixed to a thick, stringy consistency and the canal is coated with an absorbent point or root canal plugger and reamer.
- GP cone is rolled in the cement and carried into the root canal, until the buttend is even with incisal or occlusal surface.
- Radiographs are taken and the buttend is cut off with a hot instrument until it is in level with the floor of pulp chamber.
- The pulp chamber is filled with temporary cement.
- Patient is recalled after 24 hour for reevaluation.

2. LATERAL CONDENSATION TECHNIQUE

Significance

– It is a preferred technique for most of the canals as most teeth present wide canals or flares that cannot be densely filled with the single cone technique.

Technique

– This is a procedure where additional auxillary cones are inserted and condensed laterally around the primary cone.

– Tapered preparation is necessary.

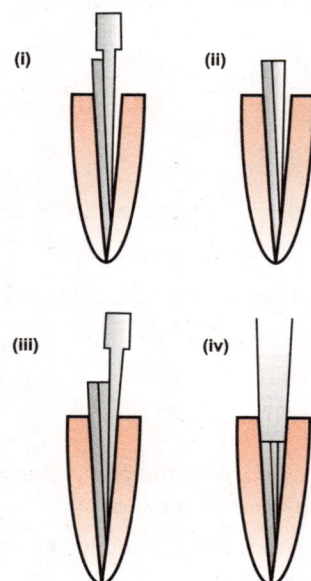

Filling the canal with gutta - percha condensed laterally against the canal wall.

Selection of master cone

– GP cone is inserted to the working length and should fit snugly and resist to removal or 'tug back'.

– A radiograph is taken to determine the apical and lateral fit of the primary cone.

– Cone is fitted in canal short of 1mm from the apex.

– Once the primary cone is accurately fitted in the root canal, it is removed to dry the canal.

– Walls are coated with thin layer of cement.

– Now the selected master cone is inserted and condensed with spreader.

– If gap is present then accessory cone is inserted and condensed.

– The process continues till the canal is filled completely.

– Cementing is not necessary for accessory canals.

– After verifying the canal by radiograph the buttend of GP in the pulp chamber is cut off with a hot instrument.

– The chamber is cleaned and temporary restoration is placed in the access cavity.

3. VERTICAL CONDENSATION OR WARM GUTTA-PERCHA TECHNIQUE

– Introduced by 'SCHILDER'.

– This technique is especially used with 'Step Back Technique'.

Indications

1. Method is specifically indicated when maximum condensation is desired.

2. They are used when reaching of conventional master cone to the apical portion of canal is impossible, as when there is ledge formation, perforation or unusual canal curvature.

3. This method can be used when other kind of treatment fail.

Advantages

1. Excellent seal of the canal apically, laterally.

2. Obturation of lateral and accessory canal.

Disadvantages

1. Complicated

2. Difficulty in length control

3. Risk of vertical root fracture

4. Overfilling of gutta-percha

Technique

– In this method, the flow property of GP to heat is utilized.

– Master cone is selected based on working length.

– The canal wall is coated with a thin layer of root canal cement.

– The selected cone is coated with cement.

– The coronal (butt) end of the cone is cut off with a hot instrument.

– A heat carrier (plugger) is heated and carried into the canal vertically and this causes the flow of gutta-percha.

– This procedure is repeated until the canal is three dimensionally filled.

– The maximum temperature is 80° C in vertical condensation and temperature at apical region is 40 - 42° C.

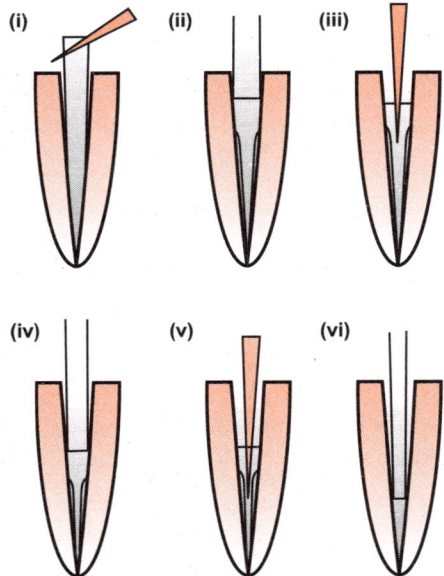

The vertical condensation technique

4. COMBINATION OF LATERAL AND VERTICAL CONDENSATIONS

Significance

– To obtain greater density and compactness.
– To force the filling material into complex configurations and ramifications of root canal system.

Technique

– Primary cone is inserted slowly and gently into the canal to the measured length.
– One or two auxillary cones inserted along with the primary cone, with or without the use of a spreader.
– A spreader is inserted apically along side the primary cone wedging it against the canal wall by applying lateral and apical pressure and creating space for additional cone.
– The spreader is removed and gutta-percha cone of corresponding size is inserted in the space just vacated by the spreader.
– The spreading process is repeated until the wedge cones block further access to the canal.
– Vertical condensation is now combined with lateral condensation.
– The spreader is heated to red hot and the butt ends of the cones are cut.
– Now the GP mass is forcibly packed apically with the preselected cold pluggers, dipped into cement powder to prevent sticking of GP.

– The whole canal is filled by the same process.
– The access cavity is filled with a temporary restoration.

5. INVERTED CONE TECHNIQUE

Significance

– Used when there is wide open apex

Technique

– GP cone is selected
– Buttend of cone is inserted first.
– Additional cones are packed around it in the usual manner.

6. ROLLED CONE TECHNIQUE

Significance

– When the root canal walls are wide and are almost parallel, rolled cones are used.

Technique

– Roll 3 to 4 GP cones and make them parallel.
– Then obturate as explained in single cone technique.

7. SECTIONAL METHOD

Significance

– This method is used when post type of crown is planned.

Advantages

1. Seals the canal apically and laterally.
2. The sealed gutta-percha is not disturbed.

Disadvantages

1. Time consuming
2. Difficult to condense the gutta-percha into a homogenous mass often resulting into voids.
3. Difficult to retrieve the section of overfilled gutta-percha.

Technique

– The selected master cone should correctly fit apically and laterally.
– The master cone is cut into sections of 3 - 4 mm of length.
– The canal is coated with cement.
– The cut master cone is inserted into the canal. The apical section is mounted on heated plugger and condensed vertically to previously measured depth.

- A radiograph is taken to check the position and fit of the condensed section.
- The next section is cut and dipped in Eucalyptol and warmed high over flame and inserted in canal and vertically condensed.
- The entire procedure is repeated until the entire canal is filled.

8. CHEMICALLY PLASTICIZED GP TECHNIQUE

- GP can be plasticized by chemical solvents, i.e.
  - Chloroform
  - Eucalyptol
  - Xylol
- These solvents make the GP more plastic and highly viscous and this can be forced into zinc, tortuous canals where other solid core fillings cannot be inserted.

Disadvantages

1. Using a chemical solvent filling material - inability to control over filling.
2. Causes periapical irritation.
3. Shrinkage of the filling material resulting in poor apical seal and lateral seal.

1. Chloropercha technique

- Not reliable technique because, excessive shrinkage of filling is seen due to evaporation of chloroform.
- This can be used in a sealer in conjunction with a well fitting cone.
- Modifications of this technique are,

  #### A. Johnson-Collahan's method
  - In this technique, canal is separately filled with 95% alcohol and dried with paper points.
  - It is then flooded with Collahan's rosin solution for 2-3 min.
  - A suitable GP cone is inserted and compressed laterally and apically with the help of pluggers and additional cones are inserted in the usual manner.

  #### B. Nygaard - Ostby method
  - Chloropercha is modified by adding a preparation made of finely-Ground GP, Canadabalsam, Colophonium, zinc oxide powder.
  - This powder is mixed with chloroform and the walls of the root canal are coated with this paste.

- The primary cone is dipped in the sealer and inserted into the root canal.
- Additional cones dipped in sealer are packed into the canal to obtain a satisfactory filling.

2. Eucapercha Method

- Eucapercha is a paste made by softening the surface of gutta-percha in warm oil of Eucalyptus.
- Eucapercha has replaced chloropercha as chloropercha is potential carcinogen.
- Apical half of primary cone is dipped in eucapercha for 1 min.
- This cone is inserted into the root canal and condensed using lateral and vertical methods.

9. THERMO MECHANICAL TECHNIQUE (COMPACTION / Mc SPADDEN TECHNIQUE)

- Introduced by Mc SPADDEN in 1978.
- This technique uses a calibrated stainless steel Mc spadden compactor.
- Method was popular for filling teeth with resorptive defects.

Mc Spadden Compactor

- This resembles a H-file with inverted blades (reverse H-files).
- Heat is created by rotating a compactor in a slow speed contra angled hand piece at 8000 - 10000 RPM along the sides of the GP Cone inside the root canal.
- Heat generated by the compactor plasticizes the GP and compacts the root canal.
- Used in straight canals only because the compactor blade breaks if it binds.

Advantages

1. Ease selection and insertion of GP
2. Rapid filling of canals.
3. Time saving

Disadvantages

1. Inability to use the technique in narrow root canals.
2. Frequent breakage of compactor blades.
3. Frequent overfilling of canal.
4. Shrinkage of the coded, set filling.

Technique

- Compactor blade is selected in according to the width and length of the prepared canal.
- Root canal is prepared following step back method. GP is inserted into canal short of root apex.

– Compactor blade is inserted between GP and the canal wall.

– The compactor blade is restricted in the canal with in 1.5mm of the root apex with the help of rubber stops.

– This prevents forcing of thermo plasticized GP through the root apex.

– The plastic GP moves laterally and apically because the reversed flutes on the compactor blade push the softened GP forward and sideways even while withdrawing the rotation of blade from the canal.

– The most important experience is the feel of the instrument backing out.

– This indicates the canal is completely filled.

10. THERMOPLASTICIZED GP INJECTION MOULDED METHOD

A. High temperature Injection Moulded Method

– The pressure apparatus contains an electrically heated syringe barrel, which is insulated and a selection of needles ranging in size from 18 - 25 guages.

– The plunger is designed to prevent backward flow of the gutta-percha.

– In this technique the canal preparation needs to be restricted apically with flaring of the body towards the access cavity.

– Thermoplasticized GP is heated to 70°C - 160°C depending on the method or material used.

– Vertical pressure is required to apply after injection of plasticized GP apically, in order to get good seal and to prevent void formation.

Advantages

1. Reduction of chair side time.

2. Produces dense homogenous obturation with minimal time.

B. Low temperature Injection Moulded Method

– In this method, low temperature, i.e. 70°C is used.

– It involves the use of a carpule containing a low temperature (70° C) GP formation.

– A special heater warms the GP sufficiently to flow under pressure, and it is discharged through a needle of suitable gauge directly into the root canal. Ex : Ultrafil.

METAL CORE OBTURATION

– It includes obturating the root canal with a silver cone, a sectioned silver cone, stainless steel (instrument blade) or amalgam.

1. SILVER CONE METHOD

Significance

– Use is restricted to teeth with fine, tortuous canals that cannot be filled properly with gutta-percha.

Technique

– Select a cone corresponding in size to the largest instrument used in the preparation of the canal.

– Sterilize the cone by alcohol flaming three times or by passing it through on open flame two or three times.

– Insert the cone in the canal using silver cone pliers or Stieglitz forceps, and press it apically.

– The cone should fit snugly and should bind at the apical foramen.

– A canal instrumented for silver cone obturation should have tapered converging walls differing in shape from a canal prepared using the step back technique.

– Take a radiograph to check the fit of the cone in the canal.

– If it protrudes beyond the apex, cut off the excess at the tip. So the final fit will terminate at 0.5 mm short of the root apex.

– If the silver cone is too short, select another that fits or reprepare the canal so the selected cone seats properly.

– Coat the canal with cement and insert the sterilized silver cone with slight pressure to the measured length.

– Take another radiograph to ensure that the filling is properly positioned.

– Laterally condense secondary gutta-percha cones around the primary silver cone.

– Wipe the walls, clean with chloroform or alcohol and fill the crown with Zinc phosphate cement.

2. SECTIONAL OR SPLIT CONE METHOD

Significance

– Designed for a tooth whose restoration may require a post and core.

Technique

- The method consists of fitting the cone snugly as described earlier.

- The cone is notched approx. 6mm from the apical tip it is sterilized and it is cemented in the root canal.

- The wedged cemented cone is rotated until it breaks at the notch, and the free end is removed to leave enough space for preparation of a post.

3. STAINLESS STEEL METHOD

Significance

- Can be used to fill fine, tortuous canals.

Technique

- Because steel files are much more rigid than silver cones, they can be inserted into a canal with greater case.

- Once the file has been cemented, its handle must be cut off with a high speed bur, 3 or 4 mm below the occlusal surface to allow space for a restoration.

REMOVAL OF ROOT CANAL FILLINGS

1. GUTTA-PERCHA

Objective

- To remove it without forcing the filling material into the periapical tissue.

Technique

- Remove the GP from the chamber by searing it with a heated excavator, or grind it out with a slowly resolving round bur.

- Flood the pulp chamber with chloroform or xylol to soften the GP

- Insert a No. 25 or 30 reamer or file into the canal along side the GP and remove the softened filling piece by piece.

- Repeat the process of softening the filling and instrumenting pieces out of the canal until all the GP has been removed.

- If an instrument binds excessively withdraw it carefully to avoid breakage, deposit another few drops of solvent to soften the GP and continue the procedure.

- As the apex is approached, insert and rotate a heated instrument so its tip is embedded in the remaining GP Allow it to cool and withdraw the remaining filling from the canal.

- A radiograph is taken to determine whether the GP has been completely removed from the canal.

2. SILVER CONES

- A silver cone is not removed as easily as a GP filling unless the butt end extends into the pulp chamber.

- In such cases chloroform or xylol is used to soften the cement and GP surrounding the butt end of the silver cone.

- An explorer tip can be used to free the silver cone of GP and cement around the canal orifice.

- First, flood the pulp chamber with chloroform to dissolve the cement.

- Grasp the projecting section of silver cone with a pair of narrow beak pliers (Stieglitz) and remove it from the canal.

- Be careful not to severe the butt end of the silver cone during this procedure.

- When the silver cone is completely in the root canal an end cutting bur or masserann instrument can be rotated along side the cone, channel the dentin around the cone so it can be grasped or elevated out of the canal.

3. PASTES

- Pastes are soluble in chloroform or xylol.
- The use of file facilitates the removal of the paste.

MISCELLANEOUS

OBTURA - II

- A second generation high temperature system capable of taking the temperature of gutta-percha in the heating chamber to 200°C.

- It consists of a delivery unit with an electrical cord connected to a temperature control box with a digital display.

- The gutta-percha is loaded into the heating chamber when the trigger of the delivery unit is squeezed, the softened gutta-percha is extruded through a 20 or 23 gauge.

Advantages

1. Well adaptation to the prepared canal.
2. Used for back filling canals after establishing an apical plug.
3. Used for filling large and irregular canals.

THERMAFIL

- It is a patented endodontic obturator consisting of a flexible central carrier, sized and tapered to match variable tapered files.
- The central carrier is uniformly coated with a layer of a refined and tested a- phased gutta-percha.

Advantages

- Significantly less strained during delivery and compaction.
- Easy flowing of GP into canal irregularities.
- Allows simple, fast, predictable filling of Root Canal.
- Especially used for small or very curved canals.

Disadvantages

- No apical stop or definitive apical constriction to prevent the GP extension beyond the Root Canal.

UNDER FILLING OF ROOT CANAL

Causes

- Natural barrier in the canal.
- A ledge created during preparation.
- Insufficient flaring.
- Poorly adapted master cone.
- Inadequate condensation pressure.

Treatment

- Removal and retreatment is preferred.

OVER FILLING OF ROOT CANAL

Causes

- Sequela of overinstrumentation through the apical foramen.
- Uncontrolled condensation forces extrude materials.
- Other causes are inflammatory resorption and incomplete development of the root.
- Extruded obturation material causes issue damage and inflammation.

Treatment

- Apical surgery may be required to remove the material from apical tissues and place a retrograde material.

CHAPTER 21

RESTORATION OF THE ENDODONTICALLY TREATED TEETH

- Restorations for endodontically treated teeth are designed to protect the remaining tooth structure from fracture and to replace the missing tooth structure.
- The final restoration includes the combination of 1. Dowel 2. Core and 3. Coronal restoration.
- Not every endodontically treated tooth needs a crown or a dowel ; some need all three components and some need only an access seal for the coronal restoration.
- The final configuration of the restored tooth includes the following,
  1. Residual tooth structure and its periodontal attachment apparatus.
  2. Dowel material
  3. Core material
  4. Definitive coronal restoration

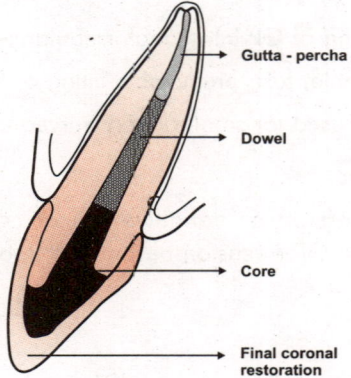

1. DOWEL (POST)

- *The Dowel is a post or other relatively rigid, restorative material placed in the root of a non vital tooth.*
- *Provides retention for the core and coronal restorations and must be designed to minimize the potential for root fracture from functional forces.*

Ideal Properties

- Dowels should provide,
1. Maximum protection of the root.
2. Adequate retention with in the root.
3. Maximum retention of the core and crown.
4. Maximum protection of the crown margin cement seal.
5. Pleasing esthetics if indicated.
6. High radiographic visibility.
7. Retrievability
8. Biocompatibility

Materials

– Include alloys of gold, stainless steel, titanium and dental amalgam.

Classification

– Based on the type of fabrication,

1. **Custom cast posts**
   1. Tapered smooth
   2. Parallel Serrated

2. **Prefabricated posts**

– Prefabricated root canal posts are classified into three main types according to the general shape of their root portion,

   i. *Parallel-sided*

   – Cylindrical in shape with rounded corners.

   – Has same diameter from one end to another.

   ii. *Taper type*

   – The sides are tapered from one end to other.

   iii. *Parallel tapered type*

   – A combination type, with the occlusal one half to two-thirds being parallel sided and the apical portion being tapered.

– Prefabricated posts are also classified according to the surface texture,

   i. *Smooth surface posts*

   – Used in a cemented technique procedure.

   – The post channel is larger in diameter than the post.

   ii. *Serrated surface posts*

   – Used in cemented technique procedure.

   iii. *Threaded Surface posts*

   – Used with a screw in procedure.

   – Post channel is slightly narrower in diameter than the post.

2. CORE

– *The core is a restorative material placed in the coronal area of a tooth which replaces carious, fractured or missing coronal structure and retains the final crown.*

– The core is anchored to the tooth by extending into the coronal portion of the root canal or through the endodontic dowel.

– The attachment between tooth, dowel, and core are mechanical or both, because of the core and dowel are usually fabricated of different materials.

Ideal Properties

– The core materials should have,
   1. High compressive strength.
   2. Dimensional stability.
   3. Ease of manipulation.
   4. Short setting time (for cement).
   5. An ability to bond to both tooth and dowel.

CORE MATERIALS

– *Include cast metal or ceramic, amalgam, composite resin and glass ionomer resin (sometimes).*

A. **Cast Core**

   – A cast metal dowel and core is a traditional way to restore endodontically treated teeth.

   – The core is an integral extension of the dowel and the cast core does not depend on mechanical means for retention to the dowel.

   – This type of construction avoids dislodgment of the core and crown from the dowel and root when minimal tooth structure remains.

   Advantages
   1. Non corrosive final restoration.
   2. Increased stiffness.
   3. Decreased dentin deformation.

   Disadvantages
   1. High rate of root fracture
   2. Not economic
   3. Technique sensitive fabrication
   4. Require two appointments

B. **Amalgam Core**

   – Has high rate of clinical success.

   Advantages
   1. High Strength
   2. Improved marginal seal
   3. Easy manipulation
   4. Rapid setting time

   Disadvantages
   1. Potential for corrosion
   2. Discoloration of the gingiva and dentin
   3. Not eco friendly

C. **Composite Resin Core**

   – To get optimum composite resin core function,
   1. There should be more than 2mm of sound tooth structure should remain at the margin.

2. The composite resin core and the bonding agent must be compatible.

Advantages

1. Ease of manipulation
2. Very rapid set
3. High compressive strength

Disadvantages

1. Polymerization shrinkage
2. Micro leakage

D. **Glass Ionomer Core**

Advantages

1. Good adhesion
2. Anti cariogenic property

Disadvantages

1. Limited to small restorations
2. Brittle
3. Low retention
4. High solubility

– Glass ionomer core is indicated in posterior teeth in which,

1. A bulk of core material is possible.
2. Significant sound dentin remains.
3. Additional retention is available with pins or dentin preparations.
4. Moisture control is assured.
5. Caries control is indicated

E. **Resin - modified glass ionomer Core**

– It is a combination of glass ionomer and composite resin technologies. They exhibit properties of both materials.

– They exhibit minimal microleakage.

3. CORONAL RESTORATION

– This is the final component of the endodontic reconstruction.

Significance

1. Re establishes function.
2. Restores esthetics.
3. Isolation of the dentin and endodontic fill materials from microleakage.
4. Distributes functional forces

– The coronal restoration for endodontically treated intact anterior teeth consists of sealing the lingual access cavity. Posterior teeth need coronal coverage to protect against fracture from occlusal forces, regardless of the amount of remaining tooth structure.

– The final coronal restoration provides added security to the tooth by consolidating the remaining cusps and prepared tooth structure and by creating a ferrule effect.

FERRULE

– It is a metal band that encircles the external dimension of the residual tooth, similar to the metal bands around a barrel or a shovel handle.

– It is formed by the walls of the crown or cast telescopic coping encasing the gingival 1 to 2 mm of the axial walls of the preparation above the crown margin.

Significance

1. Increases the fracture resistance of the tooth.
2. Increases the retention and resistance of the restoration.

Requirements of a Ferrule

1. Should have a minimum of 1 to 2mm dentin axial wall height.
2. Should have parallel axial walls.
3. Must totally encircle the tooth.
4. Must be on the sound tooth structure.
5. Must not invade the attachment apparatus of the tooth.

PRE-FABRICATED POST AND CORE SYSTEM

Advantages

1. Relatively simple to use.
2. Can be completed in single appointment.
3. Less time consuming
4. Easy to temporize
5. Cost effective
6. Strong

Disadvantages

1. Root is designed to accept the post rather than the post being designed to fit the root.
2. Chemical reactions may occur when the post and core materials are made of dissimilar metals.
3. Cannot be used if the considerable coronal tooth structure is lost.

CAST POST SYSTEMS

Advantages

1. Custom fit to the root configuration.

2. Can be adaptable to large, irregularly shaped canals and orifices.

3. Strong.

4. Adapted to be used with wrought posts and prefabricated plastic patterns.

Disadvantages

1. Expensive

2. Require two appointments

3. Less retentive

4. Difficult to temporization

5. Possible corrosion

6. Risk of casting inaccuracies

7. Require the removal of additional coronal tooth structure.

CHAPTER 22

ENDODONTIC PROCEDURAL MISHAPS

– Are those unfortunate occurrence that happen during the treatment, some owing to inattention to detail, others totally unpredictable.

CLASSIFICATION

I. Access related

1. Treating the wrong tooth
2. Missed canals
3. Damage to existing restoration
4. Access cavity perforations
5. Crown fractures

II. Instrumentation related

1. Ledge formation
2. Perforations,
   - i. Cervical canal perforations
   - ii. Mid root perforations
   - iii. Apical perforations
3. Separated instruments and foreign objects
4. Canal blockage

III. Obturation related

1. Over - or under extended root canal fillings
2. Nerve paresthesia
3. Vertical root fractures

IV. Miscellaneous

1. Post space perforation
2. Irrigant related
3. Tissue emphysema
4. Instrument aspiration and ingestion

– All the above mentioned are not discussed in detail, only the following are discussed in detail.

1. LEDGE FORMATION

– Ledges in canals can result from a failure to make access cavities that allow direct access to the apical part of the canals or from using straight or too - large instruments in curved canals.

Recognition

– Suspected when the root canal instrument can no longer be inserted into the canal to full working length.

– There is a loss of normal tactile sensation of the tip of the instrument binding in the canal.

Treatment

- Locate the position of the ledge by inserting an instrument until it is blocked and verify the depth of insertion by taking a radiograph.
- Irrigate the canal with sodium hypochlorite solution.
- Use a small file, No.10 or 15 with a distinct curve at the tip to explore the canal to the apex, in vaiven or watch winding motion.
- When the ledge is reached, the file is slightly retracted, rotated and advanced again until it by-passes the ledge.
- Once the ledge is bypassed, do not remove the instrument instead, do circumferential instrumentation of the canal before withdrawal of the instrument.
- Repeat this with larger instruments until the ledge is filed away.

Prevention

- Accurate interpretation of diagnostic radiographs before the placing of first instrument.
- Awareness to canal morphology.
- Using of pre-curving instruments.
- Using of instruments with non cutting tips.

2. PERFORATION

- They are classified into four types according to the location,
  1. Access cavity perforations
  2. Radicular Perforations
     i. Cervical
     ii. Mid - root
     iii. Apical root

1. Access cavity perforations

- In the process of searching for canal orifices, perforations of the crown occur, either, peripherally through the sides of the crown or through the floor of the chamber into the furcation.

Recognition

- *Perforation above the periodontal attachment:* The first sign is the presence of leakage either saliva into the cavity or sodium hypochlorite out into the mouth.
- *Perforation into the periodontal attachment:* First sign is bleeding into the access cavity. It is confirmed by placing a small file through the opening and taking a radiograph.

Treatment

- *Perforations above the alveolar crest :* corrected intra coronally (with out need for surgical intervention) by placing the cavit.
- *Perforations into the periodontal ligament :* Should be corrected immediately as soon as possible to minimize the injury to supporting tissues. The material used for repair should provide a good seal and should not cause further tissue damage.
- Several materials are used for the repair. Ex: Cavit, Amalgam, Calcium hydroxide, Mineral Trioxide Aggregate (MTA), GIC, etc.
- Prior to repair, bleeding should be controlled to visualize the perforation and to allow the placement of the repair material.
- It is done by irrigating with sterile water or an esthetic solution and packing a moist, sterile cotton pellet and holding it under pressure for 2 to 3 min.
- Calcium hydroxide is placed in the area of perforation and left for atleast a few days will have the area dry and allow inspection of preforation.

Prevention

- Thorough examination of diagnostic radiographs.
- Checking the long axis of the tooth and aligning the long axis of the access bur with the long axis of the tooth can prevent the perforation of a tipped tooth.
- Prevention is best accomplished by adhering to the principles of access cavity preparation.

2. Cervical canal perforations

- They are mostly occurred during the process of locating and widening the canal orifice or inappropriate use of Gates - Glidden burs.

Recognition

- By sudden appearance of blood from the periodontal ligament space.
- It is best confirmed by placing a small file into the area and taking a radiograph.

Treatment

- It includes both internal and external repair.
- A small area of perforation is sealed from inside the tooth.
- *Large perforations :* First seal from inside, then the external aspect of the tooth is opened surgically and repair the damaged tooth structure.
- Most widely used material is MTA.

3. Midroot perforations

- Occur mostly in curved canals, either as a result of perforating when a ledge has formed during initial instrumentation or along the inside curvature of the root as the canal is straightened out.

- *Stripping is a lateral perforation caused by over instrumentation through a thin wall in the root and is most likely to occur on the inside, or concave, wall of a curved canal, such as the distal wall of the mesial roots in mandibular first molars.*

- Stripping results in a fairly long perforation that severely affects the outcome of treatment.

Recognition

- Detected by the sudden appearance of hemorrhage in a previously dry canal or by a sudden complaint by the patient.

- A paper point placed in the canal can confirm the presence and location of the perforation.

Treatment

- It is repaired by both non surgical and surgical methods.

- A two - step method is used for this purpose, in this, the root canals are first obturated and then the defect is repaired surgically.

- The materials used for repair are MTA, calcium hydroxide, etc.

4. Apical root perforations

- They may be the result of the file not negotiating a curved canal or not establishing accurate working length and instrumenting beyond the apical confines.

- Perforation of a curved root is the result of ledging, apical transportation or apical zipping.

- *Transportation is the removal of canal wall structure on the outside curve in the apical half of the canal due to the tendency of files to restore themselves to their original linear shape during canal preparation.*

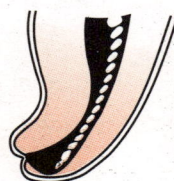

- *Apical zip is an elliptical shape that may be formed in the apical foramen during preparation of a curved canal when a file extends through the apical foramen and subsequently transports that outer wall.*

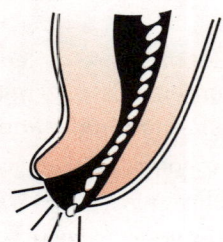

- Most common sites of Apical perforations are *maxillary lateral incisor, mesiobuccal and palatal roots of maxillary molars and the mesial root of mandibular molars.*

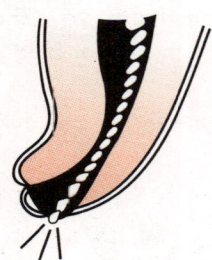

Recognition

- Suspected if the patient suddenly complains of pain during treatment, if the canal becomes flooded with hemorrhage, or if the tacticle resistance of the confines of the canal space is lost.

- If any of these occur confirmation is done by radiographically.

Treatment

- If the perforation is caused by over instrumentation, corrective treatment includes re-establishing tooth length short of the original length and then enlarging the canal, with larger instruments to that length.

- When a periapical area of rarefaction is present, a periradicular surgical procedure should be considered as an alternative.

- One can consider perforation site as the new apical opening, and obturation of the both of the foramina and main body of the canal can be done by vertical compaction technique with heat softened gutta percha.

3. SEPARATED INSTRUMENTS AND FOREIGN OBJECTS

- Most commonly, files and reamers are involved in these types of procedural mishaps.

- The causes are improper removal of binded instrument and using of a stressed instrument.

Treatment

- Ultrasonic fine instruments have proven most effective in loosing and flushing out broken fragments. Using micro scopy and special fine diamond tips, a tunnel can be created around the separated instruments which can then be vibrated and dislodged.

- Failing that, one of the following steps may be taken,

1. Fractured segment of an instrument can sometimes be removed by bypassing the segment with a hedstroem file engaging the segment and filling it out.

2. If the segment can not be removed, one should attempt to bypass it, clean and shape the root canal, and incorporate the segment into the obturation.

3. If the instrument segment is in the apical area, the root canal should be cleaned and shaped to the instrument segment, it should be obturated, and an apicoectomy should be considered.

HYPOCHLORITE ACCIDENT

Definition

- Hypochlorite accident refers to any event where sodium hypochlorite is expressed beyond the apex of a tooth and the patient immediately manifest some combination of the following symptoms.

1. Severe pain, even in areas that were previously anesthetized for dental treatment.

2. Swelling.

3. Profuse bleeding, both interstitially and through the tooth.

Causes

- Forceful injection of the irrigating solution.

- An irrigating needle wedged into a root canal.

- Irrigating a tooth with a large apical foramen.

- Apical resorption or an immature apex.

Management

- Assure and calm the patient.

- Nitrous oxide sedation can also be helpful.

- Immediate problem of pain and swelling can be relieved by regional block with a long acting anaesthetic solution.

- The tooth is monitored for next 30 minutes as a bloody exudate may discharge back into the canal.

- If drainage is persistent, then the tooth is kept open for the next 24 hours.

- To encourage further drainage from the periapical tissues, the fluid should be removed with high-volume evacuation.

- Antibiotics, i.e. Penicillin 500 mg 5 times a day, over the next 7 days are prescribed.

- NSAIDS.

- Steroids can also be prescribed as it will help minimize the ensuing inflammatory process.

- For the first 6 hours, the patient should use a cold compression followed by warm compression.

Prevention

- The irrigating needle should be bent at the center.

- Needle should never be placed deeply into the canal.

- Needle should be oscillated in and out of the canal to ensure that the tip is free to irrigate without resistance.

- Irrigation should be stopped of the needle jams.

- The hub of the needle should be checked for a tight fit to prevent any accidents.

- Irrigant should be expressed gently and slowly.

CHAPTER 23

FAILURES OF ENDODONTIC TREATMENT

- The causes for failure for endodontic treatment are classified into,

1. *Preoperative causes*
2. *Operative causes*
3. *Post operative causes.*

I. PREOPERATIVE CAUSES

1. Misdiagnosis

- It means, the endodontic treatment was initiated without identification of the true origin of the pathology.

- Consequently the pathology remains untreated and symptoms continue.

- Incorrect diagnosis usually results from a misinterpretation or lack of information either clinical or radiographic.

2. Poor case selection

- The purpose of case selection is to determine the feasibility and practicality of treatment so as to avoid treating cases that will fail regardless of the quality of treatment.

- Failures caused by poor case selection are of two types, i.e. *predictable and unpredictable.*

- **Predictable failures** result from misjudgment of the feasibility and practicality of the treatment, i.e. evaluation of the patients cooperation and of the technical difficulties in the course of treatment.

- **Unpredictable failures** are caused by conditions that are not considered to be contraindications to therapy which yet deteriorate during or following therapy, so as to cause failure i.e secondary periodontal involvement occlusal trauma or transformation of the periapical lesion to an apical cyst.

II. OPERATIVE CAUSES

- These are major cause of endodontic treatment failure,

1. Failure to obtain mechanical objectives

- Mechanical objectives are related to endodontic cavity preparation (i.e access cavity and canal shaping).

- Under extended access cavity may lead to overlooking of a canal and retention of tissue in the pulp chamber.

- Over extended access cavity results in excessive reduction of dentin which weakens the teeth and fracture may occur.

– Extreme deviation from the original canal shape or over zealous flaring of curved canals may result in perforation.

2. **Failure to attain biologic objectives**

– Biologic objectives include removal of all potential irritants from the root canal space and the control of infection and periapical inflammation.

– Remnants of pulpal debris may irritate the periapical tissues and jeopardize periapical repair.

– Periapical inflammation can be caused by over instrumentation and overextended canal filling.

III. POST OPERATIVE CAUSES

– They are trauma and fracture, superimposed non endodontic involvement, poorly designed final restoration or lack of any restoration.

– Endodontic failure can result from a non endodontic origin regardless of adequate endodontic therapy, i.e. deleterious effects from orthodontic treatment and periodontal disease.

INSTRUMENTS FOR RETRIEVING BROKEN INSTRUMENTS AND POSTS

1. Forceps

– Fine - beaked haemostats or steiglitz forceps can be used to remove a broken instrument.

– This is possible only when the end of the fractured instrument is accessible and not jammed firmly within the canal.

2. Masserann Kit

– Most comprehensive device for the removal of obstructing objects from root canals such as files, silver points or broken posts.

– It consists of an extractor into which the object to be retrieved is locked.

– An assortment of end cutting trepan burs are used in anticlockwise rotation, to provide access for the extractor.

– Frequent radiographic monitoring is mandatory and ample convenience or must be established so that the desired direction can be maintained toward the target object.

Disadvantages

1. Technique involves considerable sacrifice of radicular dentin thus making the tooth more susceptible to fracture.

2. More successful in anterior teeth than posterior teeth.

3. Can be used safely only in the coronal portions of large, straight roots.

4. Time consuming.

5. Inferior to ultrasonic technique.

3. Cancellier kit

– When the fractured file is loose but not free, a cancellier extractor may be used.

– The extractors are a set of hollow tubes, which fit into a handle; the assembly resembles a hollow plugger.

– The appropriately sized extractor is chosen to fit over the file.

– A drop of cyanoacrylate glue is placed into the hollow end of the extractor so that is adheres when fitted over the file.

– The extractors can be cleaned with a solvent like xylol and reused.

4. Post removal devices

– Many techniques have been devised to remove cemented posts.

– These include the use of ultrasound to disrupt the cement lute and loosen the post or simple drilling with burs.

– The examples for post removal devices are the post puller, Eggler post remover, Gonon post removal system.

– The principle is akin to a corkscrew in which opposing forces are created to extract the post from the root canal.

CHAPTER 24

SINGLE-VISIT ENDODONTICS

ADVANTAGES

1. Immediate familiarity with the internal anatomy facilities obturation.
2. No risk of bacterial leakage beyond the temporary coronal seal between the appointments.
3. Reduction of clinic time.
4. No additional appointments.
5. Economic.

DISADVANTAGES

1. Difficult apical access in flared-up canals.
2. Fatigue to the dentist with extended operating time.
3. Patient fatigue with extended chair side time.
4. No opportunity to place an intracanal disinfectant.

OLIET'S CRITERIA FOR CASE SELECTION

1. Positive patient acceptance.
2. Sufficient available time to complete the procedure properly.
3. Absence of acute symptoms requiring drainage via the canal and of persistent continuous flow of exudate or blood.
4. Absence of anatomical obstacles (calcified canals, fine tortuous canals, bifurcated or accessory canals) and procedural difficulties (ledge formation, blockage, perforations, inadequate fills).

INDICATIONS

1. Uncomplicated vital teeth.
2. Fractured anterior or bicuspid teeth where esthetics is a concern and temporary post and crown are required.
3. Patients who are physically unable to return for the completion.
4. Patients with heart valve damage or prosthetic implants who require repeated regimens of prophylactic antibiotics.
5. Necrotic, uncomplicated teeth with sinus draining tracts.
6. Patients who require sedation.

CONTRAINDICATIONS

1. Painful, necrotic tooth with no sinus tract for drainage.
2. Teeth with severe anatomic anomalies.
3. Asymptomatic non vital molars with periodical radiolucencies and no sirus tract.
4. Patients with acute apical periodontitis.
5. Most retreatments.

CHAPTER 25

ENDODONTIC EMERGENCIES

1. ACUTE REVERSIBLE PULPITIS (HYPEREMIA)

– Can be treated successfully by palliative procedures.

– The diagnosis and origin of the condition can be confirmed by visual, tactile, thermal and radiographic examination of the isolated tooth.

Treatment

– Premature contact point if any, in a recent restoration; recontouring this high spot will relieve the pain and will allow the pulp to recuperate.

a. If persistent painful episodes occur following cavity preparation, chemical cleansing of the cavity or leakage of the restoration, one should remove the restoration and replace it with a sedative cement such as Zinc oxide Eugenol cement.

b. The same method can be used if recurrent decay occurs under old restorations which has not caused pulp exposure.

– Following a palliative treatment such as the application of a ZOE cement as a temporary sedative fitting. The paid should disappear within several days.

– If it persists or worsen, then the pulp should be extripated.

– *The best treatment is prevention:* One should place a pulp protective base under all restorations, avoid marginal leakage, reduce occlusal trauma if present, properly contour all restorations and avoid injuring the pulp with excessive heat while preparing or polishing a metallic restoration.

2. ACUTE IRREVERSIBLE PULPITIS

– The preferable emergency treatment for both types of irreversible pulpitis is Pulpectomy.

– Teeth affected by either acute reversible pulpitis or irreversible pulpitis are abnormally responsive to cold and have many similar symptoms.

– It is therefore essential that they be distinguished from one another because the emergency procedure is different.

– If a patient describes of pain that lasts for minutes to hours or is spontaneous, or disturb sleep or occurs when bending over, most likely that patient will require pulpectomy of the affected tooth rather than palliative therapy for relief of the painful symptoms.

– On some occasions when pulpectomy cannot be complete, then emergency pulpectomy including debridement, drying and sealing of a medicated dressing in the pulp chamber usually sufficient.

– Although, this is not an effective method, it relieves the patient from pain for several days.

– The patient should be rescheduled as soon as possible for additional treatment.

3. ACUTE ALVEOLAR ABSCESS

– Place the rubber dam over the infected tooth.

– Complete the access opening painlessly by bracing the tooth with finger pressure.

– Irrigate profusely, debride the pulp chamber but avoid forcing any solution or debris into the periapical tissue.

– Using a No:10 or No:15 file or reamer as an explorer, locate the root canal within 1 mm of the root apex.

– Continue to debride and to irrigate while enlarging each root canal, but keep all instruments and irrigants within the root canals.

– Frequently, a purulent exudate escapes into the chamber and indicates that the root canal is patent and draining relief follows quickly. If no evidence of drainage appears, leave the tooth open in root canals patent and expect relief with in a short time.

– Advise the patient to use hot saline rinses for 3 min each hour.

– Prescribe analgesics and antibiotics if indicated and necessary.

– In *Mild Cases* of Acute Alveolar Abscess, the tooth may be sealed with an antiseptic, obtundent medicament after biomechanical preparation of the chamber and root canals.

– Leaving the tooth open for drainage, reduces the possibility of continued pain and swelling.

– The *open drainage technique* is preferable in which the prepared root canals are sealed followed by incision of the soft tissue and artificial fistulation by the bone to establish drainage.

– Open root canals permit drainage and frequently eliminate the need for a surgical incision as well as the routine administration of oral antibiotics and analgesics.

– The pain of acutely abscessed tooth, whether of periapical or periodontal origin is frequently accompanied by swelling.

– If the *swelling is slight* and is localized it will disappear, 24- 48 hrs after drainage has been established.

– Routinely, hot saline rinses should be prescribed to assist drainage.

– If the *swelling is extensive*, soft and fluctuant, an incision through the soft tissue to the bone may be necessary.

– One should first dry the mucosa over the affected area, then spray the tissues with a refrigerant topical anesthetic such as ethyl chloride.

– The intraoral incision is made through the soft fluctuant swelling to the cortical bone plate.

– A rubber dam or gauze drain may be inserted for several days.

– If the *swelling is hard* it can be converted to a soft fluctuant state by rinsing with hot saline solution 3 - 5 min at a time, repeated every hour.

– Antibiotics and analgesics can be prescribed as needed.

– Finally the tooth should be disoccluded slightly of it is extruded from its socket. This procedure eliminates pain caused by contact with teeth in the opposing area.

4. ACUTE PERIODONTAL ABSCESS

– It causes pain and swelling.

– It can occur with either vital or necrotic pulp, its origin is usually an exacerbation of infection with pus formation in an existing deep infrabony pocket.

i. *If the pulp is vital within the normal range*

– Treatment consists of curettage, debridement and establishment of drainage of the infrabony pocket through the sucullar crevice.

ii. *If the pulp is affected*

– It must be extripated as well.

iii. *If the pulp is abnormal and vital*

– Tooth should be treated as if for acute irrereversible pulpitis.

iv. *If the pulp is necrotic*

– The tooth should be treated as if for acute alveolar abscess.

– In any of these case, emergency periodontal treatment must be done simultaneously; otherwise, the patient will not be relieved of the pain and swelling.

5. EMERGENCIES DURING TREATMENT
Causes

– They are usually caused by instrumentation beyond the root apex, with resultant trauma to the periapical tissues or when debris and microorganisms are forced through the apical foramen into the periapical tissue and cause an infectious reaction.

— Other causes may be chemical irritants such as irrigating solutions or intracanal medicaments, penetrating the periapical tissue, incomplete or inadequate debridement of all root canals, lost or depressed access cavity seals, with resulting recontamination of root canals or overfilled root canals with subsequent periapical inflammation.

Treatment

— These emergencies can be avoided of instruments, cements, and filling materials are confined to the root canal themselves and teeth under treatment are properly sealed between visits are recontoured to prevent trauma.

— When severe periodontitis is present the patient's pain can be relieved by reopening the tooth under rubber dam isolation. Removing the sealed medicament. Carefully dry the root canals by wiping with sterile absorbent points. Reseal the root canal with a cotton pellet from which a mild obtundent such as eugenol or cresatin has been expressed. Occlusion should be adjusted if necessary. If pain or swelling occurs, the sealed medicament should be removed and the tooth opened for drainage. Analgesics should be prescribed. If indicated antibiotics may be prescribed as well. Incision and drainage of a soft, fluctuant swelling should be considered when drainage is insufficient or when severe pain persists.

— When the root canals have already been filled and discomfort is present, the occlusion should be checked and the completed treatment and root canal fillings re-evaluated.

— When relieving the occlusion has not had the desired effect after a week or so, a prescription for a corticosteroid and antibiotic may be given to the patient such as Dexamethasone (0.50 mg) and Erythromycin (250 mg) each taken 4 times a day for 4 to 5 days.

— A corticosteroid should not be prescribed for patient with hypertension, gastric or duodenum ulcers or diabetes.

— At times the root canal filling must be removed to relieve the pain and to establish drainage.

— In such cases, treatment should be as for an acute alveolar abscess.

— When a post crown restoration cannot be removed and an acute abscess is present, an incision and drainage should be considered if the swelling is soft and fluctuant and an antibiotic should be prescribed.

— If the swelling is hard, hot mouth rinses should be recommended and an antibiotic should be prescribed to control the infection.

— In some cases, if relief is not obtained, trephination of the bone over the root apex may be necessary.

6. CROWN FRACTURE

— A traumatic injury to a tooth can cause a cracked crown, a fractured crown, or a fractured root and may result in pain.

— When a visible crack is found, lateral pressure, either digital or from the handle of an operative instrument is applied along the cusp on the occlusal surface.

— If the crown segment shears off and of the pulp is not exposed, the pain will usually disappear.

— The emergency treatment is completed by covering the exposed dentin with a sedative dressing and cementing a stain steel band in place.

— If the pulp is exposed, a band should be cemented in place and a pulpectomy should be performed.

— If a greenstick fracture of the crown is present and the crown segment does not shear off under pressure one should cement a stainless steel band around the tooth.

— Adjust a provisional restoration to eliminate any occlusal trauma to the tooth.

— This procedures should eliminate the pain and should allow the dentist time to reevaluate the status of the tooth at a later date.

7. FRACTURED ROOT

— A fractured root is an endodontic emergency if the tooth is painful and especially if the incisal segment is mobile.

A. Emergency treatment for a horizontally fractured root

— Consists of stabilizing by ligation of the tooth and adjacent teeth if mobility is present.

— Treat any soft tissue lacerations.

i. When a fractured root with a necrotic pulp requires emergency care, treatment consists of ligation for stabilization and root canal therapy.

- If pain and swelling are present, the root canals may be left open for drainage.

- If the tooth is not strategic or restorable, it should be extracted as soon as possible.

ii. A horizontal fracture at the midroot level with or below the crest of alveolar bone has a guarded to poor prognosis unless it is amenable to orthodontic root extrusion.

- Usually the extra alveolar segment i.e incisal segment is mobile and requires extraction.

- When the remaining apical root segment is long enough to retain a functional post-core crown, and has sufficient bony support, the emergency treatment for this segment is pulpectomy.

- If the pulp is necrotic and the tooth causes moderate to severe pain or swelling, then the root should be treated as if for an acute alveolar abscess.

B. Treatment for a vertical or longitudinal fracture of the root

- Has hopeless prognosis.

- Usual emergency treatment is extraction.

- On occasion, a multirooted tooth with a vertical fracture of a root can be hemisected and the fractured root can be removed.

- Then the emergency treatment is removal of the fractured segment and pulpectomy of the retained segment of the tooth.

8. TOOTH AVULSION

- Refer the chapter DENTAL INJURIES AND MANAGEMENT.

CHAPTER 26

PAEDIATRIC ENDODONTICS

PULPOTOMY

Definition

- It is defined as complete removal of cornal portion of dental pulp followed by a placement of suitable dressing or medicament that will promote healing and preserve vitality of tooth.

Indications

1. Vital tooth with healthy periodontium.
2. A restorable tooth.
3. Absence of spontaneous pain.
4. Atleast 2/3 of root length should be present.
5. During pulpotomy procedure hemorrhage at amputation site should be pale red and easily controllable.

Contra Indications

1. Spontaneous pain (especially at night)
2. Swelling
3. Presence of fistula
4. Tender on percussion
5. Pathologic mobility
6. External root resorption
7. Internal root resorption
8. Periapical or inter radicular radiolucency
9. Profuse hemorrhage from amputated radicular stumps
10. Pus or exudate at exposure site
11. Presence of pulp calcifications

Material used

1. Formocresal
2. Glutaraldehyde

1. Formocresol

Buckley's formula

- *Formaldehyde 19% :* This binds with cellular proteins and helps in fixation of tissues.
- *Tricresol 35% :* Increase solubility and permeability of cell wall membrane.
- *Glycerine (25%) + water (21%) :* It acts as emulsifier and prevents conversion of formaldehyde into paraformaldehyde.

2. Glutaraldehyde (Introduced by Kopel)

- This is dialdehyde compound. It has super fixative properties, Self limiting penetration, low toxicity.

Procedure

- Radiographic interpretation.
- Administration of Local anaesthesia.
- Rubber dam application.
- Initial penetration with round bur followed by use of 169 L bur to remove roof of pulp chamber.
- Following removal of roof, coronal pulp contents are removed using long shank spoon excavators.
- The walls of coronal pulp chamber are defined.
- Following removal of coronal pulp contents the root orifices become evident (amputation site).
- The hemorrhage from pulp stumps is controlled using pressure condensation or with help of adrenalin soaked pallets.
- Cotton pellet is impregnated with formocresol.
- The pellet is placed over amputation site. The recommended time being 5 min while recent studies advocate 1 min application of same.
- A mix of formocresolised zinc oxide eugenol is lightly condensed over amputation site followed by a hard setting cement (zinc poly carboxylate) followed by silver amalgam restoration.
- As this is a pulp treated tooth a stainless steel crown is recommended.

CVEK type Pulpotomy / Shallow pulpotomy

- Administration of local anesthesia and rubberdam isolation.
- With a spoon excavator remove granulation tissue from the exposure site.
- Remove pulp tissue from the pulp proper to a depth of 1 to 2 mm with a water cooled, round diamond stone.
- Visualize the removal, layer by layer.
- Irrigate with a coolant water spray.
- After preparing the pulp tissue, bleeding is controlled by placing a cotton pellet moistened with saline.
- Wash the wound with saline.
- Apply the calcium hydroxide over the wound and cover all exposed adjacent dentin.
- An intermediate base of hard setting zinc phosphate cement or glass ionomer cement is placed.
- Restoration with composite resin.

Mineral Trioxide Aggregate (MTA)

- This is an alternative to calcium hydroxide.

- The technique for managing a traumatic pulp exposure using MTA is in many ways similar to that used with calcium hydroxide but with some minor modifications.
- Tooth is anaesthetized and isolated with rubber dam.
- Site is disinfected using Sodium Hypochlorite solution.
- A shallow pulpotomy is done.
- Removal of pulp tissue to a depth of atleast 2 mm.
- Bleeding is allowed to stop.
- Some moisture is required for the proper curing of the material.
- Mixture of MTA powder and liquid is placed on the wound surface and gently tapped with moist cotton pellet.
- Entire access into the pulp should be filled in a similar manner with small amounts of MTA.
- MTA when exposed to saliva will allow it to cure.
- A minimum of 6 hours is required for a material to adequately set.
- The tooth can then be restored with a definite restoration.

DEVITALISATION PULPOTOMY
(Pulp Mummification Procedure)

- This is a two stage procedure.
- Paraformaldehyde is used to fix the pulpal tissue.

Materials used

- Hobsons paste - contains paraformaldehyde, lignocaine, carmine, carbovax and propylene glycol.

  Mummifying agent
  - Beachwood creosote
  - Hobson's paste

Procedure

- Administration of local anesthesia.
- Initial access preparation
- Superficial layer of coronal pulp content excavation.
- Mummifying agent (Hobson's paste or Beachwood Cresote) is placed on to which a thin mix of zinc oxide eugenol is lightly condensed.
- The patient is recalled after a week during which period the mummifying procedure occurs and a routine pulpotomy is carried out.

Indications

- In cases of non negotiable radicular canals or in cases where the patient is uncooperative.

LASER PULPOTOMY

– Nd : YAG LASER has been used for pulpotomy in primary teeth with a high degree of success.

– Not very popular as it is expensive.

ELECTRO SURGICAL PULPOTOMY

– Electrocarty procedure carbonises and heat that is generated denatures the pulp and bacterial contamination.

– After the surgical amputation of coronal pulp, pulp stumps are cartriged through this method.

– This is followed by the obturation of coronal pulp chamber with zinc oxide eugenol over which a layer of hard setting restoration is placed, over which a stainless steel crown is recommended.

PULPECTOMY

– *It is a complete removal of coronal and radicular pulp and replacing the same with a suitable obturating material.*

Indications

1. In all cases of irreversible pulp disease.
2. In cases of acute pulpitis resulting from infection, injury or operative trauma.
3. In case of carious or mechanical exposure it is the treatment of choice .
4. In other cases, intentional extirpation is required for restorative and fixed prosthetic procedures.

Procedure

– Administration of local anaesthesia.

– Rubberdam application.

– Access cavity preparation.

– Roof of pulp chamber is removed followed by extirpation of radicular pulp using barbed broaches.

– Following pulp extirpation, bio mechanical preparation is carried out using suitable reamers and files.

– Radicular morphology of primary molars is characterisatic termed as *ribbon shaped* because the canals are narrower mesiodistally and broader buccolingually. Hence instrumentation may be difficult. In case of difficulty in negotiating canals one should not make an attempt to forcefully negotiate the instrument apically because of chances of perforation of root.

– Irrigation is carried out using H_2O_2 or Sodium Hypochlorite.

– Canals are dried using paper points after which a thin mix of zinc oxide eugenol or formocresolised ZOE is used to obturate canals and coronal chamber.

– Gutta percha and silver points are contraindicated in primary dentition because they are non resorbable.

– Following placement of obturating material a hard setting cement is condensed over the same followed by a silver amalgam restoration.

– As this is a pulp treated tooth, a stainless steel crown is recommended.

Other recommended materials for Root Canal Obturation in Primary Dentition

1. *Walkhoff Paste :* contains parachlorophenol camphor and menthol.
2. *KRI Paste :* contains Iodoform, camphor, parachlorophenol and menthol.
3. *Misto Paste :* Contains Zinc oxide Iodoform, Thymol, Chlorphenol, Camphor.

APEXIFICATION

– Pulpal therapy for young permanent teeth.

– *It is a method which is intended to induce further development of root apex of an immaturely developed permanent tooth by formation of osteodentin and cementum.*

Indications

1. Long standing fracture of crown involving pulp.
2. Long standing caries exposure.

Contraindications

1. All vertical and most horizontal root fractures.
2. Replacement resorption (ankylosis).
3. Very short roots.

Aim

– To obtain normal narrowing of canal and also an apical closure against which an obturation can be achieved.

Procedure

1. Radiographic interpretation to access the radiographic length and working length.
2. Working length should be maintained 1.5-2 mm short of existing radiographic length.

3. Administration of local anesthesia.

4. Application of rubberdam.

5. Pulp extirpation followed by biomechanical preparation.

6. The young permanent dentition has characteristic broad canal with a wide opened apex and hence called as `Blunder buss canals'.

7. H_2O_2 is contraindicated as an irrigating agent because of its effervescent nature and as any debris can be pushed apically, hence irrigation is limitated to use of sodium hypochlorite and normal saline.

8. Canal is obturated with a mix of calcium hydroxide and CMCP (Camphorated Para mono chlorophenol).

9. The access opening is filled with a hard setting cement.

10. The patient is recalled periodicallly for further radiographic examination to determine the presence of root closure.

11. Once the narrowing and root enclosure is achieved the existing root canal obturated material is removed and a routine root canal therapy is carried out.

– A better approach to apexification may be one in which a combination procedure,

   1. Use Calcium hydroxide for a short period of time about 2 weeks to assist in disinfection of the root canal.

2. Place Mineral Trioxide Aggregate (MTA) in the apical part of the canal to serve as an apical plug that promotes apical repair.

– After checking that the MTA has cured, complete the root canal treatment with gutta percha and a bonded resin restoration extending below the cervical level of the tooth to strengthen the root's resistance to fracture.

APEXOGENESIS

Definition

– It is defined as, Physiological root end development and formation.

– The procedure is used to initiate a full apical closure.

Indications

1. Immature tooth with incomplete root formation.

2. Damage to the coronal pulp but with a healthy radicular pulp.

Contraindications

1. Avulsed and replanted a severely luxated tooth.

2. Severe crown root fracture that requires intraradicular retention for restoration.

3. Tooth with an unfavourable horizontal root fracture.

4. Carious tooth that is unrestorable.

CHAPTER 27

DENTAL INJURIES AND MANAGEMENT

ETIOLOGY

1. Sudden impact involving the face or head.
2. Falling while running (most common).
3. Traffic accidents
4. Acts of violence
5. Sports
6. Child abuse

INCIDENCE

- The most accident prone time period is from 8 to 12 years.
- Boys tend to injure their teeth more frequently than girls in the ratio from 2:1 to 3:1.
- Most frequently involved teeth in decreasing order is maxillary central incisors, maxillary lateral incisors and mandibular incisors.
- Most commonly observed dental trauma involves fracture of enamel, or enamel and dentin but without pulp involvement

CLASSIFICATION

1. According to Ellis and Davey
   1. *Class I* : Simple fracture of crown, involving little or no dentin.
   2. *Class II* : Extensive fracture of crown, involving considerable dentin but not dental pulp.
   3. *Class III* : Extensive fracture of crown, involving considerable dentin and exposing dental pulp.
   4. *Class IV* : The traumatized tooth becomes non vital with or without loss of crown structure.
   5. *Class V* : Teeth lost as a result of trauma.
   6. *Class VI* : Fracture of root, with or without fracture of crown or root.
   7. *Class VII* : Displacement of tooth without fracture of crown or root.
   8. *Class VIII* : Fracture of crown en masse and its replacement.
   9. *Class IX* : Traumatic injuries to deciduous teeth.

2. According to WHO
   - *Modified by Andreasen and Andreasen.*
   - This classification is followed by the International Association of Dental Traumatology.
   - According to this, Dentofacial injuries are classified into,

1. *Soft Tissue Injuries*
    i.   Lacerations
    ii. Contusions
    iii. Abrasions
2. *Tooth Fractures*
    i.   Enamel fractures
    ii. Crown fractures - uncomplicated (no pulp exposure)
    iii. Crown fractures - complicated (with pulp exposure)
    iv. Crown root fractures
    v.   Root Fractures
3. *Luxation Injuries*
    i.   Tooth concussion
    ii. Subluxation
    iii. Extrusive luxation
    iv. Lateral luxation
    v.   Intrusive luxation
    vi. Avulsion
4. *Facial Skeletal injuries*
    i.   Alveolar process - maxilla / mandible.
    ii. Body of maxillary / mandibular bone.
    iii. Temporomandibular joint.

– WHO classification is followed in this chapter.

SOFT TISSUES INJURIES

– There can be lacerations, contusions or abrasions of the epithelial layer or a combination of injuries.
   Rx : Control of bleeding
       Repositioning of displaced tissues and suturing.

TOOTH FRACTURE

1. ENAMEL FRACTURES

– *Include chips and cracks confined to the enamel and not crossing the enamel dentin border.*

Classification

– According to the direction of the break in the long axis of the tooth,

a. *Horizontal :* Line of fracture is perpendicular to the long axis of the tooth.

b. *Oblique :* Line of fracture is in an inclined plane with respect to the long axis of the tooth.

c. *Vertical :* Line of fracture is parallel to the long axis of the tooth.

Diagnosis

– Can be seen by indirect light or transillumination or by the use of dyes.

– In anterior teeth, the enamel chips often involve either the mesial or distal corners of the central lobe of the incisal edge.

Treatment

– Minor smoothening of rough edges and restoring the lost tooth structure with composites.

2. CROWN FRACTURES - UNCOMPLICATED

– *Includes crown fractures involving enamel and dentin without pulp exposure.*

– They may include incisal proximal corners, incisal edges or lingual chisel type fractures in anterior teeth and cusps in posterior teeth.

– It is most common type of injury.

Diagnosis

– By clinical examination with a mirror and an explorer.

– Status of the pulp and periradicular tissues by usual examination procedures.

Treatment

– Main aim is to protect the pulp by sealing the dentinal tubules.

– Most effective method is by application of dentin bonding agents and bonded restoration.

– Placement of temporary acrylic crowns.

– Reattachment procedure can be considered if the fractured crown fragment is available.

– It is as follows,

    – Anaesthetize the tooth.

    – Rubberdam application.

    – Clean the tooth segment and fractured tooth with pumice and water.

    – Determine the reattachment path of insertion.

    – Etch the tooth and coronal segments extending 2 mm beyond the cavosurface margins. Rinse well.

    – Apply a dentinal primer followed by application of an unfilled resin.

    – Apply an light cured composite resin in a creamy consistency to both the tooth and coronal fragment.

    – Carefully reinsert the fragment onto the tooth.

- Remove the excess resin and cure it.
- Polish the resin and check the occlusion.

3. CROWN FRACTURES - COMPLICATED

- *Includes crown fractures involving enamel, dentin and pulp.*
- The degree of pulp involvement varies from a pinpoint exposure to a total unroofing of the coronal pulp.

Diagnosis

- By clinical observation.
- Pulp condition should be determined.

Treatment

- The choice of the procedure depends on the extent of exposure, the condition of the pulp, extent of development of apical foramen and extent of injury to root and supporting tissues.
- *Management - 1:* Pulp exposure within 3 hours: Direct pulp capping.
- *Management - 2:* Expsoure beyond 24 hours and within 72 hrs: Pulpotomy with calcium hydroxide or MTA.
- *Management - 3 :* Beyond 72 hours of trauma,
  - Apexification - Young permanent teeth.
  - Pulpectomy - Primary teeth.
  - Root canal therapy - Matured permanent tooth.

4. CROWN ROOT FRACTURES

- *It involves enamel, dentin and cementum,*

i. *Anterior Crown - Root fractures*

- Usually caused by direct trauma.
- This result in a chisel type fracture with the apical extent of the fracture below the lingual gingiva.
- The fragments may be single or multiple and are loose, and attached only by periodontal ligament fibers.
- Pulp may be involved, depending on the depth of fracture into dentin.

ii. *Posterior Crown - Root fractures*

- Usually caused by indirect trauma, i.e. large size restorations, thermal cycling, high speed instrumentation, pin placement and direct trauma such as accidental blows to the face and jaws.
- Pulp may be involved.

- The vertical fracture of endodontically treated tooth is an additional type of crown root fracture involving both anterior and posterior teeth.

Diagnosis

- Pain particularly when the manipulation of the loose fragments is done.
- Fragments are easy to move.
- Fracture line fills with bleeding from periodontal ligament or pulp.

Treatment

- Several treatment options are available depending on extent of the fracture,
  1. If the tooth fracture and no pulp exposure then the fragment can be reattached by bonding.
  2. If Pulp exposure has occurred,
     - i. If the tooth is still developing - shallow pulpotomy.
     - ii. If the tooth is fully developed - Root Canal Therapy.
  3. If crown root fracture extends below the alveolar crest requires surgical repositioning of the tissues to expose the level of fracture : Extrusion either surgical or orthodontic can be done for better restoration.

5. ROOT FRACTURES

- *It is the type of fracture involving the roots only, i.e. cementum, dentin and pulp.*

Etiology

A. *Iatrogenic Injuries*

1. Screw type pins
2. Inlays with posts
3. Post and core
4. Endodontic intraosseous implants
5. Obturation techniques.

B. *Traumatic Injuries*

1. Severe craniofacial Traumas
2. Industrial accidents
3. Sports
4. Habits (opening bottles with the teeth)

Classification

A. *According to Direction*

1. Horizontal
2. Oblique
3. Vertical

B. *According to Location*

1. Cervical Third
2. Middle Third
3. Apical Third

C. *According to Number*

1. Single
2. Multiple
3. Comminuted

D. *According to Extent*

1. Partial
2. Total

E. *Position of root fragments*

1. Not Displaced
2. Displaced

Diagnosis

– One additional film angulation (45 degrees or fore shortened) will, when combined with the standard 90 degree positioning reveal most of the traumatic root fractures.

Treatment

– If there is no mobility and the tooth is symptomless, the fracture is likely to be in the apical third of the root and no treatement is necessary for this.

– If the coronal fragment is mobile, the initial treatement consists of repositioning the coronal segment (if it is displaced) and the stabilization (to promote healing) of the tooth.

– Duration of stabilization : 4 to 6 weeks.

Sequelae of Root Fractures

– Provided by Andreasen and Hjorting Hansen.

– It is divided into 4 types,

1. *Healing with calcified tissue*

   – Radiographically the fracture line is discernible but the fragments are in close contact.

2. *Healing with interproximal connective tissue*

   – Radiographically the fragments appear separated by a narrow radiolucent line, and the fractured edges appear rounded.

3. *Healing with interproximal bone and connective tissue*

   – Radiographically, the fragments are separated by a distinct long bridge.

4. *Interproximal inflammatory tissue with out healing*

   – Radiographically a widening of the fracture line and / or a developing radiolucency corresponding to the fracture line become apparent.

– The first three types are considered successfully healed injuries.

– They are asymptomatic, respond to electric vitality tests, and may, over time, show only signs of coronal discoloration (yellowing) owing to coronal calcification.

– Fractures that do not heal need additional endodontic treatment.

– The following treatment options are available for cases which contain healthy, vital pulp in the apical segment and necrotic coronal pulp,

1. *RCT to both segments* : Indicated when the fracture segments are not separated, allowing the passage of files and filling materials from the coronal segment to the apical segment across the fracture site.

2. *RCT of coronal segment only* : It is current following method particularly when the apical segment contain healthy, vital pulp. CVEK modified this procedure, i.e. he used an apexification procedure in the coronal segment.

3. *Use of Intraradicular splint* : Recommended by Weine etal. Both segments are treated endodontically. Following root canal filling, a post space is prepared in the canal to extend from the coronal segment into the apical one, allowing placement of a rigid-type post to stabilize the two root segments.

4. *Root Extrusion* : Recommended for teeth with root fractures at or near the alveolar crest.

LUXATION INJURIES

– *Includes impact trauma that ranges from minor crushing of the periodontal ligament and the neurovascular supply to the pulp to more major trauma such as forceful and sometimes total displacement of teeth.*

– Tooth luxation (not including avulsion) is a frequent injury comprising the largest group of injuries in the classification of dental trauma, ranging from 30 to 44%.

Diagnosis

1. Luxated teeth that have been loosened or slightly displaced are sensitive to biting and chewing.

2. In *concussion*, it may be the only symptom and it is noted by percussion of the tooth.

3. In *subluxation and extrusive luxation*, in addition to sensitivity to percussion, sensitivity to pressure and palpation of the alveolus, mobility, dislocation and possibly bleeding from the periodontal ligament is also seen.

4. *Lateral and Intrusive Luxations* are usually firmly displaced and may not be sensitive to percussion.

1. Concussion

- It is the mildest form of luxation injury and is characterized by sensitivity to percussion only.
- There is no displacement and no mobility of the tooth.
- It is present in most cases of crown, root and crown root fractures.

Treatment

- Symptomatic treatment, i.e. allow the tooth to rest as much as possible to promote recovery of tissues from trauma.
- Monitoring of the pulp status.
- Watching clinically for tooth color changes and radiographically for resorption.

2. Sub luxation

- *When a tooth, as a result of trauma, is sensitive to percussion and has increased mobility, it is classified as subluxated.*

Treatment

- Initial treatment consists of rest to the tooth and short term stabilization for 2 to 3 weeks, to promote the recovery of tissues.
- Definitive treatment include RCT for fully developed teeth.

3. Extrusive luxation

- *It is the axial displacement of the tooth in coronal direction.*
- Tooth is highly mobile.
- Continuous trauma due to premature occlusion.

Treatment

- *Immediate treatment :* Repositioning of the tooth and stabilization by splint for 4 to 8 weeks.
- *Definitive treatment :* RCT for involving tooth except in young, developing teeth in which pulps are more prone to recover.

4. Lateral luxation

- *It is the displacement of a tooth in labial, lingual, distal or mesial directions.*
- Often very painful, especially when it is in premature occlusion.

Treatment

- *Immediate treatment :* Repositioning of the tooth and stabilization by splint for 3 to 4 weeks.
- *Definitive treatement :* RCT for involving tooth except for developing teeth.

5. Intrusive luxation

- *It is an injury in which the tooth is moved from its position in the socket, deeper into the alveolar bone.*

Treatment

1. For developing immature teeth : no need of any treatment.
2. For fully developed teeth : repositioning of the tooth either surgically or orthodontically.
3. For teeth with incomplete root formation: Apexification.

6. Tooth Avulsion (Exarticulation)

- It is the complete displacement of tooth out of its socket.
- Sports and automobile accidents are the most frequent causes for tooth avulsion.

Treatment

1. Immediate Replantation
2. Delayed replantation
- It is the treatment for teeth with more than 1 hour of extra alveolar time.
- The procedure is as follows,
1. Examine the avulsed tooth for debris remove the soft tissue pieces attached to the root surface.
2. Perform the root canal therapy in vitro and fill the canal in retrograde filling method to preserve the intactness of the crown.
3. Soak the tooth in 2.4% fluoride solution at pH 5.5. for 20min or more to slow down the resorption.
4. Prepare the tooth socket by gentle curettage and irrigate with saline.
5. Rinse the tooth thoroughly in saline, reinsert into the socket and splint it for 6 weeks.

CHAPTER 28

ENDODONTIC REPLANTATION, TRANSPLANTATION AND IMPLANTATION

REPLANTATION

Definition

- Replacement of a tooth in its socket, with the object of attaining reattachment when the tooth has been completely avulsed from its socket by an accident.
- Total luxation of avulsion of teeth is treated by Replantaiton.
- Life span of replanted tooth is less.
- Root resorption will be more in replanted tooth.

GUIDELINES FOR THE TREATMENT OF AVULSED TOOTH

- Recommended by a committee of the American Association of Endodontists.

1. **Extra oral time**
   - It is a one of the most important factor in the prognosis of an avulsed tooth.
   - The avulsed tooth should bring immediately as soon as possible to maintain the viability of root surface and periodontal ligament.

2. **Storage Media**
   - Patients saliva - Under the tongue or Buccal vestibule - most preferable.
   - Hank's balancing solution.
   - Saline
   - Bovine milk
   - Water least preferable

3. **Management of the socket**
   - The less manipulation of the socket the better the prognosis for replanted tooth.
   - Use light irrigation and gentle aspiration to remove any blood clot.
   - Do not curette or vent the socket.

4. **Management of Root Surfaces**
   - To preserve the vitality of the root surface cells do not handle, scrape, brush or remove any of the root surface.
   - If the root surface appears clean, replant as it is.
   - If the root surface is dirty, clean with tap water, wet sponge and cotton.
   - Do not apply any medicaments disinfectants or chemicals to the root surface.

5. **When to perform endodontic treatment**
   - Endodontic treatment should be initiated with in 7 to 14 days of replantation and when the tooth is in its socket.

- If the root apex is open, monitor the replanted tooth every 2 weeks for revitalization of the pulp.
- If pathologic signs are noted, then extirpate the pulp and continue with an apexification procedure until such time as endodontic treatment and root canal filling can be completed.

6. Filling materials

- Calcium hydroxide filling is given for 7 days and then permanently obturate the root canal with gutta percha.

7. Splinting

- The suggested splint is composed of acid etch resin alone or with soft arch wire, orthodontic brackets with wire arch, or large monofilament fishing line.

8. Adjunctive Drug Therapy

- Refer the patient for a tetanus consultation within the first 48 hours.
- Prescribe antibiotics if necessary.

ENDODONTIC TREATMENT: BEFORE OR AFTER REPLANTATION ?

- According to Grossman, a good rule to follow is :
  - If the periodontal ligament is still vital, replant the tooth without delay and plan an endodontic treatment at a later time.
  - If the periodontal ligament is dried out and dead, the endodontic treatment may just as well be done before replanting the tooth.

FAILURE OF REPLANTED TEETH

- Major failure in replantation is resorption of the root, frequently followed by ankylosis.

Types of Resorption (Andreasen)

1. Surface Resorption

- Occurs following trauma or orthodontic tooth movement.
- Occurs within first 2 weeks.
- Small localized areas of cemental resorption.
- Repair occurs by secondary cementum deposition.

2. Inflammatory Resorption (Infective)

- Usually results from luxation or exarticulation injury.
- Occurs after 3 weeks.
- Occurs due to the presence of micro organisms in the dentinal tubules or to necrotic tissue in the root canal that causes inflammation of bone and

destruction of both the root surface and bone with replacement by granulamatous tissue.
- Diagnosis of inflammatory root resorption is characterized radiographically by bowl like radiolucencies in the tooth and adjacent bone.

3. Replacement Resorption

- Occurs when there has been death of periodontal ligament cells.
- Seen after 6 weeks.
- Characterized by gradual root resorption including periodontal ligament, cementum and dentin of the root with replacement by bone, leading to bony ankylosis.

INTENTIONAL REPLANTATION

- *Intentional replantation is defined as, an act of deliberately removing a tooth and following examination, diagnosis, endodontic manipulation and repair returning the tooth to its original socket.*
- During this procedure, the periodontal ligament is kept viable by moistening the tooth frequently in sterile saline solution / milk / anesthetic solution.
- The planned operation can usually be performed within 15 min.
- Operation is limited to posterior teeth.
- It is not indicated when resection is possible.

Indications

1. When an instrument has been broken in the root canal and projecting out through the apical foramen.
2. When there is mechanical obstruction in the canal such as pulpstone, fractured instrument or glass bead that cannot be removed.
3. When the root canal is calcified or partly calcified and an area of rarefaction is present.
4. When the root canal is grossly overfilled and the protruding filling is irritating the periapical tissues.
5. When the root canal is sharply curved and cannot be negotiated.
6. Bifurcated root canal as it approaches the root apex and cannot be negotiated.
7. When a foreign body is lying free in the periapical tissue and is acting as an irritant such as, excess piece of guttaparcha that has broken off from the main stem or grossly overfilled canal, or root canal cement or when an absorbent point has been pushed completely through the apical foramen.

Contraindications

1. Periodontal involvement with extensive mobility of the tooth.

2. Buccal or lingual plate that is destroyed or missing.

3. Septal bone at the bifurcation and trifurcation that is destroyed or missing.

4. Likelihood that extraction of the tooth will fracture the crown.

Technique

– It is done by two persons.

– One should be given the responsibility of extraction, care of the wound and socket, the other is carrying out the necessary endodontic treatment and replacing the tooth in its socket.

– Aseptic procedure has to be carried out.

– After administering local anesthesia, tooth is cautiously extracted.

– The wound and socket will be carefully debrided.

– The wound is packed with sterile gauze.

– The endodontic procedure is started as soon as the tooth is removed from the socket.

– The tooth is wrapped in sterile gauze and root tip is protruded out of the gauge to preserve the vitality of the periodontium.

– The operator then clips about 2-3 mm from the root apice with a pair of rongeur forceps.

– Alternately the root tips can be resected using a high speed drill, sterile burs and sterile spray.

– When the root tips have been cut off a cavity is prepared in each of the resected roots with a small no. 1 or no. 2 round bur to a depth of atleast 2mm.

– The cavities are then undercut with an inverted cone bur of sizes No. 34 and 35 and varnished.

– The amalgam is packed into the cavities.

– Excess amalgam is removed with sterile cotton and the tooth is replaced in it socket.

– A splint is given to stabilize the replanted tooth and to prevent it from being displaced or dislodged.

TRANSPLANTATION

Definition

– *Removal of a tooth or tooth bud from one socket and transplanting it into another socket.*

Autotransplantaiton

– Transplanting of a tooth or tooth bud from one socket to another socket in the same person.

Allotransplantation

– Transplanting of a tooth or tooth bud from a socket of one person and inserting it into the socket of another person (of same species).

Implantation

– The insertion of an artificial tooth or stabilizer into a surgically prepared socket.

– Transplantation of teeth is not successful as intentional replantation because of the immunologic factor.

ENDODONTIC IMPLANTS

Definition

– A metallic extension of the root with the object of increasing the crown root ratio to give the tooth better stability in the arch.

Uses and Indications

1. Periodontally involved teeth requiring stabilization.

2. Transverse root fracture involving loss of the apical fragment or the presence of two fragments that cannot be aligned.

3. Pathologic resorption of the root apex due to a chronic abscess.

4. A pulpless tooth with an unusually short root.

5. Internal resorption affecting the integrity and strength of the root.

6. A tooth in which additional root length is desired for improving its alveolar support.

– Endodontic implants have a high failure rate.

Disadvantages

1. Poor apical seal resulting in periapical rarefaction around the root apex.

2. Extrusion of excessive sealer through the apical foramen into the periapical tissues with resulting irritation.

3. Limitation in the length of the osseous portion of implant by local anatomic factors in the maxilla or mandible.

4. Perforation of the lateral root surface or perforation of a curved root near the root apex.

5. A structurally weakened tooth instrumented to a much larger size than usual, to receive an inflexible implant, which may fracture during function.

TECHNIQUE

Materials

– Chrome Cobalt implants
– Titanium Implants

Equipment

– Is the same as for endodontic treatment, with the addition of a series of extra long reamers, 40mm in sequential sizes and implants of corresponding size.

Steps

– Anesthetize the tooth and involved area.
– Rubberdam application.

Access preparation

– Wider and larger in the clinical crown to accommodate rigid implant.
– Enlargement of the root canal upto 60 size.

– Irrigation of the root canal.
– A marker is then set on the 40 mm reamers at a level equivalent to the length of the tooth and the number of mm the implant will extend beyond the root apex.
– The first 40 mm reamer used to perforate the root apex should be several sizes smaller than the last sized instrument used to complete the preparation of the root canal.
– The last 40 mm reamer is used and the bone is reamed to the desired length.
– Irrigate the canal with saline or anaesthetic solution rather than sodium hypochlorite which may irritate the periapical tissues.
– Dry the canal with sterile absorbent points.
– Select an implant of equivalent size to the last instrument used and insert it into the root and bone.
– The implant must fit tightly and must penetrate the bone to the prepared length.

CHAPTER 29

BLEACHING OF DISCOLOURED TEETH

INTRODUCTION

- Normal colour of primary teeth - bluish white.
- Colour of permanent teeth - grayish yellow, Greyish white or yellowish white.
- Teeth of elderly persons are usually more yellow or grayish yellow than those of younger patients.

CLASSIFICATION OF TOOTH DISCOLOURATION

- It is classified as,
    1. Extrinsic discolouration
    2. Intrinsic discolouration.

1. Extrinsic Discolouration

- Found on the outer surface of the teeth and are usually of local origin such as tobacco stains.
- Some extrinsic discolouration, such as the *green discolouration* associated with the Nasmyth's membrane in children.
- Other types of extrinsic discolouration such as silver nitrate stains are almost impossible to eliminate without grinding as these stains penetrate the surface of the crowns.

2. Intrinsic Discolouration

- These are stains within the enamel and dentin caused by the deposition or incorporation of substances with in these structures, such as tetracycline stains.
- Intrinsic discolourations such as those occuring with amelogenesis imperfecta or dentinogenesis imperfecta are impossible to eliminate because they originate from developmental defects of the enamel and dentin.
- Stains that result from pulp necrosis can usually be removed by bleaching procedures.

CAUSES OF TOOTH DISCOLOURATION

I. 1. Local causes
    - Decomposition of pulp tissue.
    - Excessive hemorrhage following pulp removal.
    - Trauma
    - Medicaments
    - Filling materials

2. Systemic causes
    - Red or purple discolouration in congenital porphyria.
    - Violaceous as in hereditary opalescent dentin.
    - Mottled brown as in endemic flourosis.

- Grayish brown as in erythroblastosis foetalis.
- Brown as in jaundice.
- Tetracyclines cause yellow to gray or brown.

II. According to INGLE,

A. Patient related causes

1. Pulp necrosis
2. Intra pulpal hemorrhage
3. Dentin hyper calcification
4. Age
5. Tooth formation defects,
   - Developmental defects
   - Drug-related defects

B. Dentist-Related Causes

1. *Endodontically related*
   - Pulp tissue remnants
   - Intracanal medicaments
   - Obturating materials

2. *Restoration related*
   - Amalgam
   - Pins and posts
   - Composites

Prevention of tooth discolouration

- Discolouration of pulpless teeth can be prevented by detailed attention to various aspects of treatment especially debridement.
- All traces of blood should be removed by thorough irrigation.
- Any defective restorations should be replaced.
- Non staining medicaments and materials should be used.
- Root canal sealer and obturating materials should be removed from the pulp chamber beyond a level 1 to 3 mm apical to the free gingival margin.

BLEACHING AGENTS

1. SUPEROXOL

Composition

- *It is a 30% solution of hydrogen peroxide by weight and 100% by volume in pure distilled water.*
- It is *clear, colourless, odorless* liquid, stored in light proof amber bottles.

- It is *unstable* and should be kept away from heat which could cause it to explode.
- It should be stored in sealed refrigerated containers.
- It has ischaemic effect on skin and mucous membrane.
- It is painful if it comes in contact with the nail bed or, the soft tissue under the finger nail.
- It can be used alone or mixed with sodium perborate into a paste for use in the walking bleach technique.

2. CARBAMIDE PEROXIDE

- Also known as `urea hydrogen peroxide'.
- Available in the concentration range of 3 to 45%. But popular preparation contain 10% carbamide peroxide with a mean pH of 5 to 6.5.
- Solutions of 10% carbamide peroxide breakdown into urea, ammonia, carbon dioxide and approx. 3.5% hydrogen peroxide.

3. SODIUM PERBORATE

- A stable white powder, normally supplied in a granular form.
- The powder is water soluble and decomposes into *Sodium metaborate* and *Hydrogen Peroxide releasing nascent oxygen.*
- *When fresh it contains about 95% perborate, corresponding to 9.9% of the available oxygen.*

BLEACHING OF ENDODONTICALLY TREATED TEETH

Indications

1. Discolourations of pulp chamber.
2. Dentin discolourations.
3. Discolourations not amenable to extra coronal bleaching.

Contra indications

1. Superficial enamel discolourations.
2. Defective enamel formation.
3. Severe loss of dentin.
4. When caries are present.
5. Discoloured composites.

THERMO / PHOTO EXTRA CORONAL BLEACHING

1. Indications

1. Light enamel discolourations.
2. Mild tetracycline discolourations.
3. Age-related discolourations.

2. Contra indications

1. Severe dark discolourations.
2. Severe enamel loss.
3. Proximity of pulp horns.
4. Hypersensitive teeth.
5. Caries presence.
6. Large/poor coronal restorations.

TECHNIQUES FOR BLEACHING OF PULPLESS TEETH / ENDODONTICALLY TREATED TEETH / NON VITAL TEETH

TECHNIQUES

1. Walking bleach technique.
2. Ultra Violet photo oxidation / Heat and Light bleaching.
3. Thermocatalytic Technique,
   - Prior to bleaching a tooth evaluate the condition of its crown and status of its obturated root.
   - Root canal filling should be well condensed, radiopaque with no voids and it should be well adapted to the root canal walls.

WALKING BLEACH TECHNIQUE

Composition :   Superoxol

Sodium Perborate

Mechanism of Action

- When the paste is sealed into the pulp chamber, it oxidizes and discolours the stain slowly, continuing its activity over a longer period.

Procedure

1. Prepare the tooth by polishing the enamel with prophylactic paste to remove debris.
2. Apply petroleum jelly to protect against tissue irritation.
3. Adapt the rubber dam and reestablish the access cavity.
4. Remove any gutta-percha root canal filling that extends into the pulp chamber.
5. Seal the orifice of the root canal with atleast 1mm cavit over the gutta-percha to prevent percolation of the bleaching agent into the apical area.
6. Remove the smear layer, open the tubule by applying a 25% solution of citric acid or 30% solution of orthophosphoric acid to the dentinal surface.
7. Flush the surface with sodium hypochlorite or water to remove the acid.
8. Flush the pulpchamber with 95% alcohol and dry with air to dissociate the dentin.
9. Mix sodium perborate powder with superoxol to a thick paste in a dappen dish.
10. Carry the thick paste into the pulp chamber and the entire facial surface of the pulp chamber is covered with the paste.
11. Now place a small cotton pellet slightly moistened with superoxol over the bleaching paste.
12. Seal the access cavity with IRM or zinc phosphate cement.
13. Patient should return in 3-7 days for evaluation of the result.

Advantages of Walking Bleach Technique

1. Less chair side time
2. Safe
3. More comfortable for the patient

ULTRAVIOLET PHOTO OXIDATION

- After preparation of the tooth, a loose mat of cotton is placed on the labial surface and another is placed in the pulp chamber of the tooth to be bleached.
- The loose cotton mats are saturated with superoxol.
- The solution is activated by exposing it to light and heat from a powerful light.
- The tooth is subject to several, (equally 5-6 min) exposures and replenishes the bleaching solution at frequent intervals.
- On completion of the bleaching, a pellet of cotton moistened with superoxal and sodium perborate is sealed in the pulp chamber until the following appointment.

THERMOCATALYTIC TECHNIQUE

- It involves the placement of the oxidizing chemical generally 30 to 35% hydrogen peroxide (Superoxol), in the pulp chamber followed by heat application either by electric gearing devices or specially designed lamps.

Adverse effect

- Causes external cervical root resorption.

TECHNIQUES FOR BLEACHING OF VITAL TEETH

1. FLUOROSIS STAINS

- Teeth that have been discoloured as a result of ingestion of a high amount of fluoride such as

5 ppm in natural drinking water do not respond well to ordinary methods of bleaching.

- In cases of endemic fluorosis (mottled enamel) the following solution is used,

  1   Part anesthetic ether (0.2 ml)

  5   Parts hydrochlorc acid (36%) (1.0 ml)

  5   Parts hydrogen peroxide (30%) (1.0 ml)

- The anesthetic ether removes surface debris.
- The hydrochloric acid etches the enamel.
- The hydrogen peroxide bleaches the enamel.

Technique

- Polish the crown with a prophylactic paste.
- Protect the gingiva with petroleum jelly and the teeth to be bleached with a rubber dam.
- The solution should be freshly mixed and applied directly to the enamel surface for 5 min at 1 min intervals.
- On completion of the bleaching the solution is neutralized with a backing soda solution and copious irrigation with water.
- The bleached surface should be polished with cuttle discs and a prophylactic paste.
- This procedure may have to be repeated 2-3 times before the desired shade is obtained.
- Fluoride stained teeth are difficult to bleach and require longer and repeated sessions to decolourize them.

2. NIGHT / MOUTH GUARD BLEACHING (MATRIX BLEACHING)

- It is an outside the dental office bleaching procedure.
- Recently introduced bleaching technique.
- It is safe and effective procedure for mildly discoloured teeth.
- It is low cost, easy to apply and high percentage of success view.

Composition of solution

- 10% carbamide peroxide solution
- 3% H_2O
- 7% urea

Indications

1. Superficial enamel discolourations.
2. Mild yellow discolourations.
3. Brown fluorosis discolourations.
4. Age-related discolourations.

Contraindications

1. Severe enamel loss.
2. Hypersensitive teeth.
3. Caries presence.
4. Defective coronal restorations.
5. Allergy to bleaching gels.
6. Bruxism

Technique

- Shade of the natural teeth is determined with the help of shade guide.
- Alginate impression is taken and cast is poured.
- On the cast, plastic night guard is fabricated which is of 2 mm in thickness.
- Night guard should completely cover all the teeth in the arch leaving the palate uncovered.
- Patient is instructed to put 2 - 3 drops of solution in the space in which the teeth to be bleached.
- Insert the night guard in the mouth and allow the excess material to extrude out.
- Patient is asked to wear night guard during the sleep until the treatment is completed.

Complications

1. *Systemic effects*

   - Accidental ingestion of large amounts may cause irritation of gastric and respiratory mucosa.

2. Dental hard tissue damage.
3. Tooth sensitivity.
4. Pulpal damage.
5. Mucosal damage.
6. Damage to restorations.
7. Occlusal disturbances.

3. TETRACYCLINE STAINS

- The extent of tetracycline staining may be classified as, **slight, moderate or severe,**

1. Slight Tetracycline staining

- Observes as a light yellow or light gray uniform discolouration of the entire dentition.
- Slight in extent and uniformly distributed throughout the crown without `banding' or concentration of stain in localized areas such as the cervical or middle third regions; is highly amneable to vital bleaching.
- Usually requires not more than three appointments.

2. **Moderate Tetracycline staining**

   – Observes as a darker or deeper hue of uniform yellow or gray staining with out banding.

   – Usually it requires three to six appointments. `

3. **Severe Tetracycline staining**

   – Characterized by dark gray or blue to purple discolouration usually in combination with banding in which the stain is heavily concentrated in the cervical regions.

   – Veneering techniques should be followed to attain satisfactory result.

Etiology

– These discolourations are due to long term consumption of tetracycline as for the treatment of cystic fibrosis or other infections during the formative period of the teeth.

Technique

– Bleaching agent : 30% SUPEROXOL.

– Polish the crown with prophylactic paste.

– Apply petroleum jelly to protect the gingival.

– Isolation of the teeth to be bleached with rubberdam.

– The use of superoxol and heat source is applied for 20-30 sec at the temperature around 114°F .

Disadvantage

– The application of heat to the tooth structure during bleaching procedures may cause pulpal inflammation.

OTHER METHODS OF BLEACHING

– Intentional RCT, i.e. the root canals are cleaned, shaped and obturated and the teeth are internally bleached.

COMPLICATIONS OF BLEACHING

1. External root resorption

2. Chemical burns

3. Damage to restorations

CHAPTER 30

ENDODONTIC– PERIODONTIC INTER- RELATIONSHIP

CLASSIFICATION

According Oliet and Pollock

– The endodontic - periodontic lesion can be classified into 3 different treatment categories:

I. *Lesion that require endodontic treatment procedures only*

- Any tooth with a necrotic pulp and apical granulomatous tissue replacing periodontium and bone with or without a sinus tract (chronic periapical abscess).
- Chronic periapical abscess with a sinus tract draining through the gingival crevice thus passing through a section of the attachment apparatus in its entire length alongside the root.
- Root fractures, i.e. longitudinal and horizontal.
- Root perforations, i.e. pathologic and iatrogenic.
- Teeth with incomplete apical root development and inflamed or necrotic pulps, with or without periapical pathosis.
- Endodontic implants.
- Replants, i.e. intentional or traumatic.
- Transplants, i.e. autotransplants or allo transplants.
- Teeth requiring hemisection or radisectomy.
- Root submergence.

II. *Lesion that require periodontal treatment procedures only*

- Occlusal trauma causing reversible pulpits.
- Occlusal trauma plus gingival inflammation, resulting in pocket formation.
    - A. Revisable but increased pulpal sensitivity caused by trauma or possibly by exposed dentinal tubules.
    - B. Reversible but increased pulpal sensitivity caused by uncovering lateral or accessory canals exiting into the periodontium.
- Suprabony or infrabony pocket formation treated with overzealous root planing and curettage, leading to pulpal sensitivity.
- Extensive infra bony pocket formation, extending beyond the root apex and sometimes coupled with lateral or apical resorption yet with a pulp that responds with in normal limits to clinical testing.

III. *Lesions that require combined endodontic–periodontic treatment procedures*

- Any lesion in group I that results in irreversible reactions in the attachment apparatus and requires periodontic treatment.

– Any lesion in group II that results in irreversible reactions in pulp tissue and also requires endodontic treatment.

Etiologic Factors

– Examination of the etiologic factors that cause group III lesions which require combined treatment indicates that these factors originate from one of the other two groups.

– The other possible predisposing factors are may be, atypical anatomic factors:

1. Malalignment of a tooth

   – Presence of a multirooted tooth in a position usually occupied by a single rooted tooth.

   – Presence of additional canals.

   – Cervical enamel projections into the furca of multirooted teeth.

   – Large lateral canals in coronal and middle sections of roots.

2. Trauma

3. Miscellaneous errors such as perforation.

According to Weine

1. *Class I :* Tooth in which symptoms clinically and radio graphically simulate periodontal disease but are in fact due to pulpal inflammation and or necrosis.

2. *Class II :* Tooth that has both pulpal or periapical disease and periodontal disease concomitantly.

3. *Class III :* Tooth that has no pulpal problem but requires endodontic therapy plus root amputation to gain periodontal healing.

4. *Class IV :* Tooth that clinically and radiographically simulates pulpal or periapical disease but in fact has periodontal disease.

According to Cohen

1. Primary endodontic lesion.

2. Primary endodontic lesion with secondary periodontal disease.

3. Primary periodontal lesion.

4. Primary periodontal lesion with secondary endodontic involvement.

5. True combined endodontic and periodontic lesions.

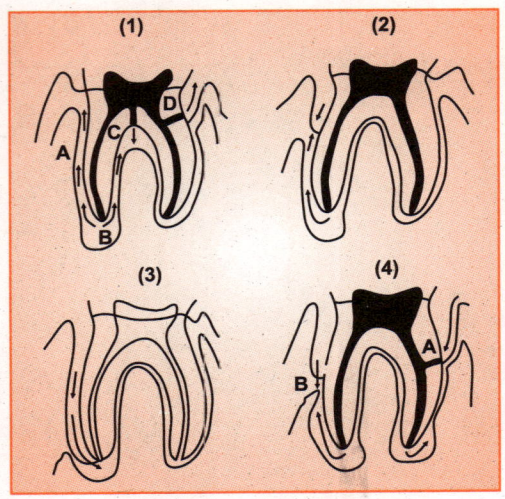

1. **PRIMARY ENDODONTIC LESIONS**
   A. *Path way extending from apex to gingival sulcus via periodontium.*
   B. *Apex to furcation.*
   C. *Lateral canal to furcation.*
   D. *Lateral canal to pocket.*
2. **PRIMARY ENDODONTIC LESION WITH SECONDARY PERIODONTAL INVOLVEMENT.**
3. **PRIMARY PERIODONTAL LESION EXTENDING TO THE APEX.**
4. **PRIMARY PERIODONTAL LESION WITH SECONDARY ENDODONTIC INVOLVEMENT.**
   Via a Lateral Canal (A)
   Combined Lesion from coalescence of separate Lesions (B)

PERFORATIONS

– These are of 2 types,

1. **Iatrogenic Root Perforations**

   – Root perforations by engine driven burs and reamers occur infrequently during post preparation.

   – Perforations of the curved root apex caused by failure to negotiate the canal curvature during instrumentation.

   – Perforation during instrumentation of a root canal with instruments that are too large or too rigid.

   – At times, with engine driven instruments, combined with chelating agents to make the dentin friable one can perforate the lateral wall or the apically curved root inadvertently.

2. **Pathologic Root Perforations**
   Causes

   – Root decay exposing the pulp cavity.

   – Internal resorption.

   – External resorption.

CHAPTER 31

SURGICAL ENDODONTICS

OBJECTIVE

– As in all endodontic procedures the objective of periapical surgery is to ensure the placement of a proper seal between the periodontium and the root canal foramina. When this seal can not be achieved satisfactorily by working through the canal system (orthograde system), a surgical procedure permits visual and manipulative control of the area and placement of the seal (retrograde filling) through the surgical site.

– The better the seal, the better the endodontic prognosis of the tooth; this feature accounts for the high percentage of healing in surgically treated teeth.

INDICATIONS

1. Any condition or obstruction that prevents direct access to the apical third of the canal. For ex: 1. Anatomic conditions like calcifications, curvatures, bifurcations, dens in dente and pulp stone etc and 2. Iatrogenic conditions like ledging, blockage from debris, broken instruments, old root canal fillings and cemented posts.

2. Iatrogenic or resorptive perforation that can not be treated with calcium hydroxide.

3. Periradicular disease associated with a foreign body.

4. Incomplete apexogenesis with blunderbuss canals or other apices that do not respond to apexification procedures and are inadequately sealed with an orthograde filling.

5. Abscess formation necessitating incision and drainage.

6. Horizontally fractured root tip with periradicular disease.

7. Periodontal lesions with furcation involvement that do not respond to periodontal treatment thus necessitating radisectomy.

8. Replantation of avulsed teeth.

9. Intentional extraction and replantation.

10. Necessity for diagnostic biopsy.

11. Predictable failure.

CONTRA INDICATIONS

A. General

1. Medcially compromised or brittle patient (i.e. a patient with an active systemic disease such as uncontrolled diabetes, TB, syphilis, nephritis, blood dyscrasias, osteoradionecrosis or in any other medical condition in which the health of the patient restricts surgical intervention.

2. Emotionally distressed patient i.e a patient unable psychologically to withstand or cope up with any surgical procedure.

3. Limitations in the surgical still and experience of the operator.

B. Local

1. Localized acute inflammation (in this condition, emergency procedure such as incision and drainage or trephination may be indicated, elective periapical surgery should be avoided).
2. Anatomic considerations (procedures that penetrate the mandibular canal, maxillary sinus, mental foramen, floor of the nares or that severe the greater palitatine blood vessel should be avoided whenever possible).
3. Inaccessible surgical sites.
4. Teeth with poor prognosis.

CLASSIFICATION OF ENDODONTIC SURGICAL PROCEDURES

A. Surgical Drainage

1. Incision and drainage
2. Cortical trephination (Fistulative Surgery)

B. Periradicular Surgery

1. Curettage
2. Biopsy
3. Root end resection
4. Root end preparation and filling
5. Corrective surgery
   i. Perforation repair
   ii. Root resection
   iii. Hemisection

C. Replacement Surgery

– Extraction / Replantation

D. Implant Surgery

1. Endodontic implants.
2. Root form osseointegrated implants.

TYPES OF INCISIONS AND FLAPS

1. HORIZONTAL INCISION

– A simple horizontal incision is often used because of the natural contours of the maxilla and mandible.

2. SEMILUNAR / CURVED / ELLIPTICAL FLAP

– It is a curved horizontal incision with the convex portion of the incision towards the gingival crest.

Indication

– Used when it is desirable to maintain the attached gingiva around the margin.
– It is important that there should be 2 to 3 mm of distance from the base of the gingival sulcus to the incision.
– A modified incision that follows the general bone contour is often used to avoid the labial frenum.

Advantages

1. Simple and easy to reflect.
2. Once reflected the operator is close to the apex of involved tooth, providing access to apex without impinging on the tissues.
3. Gingival attachment is not disturbed and marginal gingiva does not recede while healing.
4. Patient can maintain good oral hygiene.

Disadvantages

1. Restricted access with limited visibility.
2. Chances of tearing the corner of incision while attempting to improve the access.
3. If the incision is over the bony defect it may result in dehiscence and scar formation.
4. Flap use is limited by the presence of muscle attachment, canine or other bony prominence.

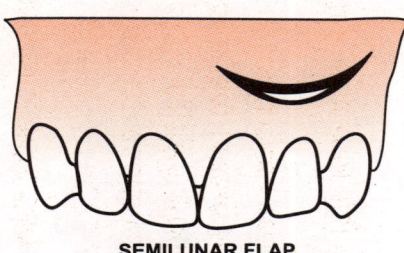

SEMILUNAR FLAP

3. SINGLE VERTICAL INCISION / TRIANGULAR FLAP

Indication

– Indicated for surgery involving the short rooted teeth (usually single).
– Incision is made with the root eminences of teeth.

Advantages

1. Provides greater access and visibilities.
2. Affords a view of periodontal defects and bony penetrations.
3. Heals with minimal scar formation.

Disadvantages

1. Difficult to retract.
2. Vertical and horizontal incision must be lengthy to gain access.

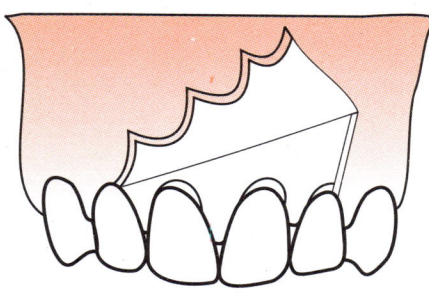

TRIANGULAR FLAP

4. DOUBLE VERTICAL INCISION / TRAPEZOIDAL FLAP

– Two oblique incisions are made and entire flap is retracted towards the vestibule.

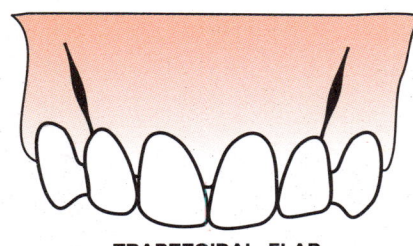

TRAPEZOIDAL FLAP

Advantages

1. Good accessibility.
2. Convenient for teeth with long roots.
3. Convenient for curetting more than one root and large lesions.

Disadvantage

– Loss of gingival attachment.

5. ENVELOPE / GINGIVAL FLAP

– Used mainly for posterior mandibular and palatal surgery.

– Greater relaxation of the flap can be achieved by giving incisions around the necks of all the teeth in a quadrant.

– A relaxing incision can be added at either end of the flap if the access is still not adequate.

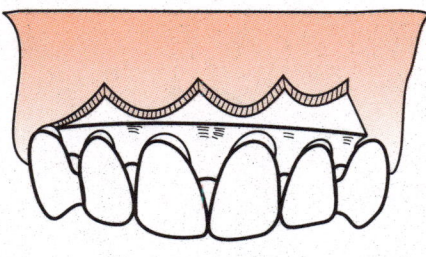

GINGIVAL FLAP

6. LUEBKE - OCHSENBEIN FLAP / SCALLOPED FLAP

– It is named after *Leuebke* an endodontist and *Ochsenbein* a periodontist who together designed the flap.

– It is a modified semilunar flap in which a scalloped horizontal incision is made in the attached gingiva with accompanying vertical incisions.

– Scalloped flap is produced by first making a continuous scalloped incision in the firm attached gingiva parallel to the free gingival groove.

– At both ends vertical oblique relaxation incisions are made.

– Scalloped incision should be 3-4 mm short of the marginal gingiva.

Advantages

1. Greater access and visibility.
2. Decreases the possibility of placing the incision over the periapical defect.
3. Flap is easily displaced and sutured.
4. Marginal gingiva is not disturbed, so there is no gingival recession.

Disadvantages

1. Misjudgement of the size of the lesion - resulting in incision crossing the osseous defect.
2. Possible scar formation.

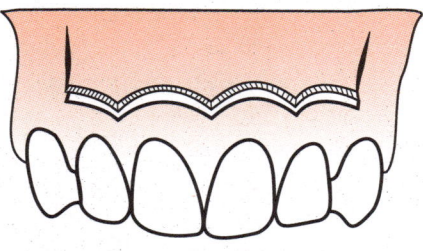

LUEBKE - OCHSENBEIN FLAP

RETROGRADE FILLING

– A retrograde filling is placed in the apically resected root when the canal is poorly sealed from the surrounding tissue.

– The technique used for resection and retrograde filling depends on the accessibility of the root tip in the operative site, the presence of hazardous anatomic structures surrounding the surgical site. The configuration, location and accessibility of the apical foramina to be used.

- The root is bevelled, to achieve the access needed to fill all the foramina present on the resected root surface.

Materials Used

- Zinc and Zinc free amalgam - widely used
- ZOE cements
- Cavit
- Polycarboxylate cement
- Glass ionomer cement
- Composite fillings
- Zinc phosphate cement
- Silver cones
- Gold Foil

Apical Seal

- The filling at the interface of the canal and periapical tissue should seal the root canal from the surrounding tissue.

Technique

- The cavity in the bevelled surface of the root is prepared for a retrograde filling with small, round burs followed by inverted cone burs.
- The ideal preparation has the smallest exposed surface at the apex while encompassing all foramina and extends about 2 mm inside the root canal.

1. Debride the operative site, wipe and dry the root tip and isolate the root tip with sterile cotton pellets to prevent any seepage into the cavity and to collect any excess amalgam particles that fall into the wound during packing and condensation.

2. Place a varnish over the prepared cavity. Pack the amalgam into the cavity using a retrofilling amalgam carrier or a plastic instrument and condense amalgam with a retrofill amalgam plugger.

3. Wipe and adapt the margins of amalgam to dentin with a moist cotton pellet.

4. Remove all the cotton pellets surrounding the root apex, cautiously to prevent amalgam particles trapped in the cotton from falling into the surrounding tissue.

5. Irrigate the wound with sterile saline or anesthetic solution and aspirate the solution thoroughly to debride the wound site.

6. Examine the root tip, filling and surrounding tissue, both visually and radiographically to that the canals have been properly sealed.

RADISECTOMY / ROOT RESECTION

Definition

- Denotes the removal of one or more roots of a molar.

Indications

- When endodontic treatment of one root is technically impossible or when such treatment has failed.
- When untreatable furcation involvement is present and removal of the root will facilitate oral hygiene in that area.
- When extensive loss of bone has occurred around one root of an upper molar.
- When a fractured root of an upper molar is present.
- When a root has been perforated and cannot be treated endodontically.
- When a root has been destroyed by extensive decay.

Contra indications

- When loss of bone involves more than one root and the remaining root would have inadequate support.
- When the bridge span is long and the abutment tooth would lend inadequate support.
- When the roots are fused.

Technique of Root Resection

- Administration of local anesthesia.
- Probe the area to determine the extent and outline of alveolar bone destruction around the root to be removed.
- Elevate the mucoperiosteal flap.
- With the contra angle hand piece and cross cut bur severe the root where it joins the crown and remove the root.
- With a stone or diamond point smooth the resected root stumps and contour the tooth.
- Scale and plane the root surface area.
- Clean the area and replace the flap and suture.
- Cover it with a periodontal pack.
- Remove the pack and suture after 1 week.

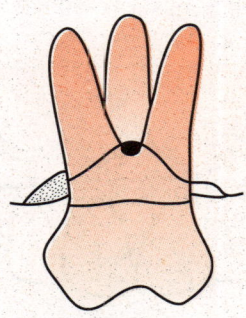

BEFORE

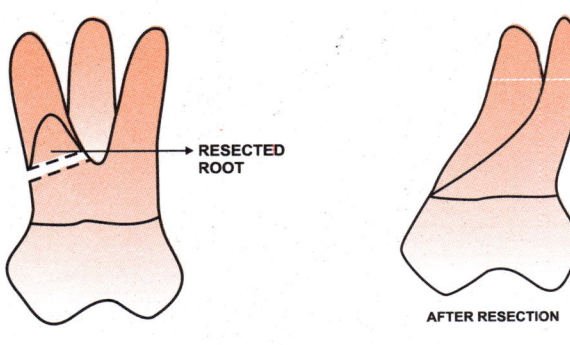

RESECTED ROOT

AFTER RESECTION

HEMISECTION

Definition

– Procedure in which one root and its corresponding crown portion is cut and removed.

Indications

– When the periodontal involvement of one root is severe.
– When loss of bone is extensive in the furcation area.
– When caries involves much of the roots.

Contraindications

– Similar to Radisectomy.

Technique

– It involves the same technique as that is used for root resection.
– In this procedure, half of the crown is removed alone with one of roots of mandibular molar.
– The retained mesial and distal halves serves as abutment for prosthesis or restoration.

BICUSPIDIZATION / BISECTION

– Molar is cut into two separate mesial and distal portion without the removal of any part of the root or crown.
– It is performed when the mandibular molars exhibit proper anatomic features and stability.
– Molar with divergent roots and bone loss restricted to furcal areas are ideal for bicuspidization.
– The tunnel like effect of the furcation involvement is eliminated by creating two separate teeth from single molar.
– The portion of the teeth will require crowns.

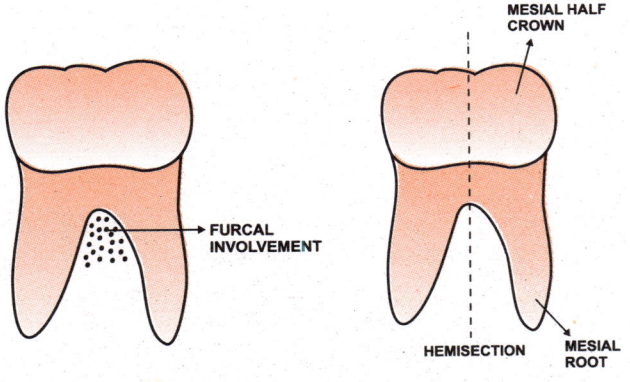

MESIAL HALF CROWN

FURCAL INVOLVEMENT

HEMISECTION

MESIAL ROOT

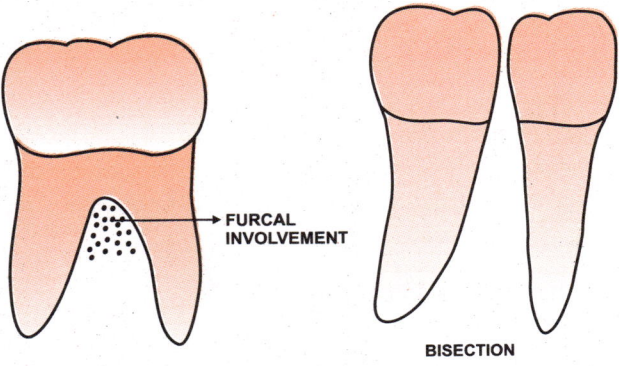

FURCAL INVOLVEMENT

BISECTION

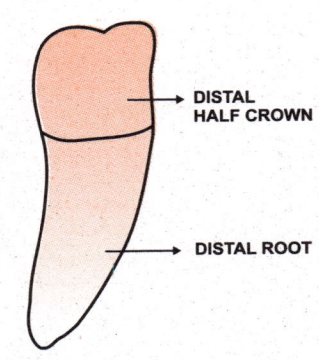

DISTAL HALF CROWN

DISTAL ROOT

AFTER HEMISECTION

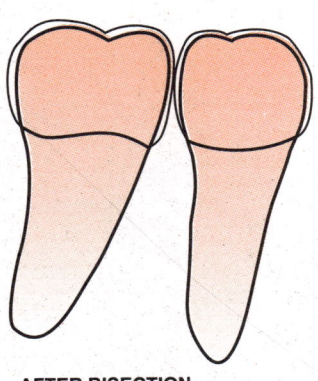

AFTER BISECTION

APICOECTOMY

– Apicoetomy is the removal of the root tip.

Indications

1. When the anatomy of the canal system has not been conductive to nonsurgical treatment.
2. When iatrogenic perforation or ledges prevent apical sealing.
3. When the root tip is resorbed or fractured.
4. When a retrograde filling must be placed in an apex because of an unremovable obstruction exists in the canal.

Procedure

– Radiograph is taken to determine the level at which the root should be amputated.
– Design the mucoperiosteal flap.
– Now the mucoperiosteal flap is raised make an opening into the periapical.
– Bony defect using a surgical bur or chisel.
– Extend the opening in the labial plate to obtain good access to the limits of the defect.
– Then with a fissured cylindrical bur amputate the root at the appropriate level.
– Apical foramen is sealed either by retrograde filling or sealing the gutta percha in the canal.
– Control hemorrhage within the defect by crushing bleeding points in bone by pressure or by cotton pledgets dipped in epinephrine.
– Suture the mucoperiosteal flap and maintain firm pressure over the area for 10 minutes.
– Obtain an immediate postoperative radiograph to check the level of root amputation and future comparison.

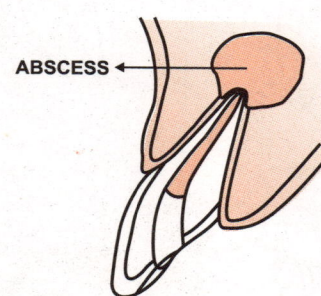

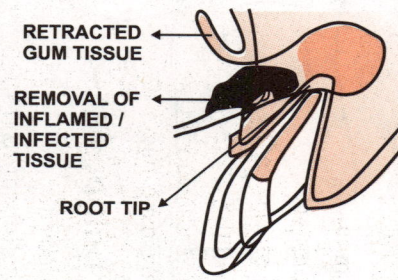

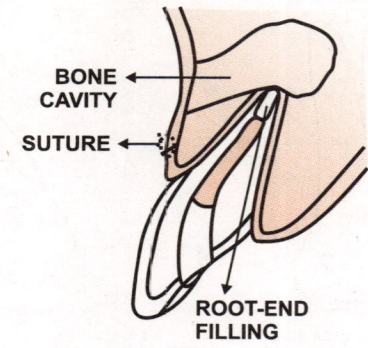

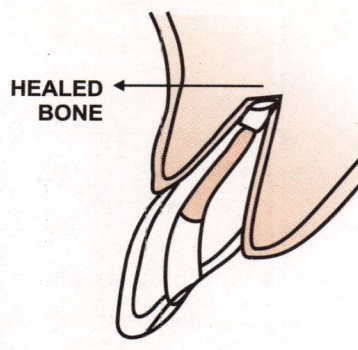

REPAIR

– Repair of the periapical tissue is usually complete within a year and progressive repair should be noticeable on a radiograph 6 months after the operation.

– According to Andreasen and Rud, three main types of repair occur following root resection,

1. Complete repair with restoration of the damaged periodontal ligament with either mild or no inflammation.

2. Repair with rear tissue adjacent to the PDL, with some degree of inflammation.

3. Sear tissue with moderate inflammation.

COMPLICATIONS OF ENDODONTIC SURGERY

1. Swelling
2. Pain
3. Ecchymosis
4. Paresthesia
5. Stitch abscess
6. Hemorrhage
7. Perforation
8. Iatrogenic damage to adjacent teeth
9. Incision failure

REFERENCES / BIBLIOGRAPHY

1. *Philip's Science of Dental Materials,* 11/e, Anusavice, 2003, Saunders, St. Louis, Missouri 63146.

2. *Restorative Dental Materials,* 11/e, Craig, Harcourt Brace and Company Asia, Singapore 238884.

3. *Notes on Dental Materials,* 6/e, E.C. Combe, A.A. Grant, 1992, Churchill-Livingstone, NY 10011.

4. McCabe, J.F. (John F) *Applied Dental Materials,* 7/e, 1990, Blackwell Scientific Publications, Oxford.

5. *Wheeler's Dental Anatomy, Physiology and Occlusion,* 8/e, Ash and Nelson, Saunders, St. Louis, Missouri 63146.

6. *Orban's Oral Histology and Embryology,* 11/e, Bhaskar, 1991, Mosby-Year Book Inc.

7. *Textbook of Oral Pathology,* 4/e, Shafer, Hine, Levy, 1993, Saunders, Philadelphia, PA 19106.

8. Shear Mervyn, *Cysts of the Oral Region,* 3/e, 1992, Wright, Linacre House, Jordan Hill, Oxford OX28DP.

9. *Dentistry for the Child and Adolescent,* 7/e, McDonald and Avery, 2001, Mosby, Harcourt Health Sciences Company, St. Louis, Missouri 63146.

10. *Clinical Pedodontics,* 4/e, S.B. Finn, 2001, W.B. Saunders Company, USA.

11. *Pediatric Dentistry : Infancy through Adolescence,* 3/e, Pinkham, 1998, W.B. Saunder's Company, USA.

12. Kennedy DB, Kapala JT. "The dental pulp : Biologic considerations of protection and treatment". In: Braham RL, Morris ME (Editors). *Textbook of Pediatric Dentistry,* 2/e, Baltimore, Williams and Wilkins, 1985.

13. *Textbook of Oral and Maxillo Facial Surgery,* G.O. Kruger, 1984, C.V. Mosby Company, St. Louis, Missouri, USA.

14. *Oral and Maxillofacial Surgery,* D.M. Laskin, Vols 1 and 2, 2003, C.V. Mosby Company, St. Louis, Missouri 63141.

15. *Clinical Periodontology,* 9/e, Newman, Takei and Carranza, 2003, Saunders, PA 19106.

16. *Tylman's Theory and Practice of Fixed Prosthodontics,* 8/e, Ishiyaku Euro America Inc, U.S.A.

17. American Association of Endodontists. *Glossary of Terms used in Endodontics,* 4/e, Chicago, Ill: 1984.

18. *Sturdevant's Art and Science of Operative Dentistry,* 4/e, T.M. Roberson, H.O. Heymann, E.J. Swift, Jr., 2002, Mosby Inc., St. Louis.

19. *A Textbook of Operative Dentistry,* 4/e, McGehee, True, Inskipp, 1989, McGraw-Hill Book Company, Inc.

20. *Operative Dentistry,* 4/e, H.W. Gilmore, M.R. Lund, Col. D.J. Bales, J.P. Vernetti, 1994, C.V. Mosby Company, St. Louis, Missouri 63141.

21. *Textbook of Operative Dentistry,* 3/e, Baum, Phillips, Lund, 1981, W.B. Saunders Company, Philadelphia, PA.

22. *Operative Dentistry : Modern Theory and Practice,* M.A. Marzouk, A.L. Simonton, R.D. Gross, 1997, Ishiyaku Euro America Inc., USA.

23. *Conservative Dentistry : An integrated approach,* P.H. Jacobsen (Editor), 1990, Churchill Livingstone, NY 10036.

24. Basrani, Enrique, *Fractures of the Teeth,* 1982, Lea and Febiger, PA 19106, USA.

25. Jordan, R.E. *Esthetic Composite Bonding : Techniques and Materials,* 2/e, 1992, Mosby-Year Book, Inc.

26. *Principles and Practice of Operative Dentistry,* 3/e, Gerald T. Charbenau, 1988, Lea and Febiger, Philadelphia, PA 19106.

27. Grossman L.I., *Endodontic Practice,* 11/e, 1988, Lea and Febiger, Philadelphia, PA, USA.

28. *Endodontics,* 5/e, Ingle, Bakland, 2002, B.C. Decker, Inc. Elsevier, Canada.

29. *Pathways of the Pulp,* 8/e, Cohen and Burns, Mosby Inc., St. Louis, Missouri 63146.

30. *Endodontic Therapy,* 5/e, Weine, 1996, Harcourt Brace and Company Asia, Singapore 238884.

31. *Harty's Endodontics in Clinical Practice,* Edited by T.R. Pitt Ford, 5/e, 2004, Wright, Elsevier Science Limited, Philadelphia, U.S.A.

32. *A Colour Atlas of Endodontics,* J.J. Messing, C.J.R. Stock, 1998, Wolfe Medical Publications Ltd, Singapore.

33. Walton R.E. *Principles and Practice of Endodontics,* 2/e, 1996, W.B. Saunders Company, PA 19106.

Relevant websites

34. www.aae.org.

35. www.ada.org.

36. www.milliondollarsmiles.com

37. www.tpub.com

38. www.hougangdental.com

39. www.uic.edu

40. www.fleshandbones.com

41. www.stropko.com

42. www.dentistry.ouhsc.edu

43. www.sci.sbsu.edu

44. www.dental.washington.edu

45. www.guidance.endo.com

46. www.endojournal.com.ar

47. www.ohsu.edu

48. www.uic.edu

49. www.rootfillings.com

INDEX

Section I
OPERATIVE DENTISTRY

A

Abfraction 113
Abrasion 138
    Types 138
    Signs and symptoms 138
    Treatment 139
Acid etching 102
Acrylic resins 99
Active caries 44
Acute caries 43
Adhesive 104
Adherend 104
Adhesion 104
Admixed alloys 18
Affected dentin 47
Agents for pulp protection 31
Air abrasion 145
Aluminous porcelain 42
Aluminium oxide 65
Amalgam
    Bonded amalgam 24
    Gallium amalgam 24
    Properties 20
Amalgapins 14, 98
Amalgamation process 19
Angle
    Line angle (axial, pulpal) 6
    Point angle 6
    Cavosurface angle 6
Angle formers 55, 66
Annealing 117
Arkansas stone 65
Arrested caries 44
ASPA 30
Attrition
    Causes 138
    Effects 137
    Treatment 138
Autoclaving 78
Automatrix 83

B

Back pressure porosity 40
Backward caries 44
Basic instrument tray setup 68
Bevels 131
    Functions 13
    Types 13
Black's matrices 83
Brushes 64
Burn out 38
Burnishing 23
    Pre carve 23
    Post carve 23
Burs
    Cylindrical/straight fissure 60
    Elliptical 60
    End cutting 60
    Inverted cone 60
    Pear shaped 60
    Round 60
    Tapered fissure 60

C

CAD CAM systems 143
Calcium hydroxide 27
Caries
    Caries activity test 45
    Criteria 45
    Diagnosis 46
    Chronic caries 43
    Prevention 49
    Zones of dentinal caries 46, 47
    Theories 45
Carvers 62
Carving 23
Cast restorations
    Advantages 130
    Contraindications 130
    Disadvantages 130
    Impression technique 135

    Indications 130
    Materials 130
    Principles of tooth preparation 130
Casting defects 39
Casting ring lining 37
Cavity
    Angles 8
    Factors affecting cavity preparation 10
    Nomenclature 6
    Objectives 10
    Stages 10
    Steps 10
    Walls 7
Cavity liners 32
Cavity varnishes 31
Cellulose wafers 70
Cement bases 32
Cemented pins 95
Ceramic materials 41
Chemical vapour pressure sterilization 78
Chisels 54, 55, 66
    Straight 54
    Monangle 54
    Binangle 54
    Triple angle 54
Clearance angle 60
Cleiod excavators 54
Cohesive gold 117
    Non cohesive gold 117
Compaction 118
Compomer 31, 100
Composites 100
    Advantages 100
    Disadvantages 100
    Composition 100
    Classification 100
    Contraindications 100
    Indications 100
Compound supported matrix 84
Condensation
    Amalgam 22

DFG 118
Conditioning of the cavity 103
Consequences of faulty reproduction of contacts
      and contours 80
Contact point 79
    Purpose of Ideal contact 79
    Purpose of breaking contact point 79
Conventional composites 101
Copper cement 26
Copy Milling process 143
Cotton roll isolation 70
Coupling agent (see composite) 100
Creep 20

D

Deewey's classification 105
Definition (s)
    Amalgam 16
    Cast 34
    Casting 38
    Cavity 10
    Cavity preparation 10
    Ceramic 40
    Convenience form 11
    Dental amalgam 16
    Dental caries 43
    Dental ceramics 40
    Dental investment 33
    Die 34
    Dry heat sterilization 78
    Operative dentistry 3
    Outline form 10
    Primary resistance form 10
    Primary retention form 11
    Restorations 14
    Sprue 317
    Veneers 111
Delayed expansion 21
Dental abrasive stones 61
    Characteristics 61
    Classification 61, 62
    Types 61
Dental adhesion 104
Dental amalgam
    Advantages 16
    Applications 16
    Classification 17
    Composition 17
    Disadvantages 17
Dental bur design 59
Dental cements 25
Dental casting procedures 35, 36
Dental ceramic 40
Dental cutting burs 58
    Classification 59
    Parts 59
Dental investments 33, 35
Dental stones 34
Dentin bonding agents 105
Dentin hypersensitivity
    Definition 140
    Causes 140
    Theories 140
    Management 141
Diastema closure 113
Diamond 65

Diamond stones 61
Dicor 41
    MGC 42
Differences between,
    Admixed high copper v/s spherical high
        copper amalgam 19
    Low copper alloys v/s high copper alloys 18
    Lathecut alloys v/s spherical alloys 18
    Class-II cavity preparation 115
        Amalgam v/s composite restorations 115
        Amalgam v/s cast restorations 136
Direct filling gold
    Advantages 116
    Disadvantages 116
    Indications 116
    Contraindications 116
    Forms/types of DFG 116
    Manipulation 118
    Characteristics 117
    Steps for insertion 120
Direct gold restorations
    Principles of tooth preparation 120
Direct posterior composites 102
Direct pulp capping 48
Direct pulp exposure 48
Discoid excavators 54, 66

E

EBA alumina-reinforced ZOE 27
Electroforming 34
Electrolytic precipitate 117
Embrasures (spillways) 79
Enamel bonding angents 104
Enamel hatchets 55
Enameloplasty 50
Enamel patterns (prisms)
    Direction 15
    Thickness pattern 15
Epoxy resins 35
Erosion 139
    Causes 139
    Signs and symptoms 139
    Treatment 139
Esthetic restorative materials 99
Ethylene oxide sterilization 78
Ethyl silica bonded investments 34
Excavators 54

F

Failures of amalgam restoration 93
Felt 64
Files 64
Fillers (see composite) 100
Finishing lines
    Chamfer 132
    Knife edge 132
    Bevelled shoulder 132
    Hollow ground bevel 133
Finishing burs 64
Finishing and polishing of restorations 146
    Amalgam 93
    Cast metal restorations 135
    Composites 110
    Direct gold restorations 128
Flares 131
Flowable composites 101

Fluoride varnish 141
Frictional lock pins 95
Frictional retention 11
Fused porcelain 99
Full veneers 112

G

Garnet 62
Gingival margin trimmers 55, 66
Gingival tissue retraction 70, 71
Glass ionomer cement 29, 99
Glass ionomer cement restorations 110
Glazing 41
Gold foil 117
Gold knife 67
Golden proportion 114
Guards 57
Gypsum bonded investments 34

H

Hand cutting instruments 52
    Advantages 56
    Classification 54
    Instrument formula 52
    Nomenclature 52
    Parts 52
Hand sharpening stones 65
Hatchet excavators 54
Height of contour 80
High copper alloys 18, 19
High volume evacuators 70
Hoe chisel 56
Hoe excavators 54
Hybrid composites 101
Hybrid layer 105

I

Idiopathic erosion 113
IN-CERAM
    Alumina 42
    Spinell 42
    Zirconia 42
Incipient or Initial carious lesion 43
Indirect posterior restorations 102
Indirect pulp capping 48
Infected dentin 47
Infected control 77
Initial cavity preparation 10
Inlay 129
Instruments (Restoring)
    Burnishing 63
    Condensing 62
    Plastic 62
    Mixing 62
Instrument design (Hand) 52, 53
Inverted pen grasp 56
Investing 38
Ionotophoresis 141
Isolation of the operating field 69
    Goals 69
    Methods 70
Ivory No. 1 83
Ivory No. 8 83

K

Knives 63

L

Lasers 144, 142
Lathecut alloys 18, 19
Local anesthesia 70
Low copper alloy 18, 19

M

Macro abrasion 144
Macro filled composites 101
Mamelon 80
Margin
   Margin outline 6
   Cavosurface margin 6
Marginal ridges 80
Matrices
   Function 82
   Specifications 82
Matrix band
   Classification 82
   For individual cavity preparations 82
   Height 82
   Materials 82
   Thickness 82
Mechanics of pin-retained restorations 96
Mechanical sharpness 65
Mercury 18
   Toxicity 23
Metal reinforced GIC 30
Methods of sterilization 78
Micro abrasion 144
Micro filled composites 101
Micro leakage 145
Model 34
Mouth Mirror 71

N

Nanoleakage 145

O

Offset hatchets 56
Onlay 129
Operators chair position 69
Operative dental instrument classification 51
Outline form 10
Overhang 80

P

Packable composites 102
Palm and thumb grasp 56
   Modified 57
Paper carried abrasives 64
Partial veneer 112
Pen grasp 56
   Modified 56
Phosphate bonded investments 34
Pickling 39
Pins 14
Pin channel preparation 96
Pin retained amalgam restoration 94
Pit and fissure caries 44
Pit and fissure sealants 49

Polishable composites 101
Poly alkenoate cement 29
Polymer reinforced ZOE 26
Positioning of,
   Dental assitant 69
   Operator 69
   Patient 69
Powdered gold 117
Primary carious lesion (see, Incipient carious
      lesion) 43
Primary resistance form 10
Primary retention form 10
Prophylactic odontotomy 50
Pulpal protection 106

Q

Quenching 39

R

Rampant caries 43
Rake angle 59, 60
   Negative 59
   Positive 59
   Zero 60
Rapid separation 81
Reaction of the pulp to irritating stimuli 141
Recurrent caries 43
Regulations of OSHA 77
Residual caries 44
Resin modified GIC (RMGIC) 30
Resin impregnation technique 141
Rests 57
Restoring instruments 63
Restorations
   Classification 14
   Indications 15
   Factors affecting placement of restorations 15
Retention
   Coves 13
   Dove tail 11
   Locks 12
   Grooves 12, 13
Reverse curve 92
Rotary instrumentation
   Characteristics 57
   Instrument design 58
   Uses and limitations 62
Rubber dam
   Anchoring clamps 72
   Forceps 73
   Frame 74
   Kit 71
   Lubricant 73
   Material 71
   Napkin 73
   Placement of rubber dam 74
   Procedure 74
   Punch 73
   Removal of rubber dam 77
   Stamp 73
   Waxed dental floss or tape 74

S

Saliva ejectors 70
Sandwich technique 114
Self threaded pins 95

Senile (root) caries 43
Separation of the teeth
   Purpose 81
   Methods 81
Sharpening
   Principles 65
   Techniques for sharpening intruments 65, 66
   Individual instruments 66
Sharpening equipment 64
Silicate cement 99
Silicon carbide 65
Silico phosphate cement 26
Sintering 41
Skirts 13
Slots 14
Slot retained amalgam restorations 97
Slow separation 81
Smear layer 104
Smear plug 105
Smooth surface caries 44
Soldered band 84
Speeds
   Low 62
   High 62
Spherical alloy 18
Spoon excavators 54, 66
Spruing 36
Stationary sharpening stones 64
Sterilization
   Burs 78
   Handpieces 78
   Impressions 78
Suck back porosity 40

T

Throat shields 71
Tofflemire matrix 83
Tooth
   Numbering systems 4
      FDI 5
      Universal 4
      Zsigmondy/palmer 5
   Surface designations 6
Tooth preparation (Amalgam)
   Class-I cavity 86
      Designs 3, 4, 5, 87
      Designs 6, 7, 8, 88
   Class-II cavity 88
      Designs 89
      Designs 3, 4, 5, 6, 7, 90
      Designs 8, 91
      Modifications 91
   Class-III cavity 92
   Class-V cavity 92
Tooth preparation (composite) 106
   Class-1 and 2, 109
   Class-III
      Conventional preparation 107
      Bevelled conventional preparation 107
      Modified Class-III tooth preparation 108
   Class-IV
      Conventional Class-IV 108
      Bevelled conventional Class-IV 108
      Modified Class-IV 108
   Class-V

Conventional 109
Bevelled conventional 109
Modified Class-V 109
Tooth preparations (cast metal inlays) 133
Class-II 133
Proximal margin designs
Box 134
Slice 134
Auxillary slice 135
Modified flare 135
Tooth preparations (DFG) 121
Class-I
Simple 121
Compound 121
Class-II
Conventional 122
Conservative 123
Class-III
Ferrier design 124
Loma Linda design 125, 126
Ingraham design 126
Class-V

Ferrier design 126
Proximal pan handle extension 127
Uni or bilateral moustable extension 127
Partial moon (crescent) shape design 128
Tradional composites 101
Triangular chiesel 56
Trituration 21
Traction method (see rapid separation)
T-shaped matrix band 84
Tungsten carbide burs 62

U

Universal matrix 83
Ultrasonic instruments 63

V

Veneers 111
Basic preparation design 112
Direct veneer technique 112
Indirect venner technique 112

Materials 111
Types 111

W

Wall
Enamel wall 7
Dentin wall 7
Subpulpal wall 7
Wedelstaedt chisels 55
Wedges 84
Classification 84
Functions 84
Types 84
Techniques 85
Wedge method (see rapid separation)
Window matrix 84

Z

Zinc oxide eugenol cement 26
Zinc phosphate cement 25
Zinc polycarboxylate cement
(Zinc polyacrylate cement) 28
Zones of operative field 68

Section II
ENDODONTICS

A

Accessory canals 154
Accessory foramina 155
Acute alveolar abscess 164, 236
Definition 164
Diagnosis 165
Differential diagnosis 165
Etiology 165
Symptoms 165
Synonyms
Treatment 165
Acute apical periodontitis 165
Clinical features 165
Definition 165
Diagnosis 165
Differential diagnosis 165
Treatment 165
Acute exacerbation of a chronic lesion 165
Definition 165
Etiology 165
Symptoms 165
Diagnosis 165
Differential diagnosis 165
Treatment 165
Acute irreversible pulpitis 235
Acute periodontal abscess 236
Acute reversible pulpitis 235
Aerodontalgia 160
AH 26, 213
Anachoresis 160

Anaerobic culturing 169
Anatomic apex 200
Anesthetic testing 174
Antibiotics 210
Apex finder 203
Apex locators 202
Apexification 241, 242
Apexogenesis 242
Apicoectomy 264
Apical closure 156, 157
Apical collar 197
Apical constriction 155
Apical foramen 155
Apical seat 155
Apical stop 155
Apical zip 230
Aseptic technique 184
Audiometric method 202
Autoclaving 186
Autotransplantation 250

B

Bacteriologic examination 168
Balanced force instrumentation 181
Barbed broach 178
Barodontalgia 160
Bicuspidization/bisection 263
Biologic indicators 188
Buckley's formula 239

C

Calcium hydroxide 209
Cancellier kit 233
Carbamide peroxide 253
Cast post systems 227
Cart 205
Carve 205
Cavit 211
Cell free zone 154
Cell rich zone 154
Central zone 154
Chemical irritation 185
Chemical sterilization 186
Chemically plasticized GP technique 220
Chemiclave 187
Chemoprophylaxis 184, 194
Chloropercha 213
Chloropercha technique 220
Chronic alveolar abscess (chronic suppurative apical periodontitis) 165
Definition 165
Etiology 166
Clinical features 166
Diagnosis 166
Differential diagnosis 166
Treatment 166
Chronic hyperplastic pulpitis 161
Circumferential/Smooth 205
Cleaning and Shaping 204
Aims 204

Motion 204
Purpose 205
Cold sterilization 186
Cold testing 174
Combination of lateral and vertical condensations 219
Comparison between reamers and files 180
Complications of bleaching 256
Complications of endodontic surgery 264
Concussion 247
Condensing osteitis 166
  Definition 166
  Etiology 166
  Diagnosis 167
  Differential diagnosis 167
  Treatment 166
Core 225
Core material 225
  Amalgam core 225
Coronal cavity preparation 195
Coronal restoration 226
Cracked tooth syndrome 163
Crown-root fracture 245
Crown fracture 237, 244, 245
CVEK pulpotomy 240

D

Dead tracts 153
Debridement 185
Debriding instruments 176
Dental injuries
  Etiology 243
  Classification 243, 244
  Incidence 243
Dentin
  Interglobular dentin 153
  Intertubular dentin 153
  Peritubular dentin 153
  Primary dentin 152
  Reparative dentin 153
  Secondary dentin 152
  Sclerotic dentin 153
Depressibility test 172
Devitalization pulpotomy 240
Diaket 213
Double vertical incision 261
Dowel (post) 224
Drainage 185
Drop test 213
Dry heat sterilization 187

E

EDTA 199
Electric pulp testing 173
Electric pulp testers 174
Electrical resistance method 202
Electrosterilization 210
Electrosurgical pulpotomy 241
Emergencies during treatment 236
Enamel fractures 244
Endodontic-periodontic interrelationship 256
Endodontic explorers 177
Endodontic implants 250
  Technique 251
Endodontic instruments
  Classification 176

Endodontic replantation 248
  Guidelines 248
  Failure 249
Endodontic treatment
  Local contraindications 193
  General contraindications 193, 194
Endodontics 151
  Defintion 151
  Aims 151
  Objectives 151
Engine driven instruments 182
Envelope flap 261
Essential oils 209
Eucapercha method 220
Eugenol 209
Eugenol sealers 212
Exploring instruments 177
External root resorption 167
Extirpating instruments 178
Extrusive luxation 247

F

Ferrule 226
Files
  K. file 178
  K. flex file 179
  Hedstroem files 179
  Uni files 179
  S. files 179
  Flexo files 179
  Niti files 179
Filing 180
Fish zones 189
Fluorosis stains 254
Follow 204
Follow withdraw 205
Forceps 233
Formocresol 208, 239
Fractured root 237
Frequency of medication 210

G

Gates glidden drill 182
Gingival flap 261
Giromatic 182
Glass bead sterilizer 187
Glutaraldehyde 209, 239
Granuloma 166
  Definition 166
  Etiology 166
  Symptoms 166
  Diagnosis 166
  Differential diagnosis 166
  Treatment 166
Grossman's method 200
Grossman's sealer 213
GT (Greater taper) hand files 179
Gutta percha cones 187
Guttapercha 216
  Removal 222

H

Halogens 209
Heat testing 174
Hemisection 263

Horizontal incision 260
Hot salt sterilizer 187
Hypochlorite accident 231

I

Immobilization 185
Implantation 250
Inflammatory resorption 249
Ingle's method 201
Instrument sterilization 186
  Classification 186
  Method 187
Intentional replantation 249
Intermediate restorative material (IRM) 211
Internal resorption 161
  Definition 161
  Etiology 161
  Clinical features 161
  Diagnosis 162
  Differential diagnosis 162
  Treatment 162
Intracanal medicaments 208
Intrinsic discolouration 252
Intrusive luxation 247
Inverted cone technique 219
Iodides 209
Irreversible pulpitis 161
  Definition 161
  Etiology 161
  Clinical features 161
  Diagnosis 161
  Differential diagnosis 161
  Treatment 161
Irrigating solutions 198

J

Johnson-Collahan's method 220

K

KRI paste 241

L

Laser pulpotomy 241
Lateral canals 154
Lateral condensation technique 218
Lateral luxation 247
Ledge formation 228
Lentulo spirals 180
Look 204
Luebke ochsenbein flap 261

M

Masserann kit 233
Master apical file determination 203
Matrix bleaching 255
Mc Spadden compactor 220
Misto paste 241
Mobility test 172
Monitoring sterilization 188
Morphology of pulp
  Pulps of maxillary teeth 156
  Pulps of mandibular teeth 156
MTA (Mineral trioxide aggregate) 240
Mummifying agent 240

N

Necrosis of pulp 162
    Definition 162
    Etiology 162
    Symptoms 162
    Diagnosis 162
    Treatment 163
Night/mouth guard bleaching 255
Non eugenol scalers 212
Nygaard Ostby method 220

O

Obtura-II 222
Obturating instruments 176, 180
Obturating materials
    Ideal requirements 215
    Classification 216
Obturation technique 217
Occlusal pressure test 172
Odontoblastic zone 152
Oliet's criteria for case selection 234
Open apex 155
Over filling of root canal 223

P

Pain 170
Palpation 172
Para chlorophenol 209
Pastes 216, 222
Patency 205
Patient response 217
PBSC 210
Peeso reamers 182
Percussion 171
Perforations 229, 258
Periradicular tissues 155
    Diseases 164
    Classification 164
Phenol 209
Phenolic compounds 209
Pluggers 180
Post removal devices 233
Predentin layer 152
Prefabricated post and core system 226
Principles of Endodontics 184
Process indicators 188
Prophylactic trephination 185
Pulp artifacts 162
Pulp cavity 154
Pulp degeneration 162
    Calcific 162
    Atrophic 162
    Fibrous 162
Pulp disease 158
    Causes 158
    Classification 159
Pulp polyp 161
Pulp vitality tests 173
Pulpectomy 241
Pulpotomy 239

Q

Quaternary ammonium 209

R

Racer 182
Radicular cyst 166
Radicular preparation 197
Radiograph test 217
Radiographic apex 200
Radiography 172
Radiovisiography 202
Radisectomy/root resection 262
Rasps/R-type files 178
RC-PREP 199
Reamers 178
Reaming 181
Recapitulation 207
Replacement resorption 249
Retrograde filling 261
Reversible pulpitis 160
    Definition 160
    Etiology 160
    Clinical features 160
    Diagnosis 160
    Differential diagnosis 160
    Treatment 160
Rickert's sealers 213
Rolled cone technique 219
Root canal 154
    Configurations 154
    Weine's classification 155
    Vertussi's classification 155
Root canal flora 168
Root canal sealers 212
Root canal shaping instruments 178, 176
Root fracture 245, 246

S

Sargentis paste 209
Scalloped flap 261
Sectional method 219
Sectional or split cone method 221
Semilunar/curved/elliptical flap 260
Series 29 files 179
Shamrock preparation 196
Silver cone method 221
Silver cones 187, 216
    Removal 222
Single cone technique 217
Single vertical incision 260
Sodium hypochlorite 190
Sodium perborate 253
Soft tissue injuries 244
Sotokawa's classification of instrument
    damage 183
Speaders 180
Stainless steel method 222
Standardization of endodontic instruments 177
Step back preparation 205
Step down technique 206
Sterilization failure 187
String test 213
Subluxation 247
Superoxol 253
Surface resorption 248
Surgical endodontics
    Objective 259

Indications 259
Contraindications 259
Classification 260

T

Tactile test 217
Temporary filling materials 211
    Definition 211
    Requirements 211
    Materials 211
Term 211
Test cavity preparation 175
Tetracycline stains 255
Thermafil 223
Thermal testing 174
Thermo/photo extra coronal bleaching 253
Thermo mechanical technique 220
Thermography 175
Thermoplasticized GP injection moulded method
    221
Tooth avulsion 238, 247
Transplantation 250
Transullumination 175
Trapezoidal flap 261
Trephination 185
Triangular flap 260
Tubiseal 214
Tumour metastasis 168
Turn and pull 181

U

Ultrasonic and sonic instruments 183
Ultraviolet photo oxidation 254
Under filling of Root canal 223

V

Vertical condensation technique 218
Visual and tactile inspection 171
Visual test 217

W

Wach's sealer 214
Walkhoff paste 241
Walking bleach technique 254
Warm gutta percha technique 218
Watch winding 181
Watch winding and pull 181
Working length determination 200
    Definition 200
    Objectives 200
    Methods 200

X

Xeroradiography 202

Z

Zones of pulp 152